SYSTEMIC PATHOLOGY / THIRD EDITION

Volume 2   Blood and Bone Marrow

SYSTEMIC PATHOLOGY / THIRD EDITION

General Editor

W. St C. Symmers

MD(Belf), PhD(Birm), DSc(Lond), FRCP (Lond, Irel, Ed), FRCS(Eng), FACP(Hon), FRCPA(Hon), FRCPath, FFPathRCPI

Emeritus Professor of Pathology, University of London; Honorary Consulting Pathologist, Charing Cross Hospital, London, UK

System Editors

M. C. Anderson   **Gynaecological and Obstetrical Pathology**

T. J. Anderson and D. L. Page   **The Breasts**

B. Corrin   **The Lungs**

M. J. Davies, R. H. Anderson, W. B. Robertson and N. Woolf   **Cardiovascular System**

I. Friedmann   **Nose, Throat and Ears**

K. Henry   **Thymus, Lymph Nodes and Spleen**

B. C. Morson   **Alimentary Tract**

K. A. Porter   **Urinary System**

R. C. B. Pugh   **Male Reproductive System**

H. A. Sissons   **Bone, Joints and Soft Tissues**

D. Weedon   **Skin**

K. Weinbren   **Liver, Biliary Tract and Pancreas**

R. O. Weller   **Nervous System, Muscle and Eyes**

S. N. Wickramasinghe   **Blood and Bone Marrow**

E. D. Williams   **Endocrine System**

SYSTEMIC PATHOLOGY / THIRD EDITION

Volume 2

Blood and Bone Marrow

EDITED BY

S. N. Wickramasinghe

ScD(Cantab), PhD(Cantab), MB BS(Ceylon), MRCPath, FIBiol

Professor of Haematology in the University of London;
Director, Department of Haematology, St Mary's Hospital Medical School;
Honorary Consultant Haematologist, Paddington and North Kensington Health Authority,
London, UK

WITH CONTRIBUTIONS BY

Barbara J. Bain
MB BS(Qld), FRACP, MRCPath
Senior Lecturer in Haematology, St Mary's Hospital Medical School,
University of London; Honorary Consultant Haematologist,
Paddington and North Kensington Health Authority,
London, UK

CHURCHILL LIVINGSTONE
EDINBURGH LONDON MELBOURNE NEW YORK AND TOKYO 1986

CHURCHILL LIVINGSTONE
Medical Division of Longman Group UK Limited

Distributed in the United States of America by Churchill
Livingstone Inc., 650 Avenue of the Americas, New York,
N.Y. 10011, and by associated companies, branches and
representatives throughout the world.

First published 1986
Reprinted 1991

ISBN 0 433 03099 5 XSO1478395

British Library Cataloguing in Publication Data

Systemic pathology.——3rd ed.
  Vol. 2: Blood and bone marrow
  1. Pathology
  I. Wickramsinghe, S. N.   II. Bain, Barbara J.
  616.07   RB111

Library of Congress Cataloging in Publication Data

Main entry under title:

Blood and bone marrow.
  (Systemic pathology; v. 2)
  Includes bibliographies and index.
  1. Blood——Diseases.   2. Marrow——Diseases.
I. Wickramasinghe, S. N.   II. Bain, Barbara J.
III. Series. [DNLM: 1. Blood.   2. Bone Marrow.
3. Bone Marrow Diseases.   4. Hematologic Diseases.
QZ 4 S995 v. 2]
RB111.S97   vol. 2 [RC633]   616.07 s [616.1'5]   85-19489

Produced by Longman Group (FE) Ltd
Printed in Hong Kong

Preface

In the first two editions of Systemic Pathology, published in 1966 and 1976–1980, the chapter on Blood and Bone Marrow was contributed by Professor W. M. Davidson of the Department of Haematology at King's College Hospital Medical School, London, with the collaboration for the second edition (1978) of two colleagues in his Department, Dr K. G. A. Clark and Dr M. L. Lewis. Professor Davidson's clear, concise and scholarly chapter was appreciated warmly by the readers and reviewers of both editions and set a fresh standard for the presentation of blood diseases in text books of systemic pathology. Since 1978, knowledge of the pathology of blood and bone marrow has advanced at an impressive pace and as a result the account in the second edition needed to be completely rewritten. When I was invited by Professor Symmers and the publishers, Churchill Livingstone, to become the System Editor of the section on Blood and Bone Marrow in the Third Edition of *Systemic Pathology* I was advised that the length of this section should be commensurate with a comprehensive account which would serve the practising pathologist and haematologist as a reference work: this requirement could be met only by devoting an entire volume to the subject. In preparing this volume I enlisted the participation of my colleague, Dr Barbara J. Bain, who wrote three of the chapters and substantial parts of others.

It has been a particular pleasure to work with Professor Symmers, who as the General Editor of this edition read carefully through the manuscript and made numerous helpful suggestions, for which I am most grateful. I should also like to thank the staff of Churchill Livingstone for their encouragement and assistance throughout this project.

During the preparation of this volume, the authors have been helped by several members of the Haematology Department as well as of other departments of our Medical School and we are very grateful for their assistance. Specific contributions made by colleagues are acknowledged individually in the relevant figure legends.

We are especially grateful to Professor P. L. Mollison FRS and Dr N. C. Hughes-Jones FRS for reading through Chapter 2 and suggesting several improvements. We are grateful to Dr S. Wilson and other members of the Histopathology Department for providing several histological sections for our use, and to Dr Oscar Craig, Director of the Radiology Department, and Dr P. N. Cardew, Director of the Audio-Visual Department, for permission to reproduce some of the radiographs and photographs held in their departments. We are also indebted to Mrs Anne-Marie Colbert, Ms Madeleine Hughes and Mr Richard Litwinczuk for their painstaking work in the production of many of the illustrations for this book. Finally, we wish to thank Mrs Janet Williams for her very skilful typing of the manuscript.

London, 1986   S. N. W.

Contents

Units and Abbreviations

SI units (*Système international d'unités*) are used whenever possible. However, in accordance with current practice, the concentration of haemoglobin is expressed not in SI units but in grams per decilitre (g/dl). Most abbreviations are defined when first used in a chapter but, for convenience, commonly used abbreviations are listed below. When the *British Journal of Haematology* has recommended an abbreviation, this has been used (Editorial Board, Br J Haematol 1978; 40: 1).

ADP	adenosine-5'-diphosphate
AIDS	acquired immunodeficiency syndrome
AIHA	autoimmune haemolytic anaemia
ALL	acute lymphoblastic leukaemia
AML	acute myeloid leukaemia
ATLL	acute T-cell leukaemia/lymphoma
ATP	adenosine-5'-triphosphate
B-cell	B-lymphocyte
BFU-E	erythroid burst-forming unit
BJP	Bence Jones protein
C	complement
cALL	common acute lymphoblastic leukaemia
CFU-C	colony-forming unit in culture
CFU-E	erythroid colony-forming unit
CFU-Eo	eosinophil colony-forming unit
CFU-GM	granulocyte/macrophage colony-forming unit
CFU-Meg	megakaryocyte colony-forming unit
CFU-S	colony-forming unit in spleen (multipotent haemopoietic stem cell)
CGL	chronic granulocytic leukaemia
CHAD	cold haemagglutinin disease
CLL	chronic lymphocytic leukaemia
CML	chronic myeloid leukaemia
CNS	central nervous system
CSF	cerebrospinal fluid
CSF	colony-stimulating factor
DAGT	direct antiglobulin test
DIC	disseminated intravascular coagulation
DNA	deoxyribonucleic acid
EBV	Epstein-Barr virus
ERC	erythropoietin-responsive cell
ERFC	sheep-erythrocyte rosette-forming cells
E-rosettes	rosettes with sheep erythrocytes
ESR	erythrocyte sedimentation rate
FDP	fibrin/fibrinogen degradation products
G6PD	glucose 6-phosphate dehydrogenase
H&E	haematoxylin and eosin stain
Hb	haemoglobin
HbA	adult haemoglobin ($\alpha_2\beta_2$)
HbF	fetal haemoglobin ($\alpha_2\gamma_2$)
HCD	heavy chain disease
HCL	hairy cell leukaemia
HDN	haemolytic disease of the newborn
HES	hypereosinophilic syndrome
HLA	human leucocyte antigen
HTLV	human T-cell lymphotropic virus

IAGT	indirect antiglobulin test	NK cell	natural killer cell
IATP	idiopathic autoimmune thrombocytopenic purpura	PAS	periodic acid-Schiff
ITP	idiopathic thrombocytopenic purpura	PCH	paroxysmal cold haemoglobinuria
Ig	immunoglobulin	PCV	packed cell volume
IgG, IgM etc.	immunoglobulin of class G, class M, etc.	PEM	protein-energy malnutrition
K cell	killer cell	Ph^1	Philadelphia chromosome
LDH	lactate dehydrogenase	PLL	prolymphocytic leukaemia
MAHA	microangiopathic haemolytic anaemia	PNH	paroxysmal nocturnal haemoglobinuria
MCH	mean corpuscular haemoglobin	PRV	polycythaemia rubra vera
MCHC	mean corpuscular haemoglobin concentration	RAEB	refractory anaemia with excess of blasts
MCV	mean corpuscular volume	RBC	red blood cell count
MGG	May-Grünwald-Giemsa stain	RNA	ribonucleic acid
MM	multiple myeloma	s.d.	standard deviation
mRNA	messenger ribonucleic acid	SLE	systemic lupus erythematosus
MRFC	mouse-erythrocyte rosette-forming cells	SmIg	surface membrane immunoglobulin
M-rosettes	rosettes with mouse erythrocytes	T-cell	T-lymphocyte
MW	molecular weight	$T_{\frac{1}{2}}$	half life
NAD	nicotinamide-adenine dinucleotide	TdT	terminal deoxynucleotidyl transferase
NADH	reduced nicotinamide-adenine dinucleotide	TIBC	total iron-binding capacity
NADP	nicotinamide-adenine dinucleotide phosphate	VWD	von Willebrand's disease
		VWF	von Willebrand's factor
NADPH	reduced nicotinamide-adenine dinucleotide phosphate	WBC	white blood cell count
		WM	Waldenström's macroglobulinaemia
NAP	neutrophil alkaline phosphatase	2,3-DPG	2,3-diphosphoglycerate
		5HT	5-hydroxytryptamine (serotonin)

S. N. Wickramasinghe

Composition and functions of normal blood: normal haematological values

Blood consists of a pale-yellow, coagulable fluid called plasma in which various types of blood cells are suspended. The cells comprise the erythrocytes, granulocytes, monocytes, lymphocytes and platelets.

BLOOD PLASMA

This fluid contains about 9% of solids, about four-fifths of which consists of protein. There are many different plasma proteins and these have been separated into various fractions using techniques such as salt precipitation, electrophoresis and ultracentrifugation. Plasma proteins are classically divided into three main fractions: fibrinogen, albumin and globulin. On the basis of their electrophoretic mobility the globulin fraction is divided into α_1, α_2, β_1, β_2 and γ globulins (see Figs 8.4 and 8.5, p. 292). In clinical practice, proteins are usually studied in serum rather than plasma as fibrinogen may be converted to fibrin and cause blockages in automated analysers. Total protein is most often measured by a modified biuret reaction since the rapidity of this reaction makes it suitable for automation. Albumin is measured by a dye-binding method (bromcresol green or bromcresol purple). The globulins are investigated by zone electrophoresis of serum on filter paper, cellulose acetate or agarose gel using a barbitone buffer (pH 8.6, ionic strength 0.05 – 0.1 mol/l). If plasma rather than serum is electrophoresed, fibrinogen moves between β and γ globulins. At a pH of 8.6, the proteins (except the immunoglobulins) become negatively charged and migrate towards the anode. Albumin moves fastest followed by α_1, α_2 and β globulins, in that order. The γ globulins are electrically neutral but move towards the cathode because of the effect of electroendosmosis. The serum protein electrophoretic pattern remains remarkably constant in a healthy individual but the 95% confidence limits for the concentrations of the various protein fractions in a healthy population are fairly wide (Table 1.1).

sible for about 80% of the total colloid osmotic pressure of plasma partly because of its abundance and partly because, owing to its low molecular weight, it exerts 2–3 times the osmotic pressure of globulins per unit weight.

The plasma contains blood coagulation proteins and their inhibitors (Chapter 9), proteins of the fibrinolytic system and their inhibitors (Chapter 9), precursors of kinins (Chap-

Table 1.1 Concentration of serum proteins in g/l at various ages[1]. Values represent 95% confidence limits

Age	Total Protein	Albumin	α_1 globulin	α_2 globulin	β globulin	γ globulin
Birth	46–70	32–48	1–3	2–6	3–6	6–12
3 months	45–65	32–48	1–3	3–7	3–7	2–7
1 year	54–75	37–57	1–3.4	2.8–11	3.8–10	2–9
2 years–Adult	53–80	33–58	1–3	4–10	3–12	4–14
Adult	64–78	36–52	1–4	4–8	5–12	7–15

Increased or decreased levels of many serum proteins can be detected on an electrophoretic pattern. Individual proteins can also be quantified by immunochemical methods, such as radial immunodiffusion (e.g. haptoglobin, antithrombin III), electroimmunodiffusion (factor VIII related antigen), immunoprecipitation followed by nephelometry (immunoglobulins, C3, C4, haptoglobin, caeruloplasmin) or radioimmunoassay (e.g. ferritin).

Fibrinogen (MW 330 000) is formed almost exclusively in the liver and is the precursor of the fibrin of a blood clot. Its role in blood coagulation is described on page 320. Fibrinogen is also largely responsible for the viscosity of the plasma; solutions of fibrinogen are about six times as viscous as solutions of albumin of the same concentration.

Albumin (MW 68 000) is the most abundant plasma protein and is synthesized mainly in the liver. It has a $T_{\frac{1}{2}}$ of 26d in the circulation.

The major classes of plasma protein pass through the capillary walls with difficulty and, by virtue of their colloidal osmotic pressure (of about 25 mmHg), play an important role in maintaining the distribution of water between the blood and the tissue fluids. Albumin is respon-

ter 9), immunoglobulins (Chapter 8) and complement components (Chapter 2). Plasma is the medium in which numerous substances such as hormones, minerals, vitamins, amino acids, sugars and excretory products are transported to and from various parts of the body. Specific plasma proteins transport some of these substances. For example, iron is transported by transferrin (a β_1 globulin), copper by caeruloplasmin, free haemoglobin (from lysed red cells) by haptoglobin, and vitamin B_{12} by transcobalamins I, II and III.

Disease processes are often reflected in changes in plasma proteins. A common, non-specific change is the 'acute phase response' to tissue inflammation and damage. Within one to two days a rise occurs in α_1 globulins (orosomucoid, α_1 antitrypsin and α_1 antichymotrypsin), α_2 globulins (α_2 macroglobulin, haptoglobin), fibrinogen, and C-reactive protein (γ mobility). Subsequently C3, C4 and caeruloplasmin rise followed by immunoglobulins. Albumin, prealbumin and transferrin fall. The acute phase response is reflected in a rise in the erythrocyte sedimentation rate (ESR) which is largely caused by a rise in fibrinogen and α_2 macroglobulin. The normal range (95% confidence limits) for the ESR measured by the Westergren method in people aged 18-65 years is 0-10 mm/h for men and 1-20 mm/h for women.[2]

BLOOD CELLS

ERYTHROCYTES

Morphology

Erythrocytes are highly differentiated cells which have no nuclei or cytoplasmic organelles. Although these cells are responsible for the red colour of blood, single erythrocytes are pale reddish-yellow when examined in transmitted light. Normal erythrocytes are circular biconcave discs with a mean diameter of 7.2 μm (range 6.7-7.7 μm) in dried fixed smears and about 7.5 μm in the living state. They are eosinophilic and consequently appear red with a central area of pallor in smears stained by a Romanowsky stain (Fig. 1.1).

Red cell parameters[3]

The three basic parameters which can be measured in relation to the red cell population are: 1) the concentration of haemoglobin per unit volume of blood after lysis of the red cells (haemoglobin concentration); 2) the number of

(a) (b) (c)

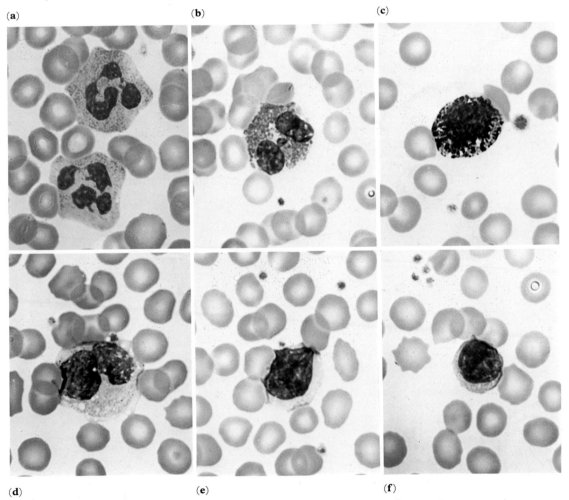

(d) (e) (f)

Fig. 1.1a–f Cells from peripheral blood smears of normal individuals. May-Grünwald-Giemsa stain.
a. Two neutrophil granulocytes; **b.** eosinophil granulocyte; **c.** basophil granulocyte; **d.** monocyte; **e.** large lymphocyte; **f.** small lymphocyte. Red cells and platelets are seen in all the photomicrographs.

×940

red cells per unit volume of blood (red cell count); and 3) the haematocrit. The haemoglobin concentration is usually determined spectrophotometrically, after conversion to cyanmethaemoglobin. The red-cell count was previously determined visually using counting chambers but is now determined more precisely using electronic cell counters. The haematocrit (packed cell volume) is determined after centrifugation of the blood in tubes of standard specification under a fixed centrifugal force and for a fixed time. It is defined as the length of the column of resulting packed red cells expressed as a fraction or percentage of the length of the column of cells plus plasma. The value obtained for the packed cell volume includes the volume of some plasma trapped between the red cells. From the values obtained for the haemoglobin concentration, red cell count and packed cell volume, it is possible to calculate the mean cell volume (MCV), mean

Table 1.2 Calculation of red cell indices

MCV (in fl)	$= \text{PCV*} \div \text{RBC per litre} \times 10^{15}$
MCH (in pg)	$= \text{Hb†} \div \text{RBC per litre} \times 10^{13}$
MCHC (in g/dl)	$= \text{Hb†} \div \text{PCV*}$

*Expressed as a fraction.
†In g/dl.

cell haemoglobin (MCH) and mean cell haemoglobin concentration (MCHC) as shown in Table 1.2. The Coulter S and Coulter S Plus series of automatic blood-counting machines determine the MCV electronically and calculate the PCV from the measured MCV and red cell count. The normal values for various red-cell parameters at different ages are given in Tables 1.3 and 1.4. Between the age of 2 years and the onset of puberty there is a gradual rise in the haemoglobin concentration in both sexes. In the next few years there is a further rise in males but not females with the result that the mean haemoglobin value

Table 1.3 95% confidence limits for some haematological parameters in healthy Caucasian adults; the data were derived in the Haematology Department of St Mary's Hospital, London, by Drs H. Dodsworth* and B.J. Bain§. When no difference was found between men and women, results were pooled

	Men	Women
Haemoglobin* (g/dl)	13.4–17.0 (n=271)	11.9–15.3 (n=188)
Red cell count* (10^{12}/l)	4.4–5.8 (n=271)	4.1–5.2 (n=188)
Packed cell volume* (PCV)	0.40–0.51† (n=271) 0.41–0.53‡	0.36–0.46† (n=188) 0.37–0.47‡
Mean corpuscular volume (MCV)	81–96 fl*† (n=459) 84–99 fl§ (n=149)	
Mean corpuscular haemoglobin* (MCH)	27–32 pg (n=459)	
Mean corpuscular haemoglobin concentration* (MCHC)	32–36 g/dl (n=459)	
Platelet count (10^9/l)§	170–410 (n=150)	185–450 (n=229)
Erythrocyte sedimentation rate (mm/h)‖	0–20 (n=311)	1–20 (n=226)

* data for non-smokers determined on a Coulter counter model S.
† determined on a Coulter counter model S with a 3% correction for plasma trapping.
‡ equivalent figures if no correction is applied for plasma trapping.
§ data for smokers plus non-smokers determined on a Coulter counter S Plus III or IV. MCV has 3% correction for plasma trapping.
‖ for subjects aged 18–60 years[2].

Table 1.4 Age-dependent changes in the mean values (and 95% confidence limits) for red cell parameters in normal individuals. The data from cases in which iron deficiency was excluded are marked with an asterisk

Age	n	Hb (g/dl)	RBC (x 10^{12}/l)	MCV (fl)	Reference and other details
Cord blood	59	17.1 (13.5–20.7)	4.6 (3.6–5.6)	113 (101–125)	a
1 day	59	19.4 (15.1–23.7)	5.3 (4.2–6.4)	110 (99–121)	a
1 month*	240	13.9 (10.7–17.1)	4.3 (3.3–5.3)	101 (91–112)	b
2 months*	241	11.2 (9.4–13.0)	3.7 (3.1–4.3)	95 (84–106)	b
4 months*	52	12.2 (10.3–14.1)	4.3 (3.5–5.1)	87 (76–97)	b
6 months*	52	12.6 (11.1–14.1)	4.7 (3.9–5.5)	76 (68–85)	b
12 months	56*	12.7 (11.3–14.1)	4.7 (4.1–5.3)	78 (71–84)	b
	51	11.1 (7.7–14.5)	4.8 (3.8–5.8)	73 (58–88)	a
	163	10.1 (7.5–12.7)	4.7 (3.5–5.5)	72 (58–86)	c
10–17 months*	59			77 (70–84)	d
3 years	103	12.4 (10.1–14.7)	4.7 (3.9–5.5)	78 (68–88)	a
	128	11.0 (8.6–13.4)	4.5 (3.5–5.5)	78 (64–92)	c
18 months–4 years*	26			80 (74–86)	d
5 years	97	12.7 (10.7–14.7)	4.7 (3.7–5.6)	80 (72–88)	a
	24	11.8 (9.2–14.4)	4.4 (3.7–5.1)	83 (69–97)	c
4–7 years*	42			81 (76–86)	d
7 years	103	12.9 (9.2–16.6)	4.8 (3.8–5.8)	79 (61–97)	a
7–8 years	151	12.5 (10.3–14.7)	4.6 (4.0–5.2)	81 (72–89)	e
10 years	111	13.2 (10.8–15.6)	4.8 (3.9–5.7)	81 (68–94)	a
14 years	45	13.6 (10.7–16.5)	4.9 (3.9–5.9)	81 (66–96)	a
20 years male	–	15.9 (13.7–18.3)	5.3 (4.6–6.2)	89 (78–99)	f
20 years female	–	13.8 (11.7–15.8)	4.6 (4.0–5.4)	89 (76–99)	f
60 years male	–	15.9 (13.8–18.4)	5.0 (4.3–5.9)	93 (82–103)	f
60 years female	–	13.9 (11.8–15.9)	4.6 (3.9–5.3)	90 (77–100)	f

a = Healthy and sick American Whites; used microhaematocrit and counting chambers.[4]
b = Healthy full-term infants from Finland; continuous iron supplementation; normal transferrin saturation and serum ferritin level; used Coulter counter model S.[5]
c = Healthy Jamaican Blacks; cohort study; HbS and β-thalassaemia excluded; used Coulter ZBI 6.[6]
d = Healthy Caucasian, Asian and Black children in America; Hb > 11.0 g/dl, transferrin saturation ≥ 20%, normal serum ferritin; haemoglobinopathy and β-thalassaemia trait excluded; used Coulter counter model S.[7]
e = Healthy individuals; mostly American Blacks; used Coulter counter model S.[8]
f = Reference intervals derived from 1744 healthy Americans (ethnic origin not stated) aged 16–89 years using Hemac 630 laser cell counter.[9]

is higher in adult males than in adult females (also see p. 183). In healthy infants aged 4 months and over, and in healthy young children, the average MCV is lower than in healthy adults. As this difference is evident even in children in whom subclinical iron deficiency is excluded, a low MCV appears to be an intrinsic feature of erythropoiesis in childhood.[5, 7, 10] Whereas the lower limit for the MCV in unselected healthy adults is 82 fl, the corresponding figure for children between 1 and 7 years (who show no biochemical evidence of iron deficiency) is about 70 fl. The MCV increases progressively with age both in children and, to a much lesser extent, in adults.

Red cell life-span[11, 12, 13]

As red cells do not contain ribosomes, they cannot synthesize new protein to replace essential molecules (e.g. enzymes, structural proteins) which become denatured in the course of time. Red cells therefore have a limited life-span of 110–120 days, at the end of which they are ingested and degraded by the phagocytic cells of the marrow, spleen, liver and other organs. A variety of changes affect red cells as they age within the circulation. These include a progressive decrease in MCV and in surface area, a progressive increase in density and osmotic fragility, a decrease in deformability, a decreased ability to reduce methaemoglobin and a decrease in the rate of glycolysis. Recent studies suggest that the critical change which causes a red cell to be destroyed at the end of its life-span could be the desialation of the glycophorin of the red cell membrane. Normal plasma contains an antibody against asialoglycophorin and the antibody-coated aged erythrocytes appear to be recognized and phagocytosed by macrophages.[14]

Functions of red cells[15, 16, 17]

Normal function of the erythrocyte requires a normal red cell membrane, and normal enzyme systems providing energy and protecting against oxidant damage. The erythrocyte membrane is composed of a lipid bilayer (containing integral proteins) and is bound to a submembranous cytoskeletal network of protein molecules including spectrin, actin and the proteins constituting bands 4.1a and 4.1b.[18] This cytoskeletal network is responsible for maintaining the biconcave shape of a normal red cell. The membrane also contains ATP-dependent cation pumps which continuously pump Na^+ out of and K^+ into the red cell, against concentration gradients, thereby counteracting a continuous passive diffusion of ions across the membrane in the opposite direction. Mature erythrocytes derive their energy from glycolysis by the Embden-Meyerhof pathway (p. 120). They can also metabolize glucose through the pentose phosphate shunt, which generates the reduction potential of the cell and protects the membrane, the haemoglobin and erythrocyte enzymes from oxidant damage (p. 120). Both a normal cell membrane and normal energy production are required to enable the biconcave red cells to repeatedly and reversibly deform during numerous transits through the microcirculation.

The prime function of the red cell is to combine with oxygen in the lungs and to transport and release this oxygen for utilization by tissues. The red cells also combine with CO_2 produced in tissues and release this in the lungs.

The function of oxygen transport resides in the haemoglobin molecule which is ideally structured for this purpose. Most of the haemoglobin (Hb) of an adult is HbA which is a tetramer consisting

of two α-globin chains and two β-globin chains. Each of these globin chains is associated with a haem molecule which is inserted deeply within a pocket which excludes water but allows O_2 to enter and interact with the iron atom at the centre of the haem molecule. In the deoxygenated state, the iron atom is in the ferrous state (Fe^{++}) and has a 'spare' electron. In the oxygenated state there is a weak ionic link between the oxygen molecule and the iron atom as a result of the 'sharing' of the 'spare' electron, but the iron remains in the ferrous state. This reaction between the oxygen molecule and the iron atom of the haem ring is reversible and the oxygen is readily released at the low oxygen concentrations found in tissues. The importance of excluding water from the haem pocket is that the water could oxidise the iron atom to the ferric state by accepting the spare electron. Haemoglobin in which the iron atoms are in the ferric state is called methaemoglobin and does not combine with oxygen.

The ability of red cells to combine with and release oxygen is illustrated in the oxygen dissociation curve shown in Figure 1.2. The shape of the oxygen dissociation curve of HbA is sigmoid and this is a function of the interaction of the four monomers which make up its tetrameric

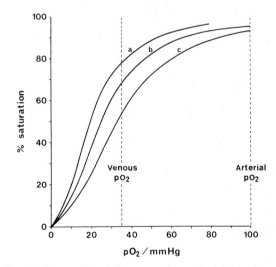

Fig. 1.2 Oxygen dissociation curve of normal adult blood and the effect of varying the pH. P_{O_2} and P_{CO_2} = partial pressure of O_2 and CO_2 respectively.

a = pH 7.6 (P_{CO_2} 25 mmHg); b = pH 7.4 (P_{CO_2} 40 mmHg); c = pH 7.2 (P_{CO_2} 61 mmHg).

structure; the shape of the oxygen dissociation curve of the monomer, myoglobin, is hyperbolic. The advantage of the sigmoid curve over the hyperbolic curve is that much more oxygen is released from the haemoprotein at the low Po_2 values obtained in tissues (35–40 mmHg) with the former than with the latter. The percentage saturation of haemoglobin at this Po_2 is about 70%. The biochemical basis of the interaction between the four haem groups of the globin chains of the haemoglobin molecule (haem–haem interaction), which determines the sigmoid shape, appears to be related to conformational changes resulting from the combination of oxygen with haem and is dependent on movement at the $\alpha_1-\beta_2$ contact. The changes are such that the combination of O_2 with one haem moiety facilitates combination with the other haem moieties. The capacity of haemoglobin to combine with O_2 at a given Po_2 is referred to as its oxygen affinity and is expressed as the Po_2 required to cause 50% saturation (P_{50}). A decrease in pH leads to a shift of the oxygen dissociation curve to the right and a decrease in oxygen affinity. This effect, which is known as the Bohr effect, facilitates the release of oxygen at the low pH of tissues. A shift of the oxygen dissociation curve to the right also results from the combination of haemoglobin with 2,3-diphosphoglycerate which is produced as a result of the metabolism of glucose via the Rapoport–Luebering shunt of the Embden–Meyerhof pathway (Fig. 5.8, p. 120).

The CO_2 produced in the tissues enters the blood. Most of this CO_2 enters the red cells and is converted there to carbonic acid by the enzyme carbonic anhydrase. The hydrogen ions released from the dissociation of this weak acid combine with the haemoglobin, and are largely responsible for the Bohr effect referred to above. A small proportion of the CO_2 entering red cells combines with haemoglobin to form carbaminohaemoglobin. When the blood circulates through the lungs, where the Pco_2 is lower than that in the blood, the CO_2 is released from the red cells into the alveolar air. The release of CO_2 from red cells results in a reversal of the Bohr effect (i.e. a shift of the oxygen dissociation curve to the left) and the uptake of considerable amounts of O_2. The

oxygen saturation and Po_2 of arterial blood is greater than 95% and 100 mmHg respectively.

The biconcave shape of normal erythrocytes facilitates the diffusion of gases in and out of the cytoplasm and also imparts adequate flexibility and deformability to enable these cells to repeatedly traverse the microcirculation.

RETICULOCYTES

These are the immediate precursors of the red cells. They are rounded anucleate cells which are about 20% larger in volume than mature red cells and appear faintly polychromatic when stained by a Romanowsky method. When stained supravitally with brilliant cresyl blue, the diffuse basophilic material responsible for the polychromasia (i.e. ribosomal RNA) appears as a basophilic reticulum (Fig. 1.3). Electron-microscope studies[19] have shown that reticulocytes are rounded cells with a tortuous surface and that in addition to ribosomes they contain mitochondria and autophagic vacuoles (Fig. 1.4). Circulating

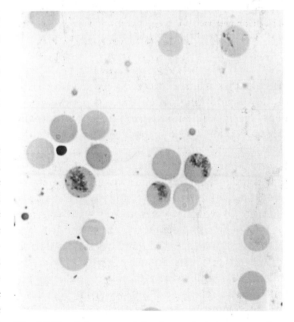

Fig. 1.3 Blood smear containing four reticulocytes, one of which is more mature and contains much less basophilic reticulum than the others. The blood was stained supravitally with brilliant cresyl blue at 37°C for 20 minutes prior to the preparation of the smear. × 940.

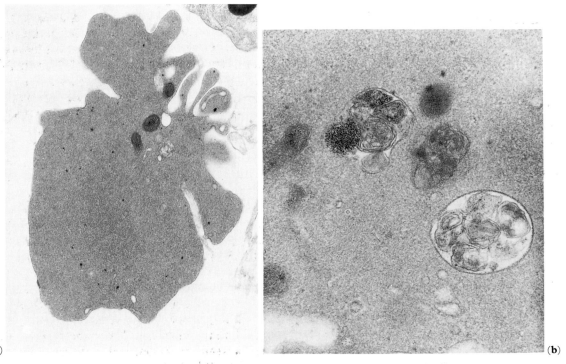

(a)   **(b)**

Fig. 1.4a,b Electron micrographs of two normal reticulocytes. Uranyl acetate and lead citrate.
a. The reticulocyte profile has an irregular outline and contains three mitochondria.

$\times$ 14 400.

b. Higher power view of part of another reticulocyte showing three autophagic vacuoles. These vacuoles contain structures which may represent mitochondria in the process of degradation.

$\times$ 19 180.

reticulocytes mature into red cells over a period of 1–2 days during which there is a progressive degradation of ribosomes and mitochondria and the acquisition of the biconcave shape. Reticulocytes actively synthesize haemoglobin and non-haemoglobin proteins. They contain enzymes of the Embden-Meyerhof pathway and the pentose phosphate shunt and, unlike the mature red cells, can also derive energy aerobically via the Krebs cycle which operates in the mitochondria and oxidizes pyruvate to CO_2 and water. In normal adults, reticulocytes comprise 0.8–2.6% of the total circulating erythrocyte plus reticulocyte population in males and 1.0–3.7% in females.[20] Although most laboratories still express reticulocyte counts as a percentage, it is more useful to express them as the total number per litre of blood, i.e. as an absolute reticulocyte count. The latter is directly proportional both to the rate of effective erythropoiesis and to the average matur-ation time of blood reticulocytes.[21] In normal adults the absolute reticulocyte count is 18–158 $\times$ 10^9/1.[22]

GRANULOCYTES (POLYMORPHONUCLEAR LEUCOCYTES)

These cells contain characteristic cytoplasmic granules and a segmented nucleus. The latter consists of two or more nuclear masses (nuclear segments) joined together by fine strands of nuclear chromatin.

The nuclear masses contain moderate quantities of condensed chromatin. The granulocytes are subdivided into neutrophil, eosinophil and basophil granulocytes according to the staining reactions of the granules.

Neutrophil granulocytes

Morphology and composition

Neutrophil granulocytes have a mean volume of 500 fl and, in dried fixed smears, have a diameter of 9–15 μm. Their cytoplasm is slightly acidophilic and contains many very fine granules which stain with neutral dyes; the granules stain a faint purple colour with Romanowsky stains (Fig. 1.1a). The nucleus usually contains two to five nuclear segments; the average values for the proportions of cells with two, three, four and five or more segments are 32, 46, 19 and 3% respectively. In the female, 1–17% of cells contain a drumstick-like appendage attached by a fine strand of chromatin to one of the nuclear masses; these appendages correspond to Barr bodies (inactivated X chromosomes).

Neutrophil granules show a considerable heterogeneity with respect to their ultrastructure[19] (Fig. 1.5). Some granules are electron-dense and ellipsoidal; they are referred to as primary granules. Others are less electron-dense and are very pleomorphic; they are termed specific granules. The primary granules, which are formed at the promyelocyte stage, are 0.5–1.0 μm in their long axis and contain myeloperoxidase, acid phosphatase, β-galactosidase, esterase, elastase, collagenase and cationic proteins. The specific granules are formed in the myelocyte and metamyelocyte stages. They vary considerably in size being frequently quite small (0.2–0.5 μm long) and contain lysozyme (muramidase), aminopeptidase and lactoferrin. The enzyme muramidase is capable of lysing the walls of certain bacteria. The alkaline phosphatase activity of neutrophils appears to be present within membrane-bound intracytoplasmic vesicles which have been called phosphosomes. In addition to the various organelles mentioned above, the cytoplasm contains a centrosome, a poorly-developed Golgi apparatus (Fig. 1.6), microtubules and microfilaments, a few small mitochondria, a few ribosomes, a little endoplasmic reticulum and numerous glycogen particles (Fig. 1.6).

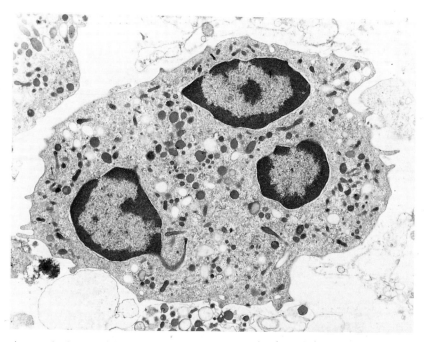

Fig. 1.5 Electron micrograph of a neutrophil granulocyte. The three nuclear segments contain a large quantity of condensed chromatin at their periphery. The cytoplasmic granules vary considerably in size, shape and electron-density. Uranyl acetate and lead citrate.

$\times$ 7 000.

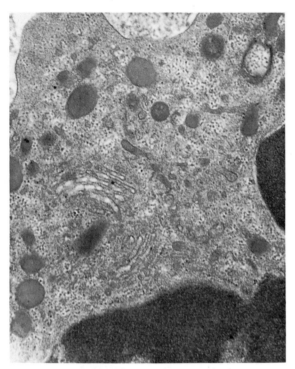

Fig. 1.6 Electron micrograph of part of a neutrophil granulocyte showing the flattened saccules of the Golgi apparatus. The numerous electron-dense particles scattered within the cytosol consist of glycogen. Uranyl acetate and lead citrate.

× 33 400.

Number and life-span

In the blood, the neutrophil granulocytes are distributed between a circulating granulocyte pool (CGP) and a marginated granulocyte pool (MGP).[23] The latter, which is in a rapid equilibrium with the CGP, consists of cells which are loosely associated with the endothelial cells of small venules. The CGP accounts for 16–99% (mean 44%) of the total blood granulocyte pool in healthy subjects. Exercise and adrenaline cause a rapid shift of cells from the MGP to the CGP and bacterial endotoxin causes a shift from the CGP to the MGP. The concentrations of neutrophil granulocytes in the peripheral venous blood of healthy Caucasians of different ages and sexes are given in Tables 1.5 and 1.6. Healthy Blacks

Table 1.5 95% confidence limits for the concentrations of circulating leucocytes in the peripheral venous blood of healthy adults

	Caucasians*		Blacks	
	Male (n = 100)	Female (n = 100)	Female (West Indian plus African)* (n = 158)	Male plus female (American)‖ (n = 226)
White cell count (WBC) (10⁹/l)	3.5–9.5†	4.1–10.9†	3.1–8.7‡	3.6–10.2
Neutrophil count (10⁹/l)	1.6–6.0†	2.0–7.3†	1.1–6.1‡	1.3–7.4
Lymphocyte count (10⁹/l)	1.2–3.5		1.0–3.6	1.45–3.75
Monocyte count (10⁹/l)	0.2–0.8		0.14–0.77	0.21–1.05
Eosinophil count (10⁹/l)	0.02–0.59		0.01–0.82	0.03–0.72
Basophil count (10⁹/l)	0–0.15		0–0.08	0–0.16

* Based on total WBCs determined on a Coulter S Plus and 500-cell differential counts (confidence limits based on a 100-cell differential count are broader).
† Men have WBC and neutrophil counts significantly lower than women ($p < .001$).[24]
‡ Black women[25] and men have WBC and neutrophil counts significantly lower than Caucasian women ($p < .001$) and men.
‖ Based on total WBCs determined on a Coulter counter A or F and 200-cell differential counts. Only 22 cases were female.[26]

Table 1.6 Age-dependent changes in the mean values (and observed ranges) for the concentration of circulating white blood cells ($\times 10^9$/l) in normal individuals. From Dittmer[27]

Age	WBC	Neutrophils			Eosinophils	Basophils	Lymphocytes	Monocytes
		Segmented	Band*	Total				
Birth	18.1(9.0–30.0)†	9.4	1.65	11.0(6.0–26.0)	0.40(0.02–0.85)	0.10(0–0.64)	5.5(2.0–11.0)	1.05(0.40–3.1)
12 hours	22.8(13.0–38.0)	13.2	2.33	15.5(6.0–28.0)	0.45(0.02–0.95)	0.10(0–0.50)	5.5(2.0–11.0)	1.20(0.40–3.6)
24 hours	18.9(9.4–34.0)	9.8	1.75	11.5(5.0–21.0)	0.45(0.05–1.00)	0.10(0–0.30)	5.8(2.0–11.5)	1.10(0.20–3.1)
7 days	12.2(5.0–21.0)	4.7	0.83	5.5(1.5–10.0)	0.50(0.07–1.10)	0.05(0–0.25)	5.0(2.0–17.0)	1.10(0.30–2.7)
2 months	11.0(5.5–18.0)	3.3	0.49	3.8(1.0–9.0)	0.30(0.07–0.85)	0.05(0–0.20)	6.3(3.0–16.0)	0.65(0.13–1.8)
6 months	11.9(6.0–17.5)	3.3	0.45	3.8(1.0–8.5)	0.30(0.07–0.75)	0.05(0–0.20)	7.3(4.0–13.5)	0.58(0.10–1.3)
1 year	11.4(6.0–17.5)	3.2	0.35	3.5(1.5–8.5)	0.30(0.05–0.70)	0.05(0–0.20)	7.0(4.0–10.5)	0.55(0.05–1.1)
2 years	10.6(6.0–17.0)	3.2	0.32	3.5(1.5–8.5)	0.28(0.04–0.65)	0.05(0–0.20)	6.3(3.0–9.5)	0.53(0.05–1.0)
4 years	9.1(5.5–15.5)	3.5(1.5–7.5)	0.27	3.8(1.5–8.5)	0.25(0.02–0.65)	0.05(0–0.20)	4.5(2.0–8.0)	0.45(0–0.8)
6 years	8.5(5.0–14.5)	4.0(1.5–7.0)	0.25	4.3(1.5–8.0)	0.23(0–0.65)	0.05(0–0.20)	3.5(1.5–7.0)	0.40(0–0.8)
10 years	8.1(4.5–13.5)	4.2(1.8–7.0)	0.24	4.4(1.8–8.0)	0.20(0–0.60)	0.04(0–0.20)	3.1(1.5–6.5)	0.35(0–0.8)
14 years	7.9(4.5–13.0)	4.2(1.8–7.0)	0.24	4.4(1.8–8.0)	0.20(0–0.50)	0.04(0–0.20)	2.9(1.2–5.8)	0.38(0–0.8)
18 years	7.7(4.5–12.5)	4.2	0.23	4.4(1.8–7.7)	0.20(0–0.45)	0.04(0–0.20)	2.7(1.0–5.0)	0.40(0–0.8)

*Includes a small percentage of myelocytes during the first few days after birth.
†Includes a small percentage of erythroblasts.

have lower neutrophil counts than Caucasians (Table 1.5); Chinese and Indians have similar counts to those in Europeans.[25] Considerably lower total white cell and neutrophil counts have been reported from East Africa than those shown in Table 1.5 for American Blacks, and West Indian and African Blacks living in England. However, the former studies have not allowed for the skewed distribution of leucocyte numbers in calculating reference ranges, and thus have exaggerated the difference between Blacks and Caucasians.[28] Despite this, total white cell and neutrophil counts are probably genuinely lower in Africans living in African countries, particularly if taking an African diet, than in Africans living in Western countries.[29] Neutrophil granulocytes leave the circulation in an exponential fashion with a $T_{\frac{1}{2}}$ of 2.6–11.8 h (mean 7.2 h)[23] and appear in normal secretions (saliva, secretions of the respiratory and gastrointestinal tracts and urine) and in various tissues. They probably survive outside the blood for up to 30 h.

Functions of neutrophils[30]

These cells are highly motile. They move towards, phagocytose and degrade various types of particulate material such as bacteria and damaged tissue cells. Neutrophils are attracted to sites of infection or inflammation as a result of chemotactic gradients generated around such sites. The chemotactic factors include activated complement components (C3a, C5a, C567) (see Chapter 2), lymphokines released from activated lymphocytes, kallikrein (see p. 320), products of certain bacteria and a factor released by neutrophils containing phagosomes. The arrival of neutrophils is probably facilitated by an increased permeability of adjoining blood vessels as a result of the action of anaphylatoxins such as C3a.

The first stage in the phagocytosis of a particle such as a bacterium is the adherence of the neutrophil to the particle. The adherence is mediated through specific receptors on the neutrophil cell membrane: these include Fc (IgG_1, IgG_3) and C3 receptors. Both the adherence and the subsequent ingestion of such particles are enhanced by their interaction with opsonizing factors such as C3 generated via the classical or alternative complement activation pathway, antibody, C-reactive protein and serum α_2 glycoprotein. Following adhesion, pseudopodia form around the particle and progressively encircle it, probably via a zipper-like mechanism dependent on the interaction between receptors on the cell membrane and opsonizing factors present all over the particle. Both the movement of neutrophils towards a particle and the act of phagocytosis may be dependent on the activity of intracytoplasmic microfilaments composed of actin. The act of phagocytosis is associated with a burst of oxygen consumption (respiratory burst) and the production of hydrogen peroxide.

The ingestion of a particle is followed by the fusion of both primary and specific granules with the membrane of the phagosome and the discharge of granule contents into the phagocytic vacuole. Neutrophils contain considerable quantities of glycogen which can be converted to glucose. They obtain much of their energy by breaking down glucose anaerobically via the Embden-Meyerhof pathway but can oxidize some glucose aerobically through the Krebs cycle. The killing of certain bacteria (e.g. *Staphylococcus aureus*, *Escherichia coli*, *Salmonella typhimurium*, *Klebsiella pneumoniae*, *Proteus vulgaris*) is oxygen-dependent and the killing of others (e.g. *Pseudomonas aeruginosa*, *Staphylococcus epidermidis*, 'viridans' streptococci, various anaerobes) oxygen-independent.

The mechanisms responsible for the killing of bacteria are still under investigation. It is possible that NADH and NADPH serve as the electron donors in the biochemical processes leading to oxygen-dependent killing; a membrane-associated electron transport system which includes cytochrome b_{-245} has been implicated in the electron transfer. The substances proposed as the killing agent in oxygen-dependent killing include singlet oxygen (i.e. activated O_2), superoxide radicals, hydrogen peroxide and free halogens generated from halides by hydrogen peroxide in the presence of the enzyme myeloperoxidase. The mechanisms underlying oxygen-independent killing are uncertain. They may include reductions in intravacuolar pH and damage to bacteria by various granule components, either by a direct effect (e.g. lysozyme, esterase, cationic proteins) or indirectly by the limitation of growth factors. For example, lactoferrin is bacteriostatic as it binds iron at a low pH and thus deprives bacteria of this growth factor.

Eosinophil granulocytes[31]

Morphology and composition

Eosinophil granulocytes have a diameter of 12–17 μm in fixed smears. Their cytoplasm is packed with large rounded granules which stain reddish-orange with Romanowsky stains (Fig. 1.1b). The proportions of cells with one, two, three and four nuclear segments are 6, 68, 22 and 4%, respectively.

Two types of eosinophil granules can be distinguished by electron microscopy: a few rounded homogeneously electron-dense granules and many rounded, elongated or oval crystalloid-containing granules[19] (Fig. 1.7). The homogeneous granules contain a sulphated acid muco-substance and high levels of acid phosphatase. Both homogeneous and crystalloid-containing granules contain an arginine- and zinc-rich basic protein, a peroxidase (distinct from neutrophil peroxidase) and aryl sulphatase. Eosinophil granules also contain phospholipase B and D, β-glycerophosphatase, histaminase, kininase, ribonuclease, β-glucuronidase, cathepsin, PGE_1 and PGE_2 but probably not lysozyme. Eosinophils possess surface receptors for IgG-Fc, C4, C3b and C3d.[32]

Number and life-span

The 95% confidence limits for the eosinophil count in normal adult venous blood is given in Table 1.5. Contrary to earlier reports, eosinophil counts are the same in healthy Blacks, and in

(a)
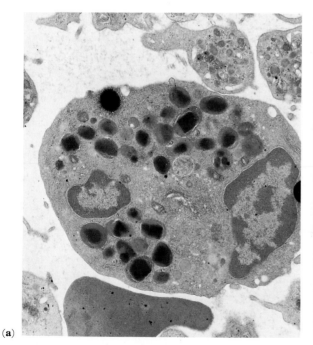

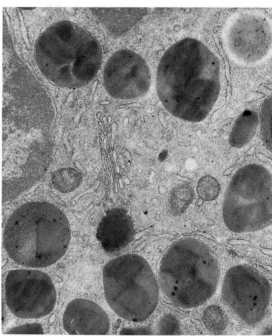
(b)

Fig. 1.7a,b Electron micrographs of normal eosinophil granulocytes. Uranyl acetate and lead citrate.

a. The two nuclear segments contain a large quantity of condensed chromatin at their periphery. One homogeneous granule and several crystalloid-containing granules are present in the cytoplasm. There is a small Golgi apparatus at the centre of the cell (this apparatus is usually somewhat better developed in eosinophils than in neutrophils).
× 10 000.

b. Higher power view of part of another eosinophil granulocyte showing the Golgi apparatus and strands of rough endoplasmic reticulum.
× 24 650.

people whose origins are in the Indian subcontinent, as in Caucasians.[25] Eosinophil granulocytes leave the circulation in a random manner with a $T_{\frac{1}{2}}$ of about 4.5–8 h; they probably survive in the tissues for 8–12 days.

Functions[33, 34]

Eosinophils share several functions with neutrophils: both cell types are motile, respond to specific chemotactic agents and phagocytose and kill similar types of microorganisms. Eosinophils tend to be somewhat slower at ingesting and killing bacteria than neutrophils but appear to be metabolically more active than these cells. Recent work suggests that eosinophils, but not neutrophils, function as the effector cell (killer cell) in antibody-dependent damage to metazoal parasites. The killing of metazoal parasites is associated with the degranulation of eosinophils around the parasite and appears to be caused by the major basic protein of the eosinophil granules. Eosinophils also have a role in regulating immediate-type hypersensitivity reactions. In these reactions chemical mediators of anaphylaxis are released from mast cells and basophils as a result of the interaction between specific antigen and IgE on the surface of these cells. The three best-known chemical mediators are histamine, slow-reacting substance of anaphylaxis and an eosinophil chemotactic factor. The latter, and probably also histamine, attracts eosinophils to the site of the activated mast cells or basophils. The eosinophils then release a substance which inhibits further histamine release. Eosinophils also release histaminase and arylsulphatase which inactivate histamine and slow-reacting substance, respectively.

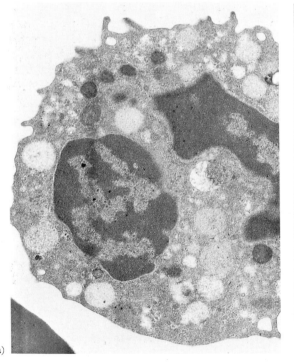

(a)

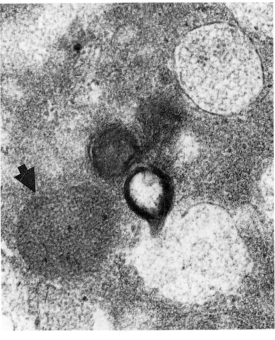

(b)

Fig. 1.8a,b Ultrastructure of basophil granulocytes from normal peripheral blood. Uranyl acetate and lead citrate.

a. There are several large distinctive granules within the cytoplasm. Most of the granules have been partially or completely extracted during the processing for electron microscopy.

× 18 275.

b. Higher power view of part of another basophil granulocyte showing a well-preserved cytoplasmic granule (arrowed) and two virtually completely extracted granules. The unextracted granule shows a characteristic particulate substructure.

× 36 550.

Basophil granulocytes[35]

In Romanowsky-stained blood smears, basophil granulocytes have an average diameter of about 12 μm and display large rounded purplish-black cytoplasmic granules (Fig.1.1c). Some of these granules lie over the nucleus. The nucleus usually has two segments. The granules stain metachromatically (i.e. reddish-violet) with toluidine blue or methylene blue. They appear to undergo varying degrees of extraction during processing for electron microscopy and characteristically show a particulate substructure with each particle measuring about 20 nm in diameter[36] (Fig. 1.8). The granules contain histamine (which is synthesized by the cell), kallikrein, peroxidase, neutral esterases and proteases, serine hydrolase and three sulphated mucopolysaccharides (chondroitin sulphate, dermatin sulphate and heparin sulphate). The mucopolysaccharides account for the metachromatic staining of the granules. Basophils possess receptors for IgE, IgG, C and histamine at their cell surface and contain platelet-activating factor (which causes platelets to aggregate and release their contents) and an eosinophil chemotactic factor (ECF-A). Both basophils and mast cells play a key role in immediate-type hypersensitivity reactions. When IgE-coated basophils react with specific antigen, they rapidly degranulate (by exoplasmosis), release histamine and ECF-A and generate and release slow-reacting substance of anaphylaxis. The response of eosinophils to basophil degranulation is discussed on page 14. Apart from participating in immediate-type hypersensitivity reactions, basophils accumulate at sites of resolving inflammation and may modulate inflammatory responses by releasing heparin (which prevents further fibrin deposition) and proteases (which may inhibit coagulation and promote fibrinolysis). Basophils may also be involved in the histamine-mediated killing of intestinal parasites and, by virtue of their heparin content, in triglyceride metabolism.

Basophils represent the most infrequent type of leucocyte in the blood. The normal ranges for the basophil count in venous blood at different ages are given in Tables 1.5 and 1.6.

MONOCYTES[37] (Figs 1.1d and 1.9)

These are the largest leucocytes in peripheral blood. In stained smears, they vary considerably in diameter (15–30 μm) and in morphology. The nucleus is large and eccentric and may be rounded, kidney- or horseshoe-shaped or lobulated. The nuclear chromatin has a skein-like or lacy appearance. The cytoplasm is plentiful, stains greyish-blue and contains few to many fine azurophilic granules. One or more intracytoplasmic vacuoles may be present. Cytochemical studies with the light microscope have shown the presence of many hydrolytic enzymes, including acid phosphatase, NaF-resistant esterase, lysozyme and galactosidases. Monocytes also have membrane receptors for IgG-Fc and C3. Under the electron microscope, monocyte granules are seen to vary considerably in size and shape and to be more or less homogeneously electron-dense. Some of these granules contain acid phosphatase and peroxidase; the composition of the remainder is unknown. The peroxidase-positive granules are characteristically smaller than those of neutrophils. In thin sections, monocytes display finger-like projections of their cell membrane. Their cytoplasm contains appreciable amounts of rough endoplasmic reticulum, moderate numbers of dispersed ribosomes, a well-developed Golgi apparatus, several mitochondria and bundles of microfibrils. The nucleus has moderate quantities of heterochromatin and although nucleoli are not usually detectable by light microscopy, they are frequently seen by electron microscopy.

Blood monocytes are distributed, as are neutrophils (see p. 10), between a circulating and a marginated pool; there are, on average, 3.6 times more marginated than circulating cells. The concentration of circulating monocytes in the peripheral venous blood of healthy adults is given in Table 1.5. Monocytes leave the circulation in an exponential manner, with an average $T_{\frac{1}{2}}$ of 71 h. They transform into macrophages in various tissues and may survive in this form for several months.

Monocytes are actively motile cells which respond to chemotactic stimuli and phagocytose particulate material in a manner similar to that described for neutrophil granulocytes (p. 12).

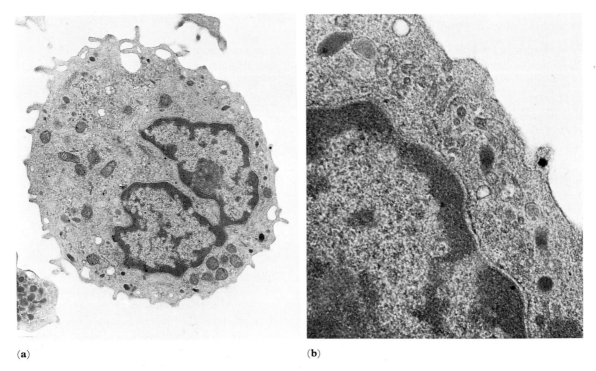

(a)   (b)

Fig. 1.9a,b Electron micrograph of a monocyte from normal peripheral blood. Uranyl acetate and lead citrate.

a. The cytoplasm contains numerous mitochondria, several typical pleomorphic electron-dense granules and short strands of rough endoplasmic reticulum. The nucleus has an irregular outline. It contains moderate quantities of condensed chromatin and a prominent nucleolus.

× 11 325.

b. Higher power view of part of the cell shown in **a.** The electron-dense granules are clearly seen as are a large number of small vesicular structures. These vesicles are typically found around the Golgi apparatus.

× 25 270.

Monocytes and monocyte-derived macrophages are particularly conspicuous in sites of chronic inflammation. Macrophages appear to play important roles in various aspects of the immune response, including the processing of antigen to a form recognizable by lymphocytes and the degradation of excess antigen. The macrophages of the liver, spleen and bone marrow destroy senescent red cells and those in the marrow may produce factors regulating various aspects of haemopoiesis (see p. 66).

LYMPHOCYTES

Most of the lymphocytes in normal blood are small (Fig. 1.1f). Lymphocytes have an average volume of approximately 180 fl[38] and in stained smears have a diameter which varies from about 7 to 12 μm. In Romanowsky-stained preparations they have scanty bluish cytoplasm; the nucleus is round or slightly indented and there is considerable condensation of nuclear chromatin.

The cytoplasm, which sometimes merely consists of a narrow rim around the nucleus, may contain a few azurophilic granules. Ultrastructural studies reveal that small lymphocytes contain a few scattered monoribosomes, an inactive Golgi apparatus, a few mitochondria, a few lysosomal granules and a small nucleolus (Fig. 1.10). In Romanowsky-stained smears, large lymphocytes are about 12–16 μm in diameter and contain more cytoplasm and less condensed chromatin than small lymphocytes (Fig. 1.1e).

The concentration of lymphocytes in the blood is age-dependent: normal values are given in

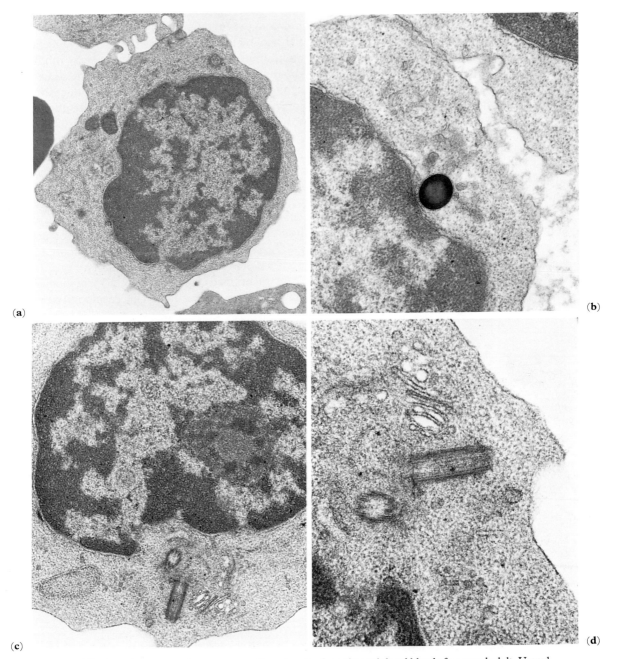

(a)

(b)

(c)

(d)

Fig. 1.10a-d Various ultrastructural appearances of lymphocytes from the peripheral blood of a normal adult. Uranyl acetate and lead citrate.

a. Typical lymphocyte with a high nucleus:cytoplasm ratio, a rounded nuclear outline and large quantities of nuclear-membrane-associated condensed chromatin. The cytoplasm lacks granules but has a few mitochondria and a few moderately long strands of rough endoplasmic reticulum.   × 14 200.

b. Part of a lymphocyte showing a large electron-dense intracytoplasmic inclusion (Goll body) of uncertain nature. The cytoplasm contains numerous monoribosomes and there is a cluster of small membrane-bound granule-like structures adjacent to the Goll body.   × 34 700.

c. Small lymphocyte with a nucleus containing a nucleolus as well as large quantities of condensed chromatin. There is a slight indentation of the nucleus adjacent to two centrioles and the Golgi apparatus.   × 22 075.

d. Higher power view of the centrioles and Golgi apparatus shown in **c.**   × 44 000.

Table 1.5 and 1.6. Lymphocytes recirculate: they leave the blood through the endothelial cells of the post-capillary venules of lymphoid organs and eventually find their way back into lymphatic channels and re-enter the blood via the thoracic duct. The life-span of lymphocytes varies considerably. The average life-span in humans appears to be about four years but some cells survive for over 10 years.

Although mature lymphocytes are morphologically similar to one another they can be divided into two major functionally dissimilar groups, designated B-lymphocytes (B-cells) and T-lymphocytes (T-cells). Some characteristics of these two types of cell, including their various functions, are summarized in Table 1.7. T-cells are further divided into several functionally different groups, including helper cells (which promote the functions of B-cells and are required for the maturation of other kinds of T-cells) and suppressor/cytotoxic cells (which inhibit the functions of other lymphocytes and also have cytotoxic capability against foreign or virus-infected cells). Although cytotoxic and suppressor T-cells share certain well-characterized surface markers, recent evidence indicates that it is possible to distinguish between the cytotoxic and suppressor subpopulations. Lymphocytes which are neither B-cells nor T-cells also exist. For example, K (killer) cells, which have Fc receptors but not the other surface receptors of B-cells, lyse antibody-coated cells, and NK (natural killer) cells are thought to play a role in the body's defence against certain tumours.

As mentioned in Chapter 3, T-lymphocytes participate in the regulation of eosinophil gran-

Table 1.7 Some characteristics of T- and B-lymphocytes

		T-lymphocyte	B-lymphocyte
Identifying characteristics		Form rosettes with sheep red blood cells (ERFC)	Surface membrane immunoglobulin (SmIg) Receptors for complement components—C3b, C3d, C4 Receptors for Fc end of immunoglobulin molecule in immune complex or in aggregated immunoglobulin (FcR) Receptors for EB virus (some cells only)
Origin (also see page 60)		Derived from a lymphoid stem cell initially detectable in fetal liver and subsequently in bone marrow; develop under the influence of thymic epithelium	Derived from a lymphoid stem cell initially detectable in fetal liver and subsequently in bone marrow
Relative distribution	Peripheral blood	≃ 70%	≃ 20–30%
	Bone marrow	≃ 20%	≃ 80%
	Lymph node	≃ 75% Paracortical distribution; medullary sinuses	≃ 25% Follicles; medullary cords
	Lymph	≃ 75%	≃ 25%
	Spleen	≃ 50% Periarteriolar lymphoid sheath	≃ 50% Follicles; marginal zone between T zone and red pulp; cords of red pulp
Function		Cellular immunity (e.g. against viruses, fungi, low-grade intracellular pathogens such as mycobacteria) Graft rejection Tumour rejection Delayed hypersensitivity Interaction with B-cells in production of antibodies against certain antigens Suppression of B-cell function Production of eosinophilia	Maturation into plasma cells for the production of antibodies (immunoglobulin)

ulocytopoiesis *in vivo* (p. 55). There is also some (albeit still controversial) evidence that T-lymphocytes may regulate (augment) erythropoiesis both in experimental animals *in vivo* and in human marrow cultures.[39] In man, specific abnormalities in T-cell subpopulations seem to play a role in the pathogenesis of the cytopenias in some cases of aplastic anaemia, pure red cell aplasia associated with chronic lymphocytic leukaemia and chronic idiopathic neutropenia (pp. 188, 190, 214). It appears that T-cells which are suppressors or helpers of immune functions may also be suppressors or helpers of haemopoiesis.

PLATELETS

Morphology and composition[40]

Platelets are small fragments of megakaryocyte cytoplasm with an average volume of 7–8 fl. When seen in Romanowsky-stained blood smears, most platelets have a diameter of 2–3 μm. They may be found lying singly but show a tendency to form small clumps. Platelets have an irregular outline, stain light blue and contain a number of small azurophilic granules which are usually concentrated at the centre. Newly-formed platelets are larger than more mature ones.

Ultrastructural studies have revealed that non-activated (resting) platelets are shaped like biconvex discs and contain mitochondria, granules, two systems of cytoplasmic membranes (a surface-connected canalicular system and a dense tubular system), microfilaments, microtubules and clumps of glycogen molecules (Fig. 1.11). The discoid shape is actively maintained by a cytoskeleton consisting of many short contractile microfilaments composed of actomyosin and an equatorial bundle of microtubules composed of tubulin. The microfilaments are situated between various organelles and may be attached to specific proteins at the inner surface of the cell membrane. In addition to maintaining cell shape the microfilaments are probably involved in clot retraction. The equatorial bundle of microtubules is situated in an organelle-free sol-gel zone just beneath the cell membrane and appears to be connected to this membrane by filaments. When platelets change shape during activation, the microtubules break their connections with

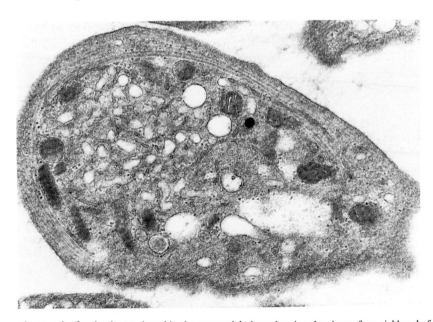

Fig. 1.11 Electron micrograph of a platelet sectioned in the equatorial plane showing the circumferential band of microtubules. Many electron-lucent vesicles belonging to the surface-connected canalicular system, a few mitochondria and some platelet granules (including one dense body) can be seen. The dense tubular system is present between the vesicles of the surface-connected canalicular system, but is only just visible at the present magnification. Uranyl acetate and lead citrate.   × 24 325.

the cell membrane and contract inwards; the platelet granules also become concentrated at the centre of the cell. The cell membrane of the platelet is extensively invaginated to form a surface-connected canalicular system. This canalicular system provides a large surface area through which various substances, including the contents of platelet granules, can be released to the exterior. It is thought that the contraction of the microfilaments during platelet activation brings the platelet granules close to special areas of this canalicular system which are capable of fusing with granules. The contraction of microtubules may also play a role in this process. Adjacent to the bundle of microtubules is a specialized form of endoplasmic reticulum known as the dense tubular system. This system is the main site of synthesis of thromboxane A_2 which plays an important role in the reactions leading to the release of the contents of platelet granules. The dense tubular system also contains a high concentration of calcium ions when compared with that elsewhere in the cytoplasm and may regulate the activity of several calcium-dependent reversible cytoplasmic processes such as the activation of actomyosin, depolymerization of microtubules and glycogenolysis.

On the basis of the ultrastructural appearances and ultrastructural cytochemistry of the granules, and of studies of patients with a selective lack of one type of granule, the platelet granules can be divided into four types (Table 1.8).[19] Dense bodies are very electron-dense, usually show a bull's eye appearance because of the presence of an electron-lucent zone between the central electron-dense material and the limiting membrane and contain the storage pool of ADP and ATP which is concerned with secondary platelet aggregation. They also contain calcium and adrenaline as well as 5HT (which causes both vasoconstriction and platelet aggregation). The α granules and lysosomal (λ) granules are slightly larger than dense granules, and are moderately electron-dense. The peroxisomes are smaller than α and λ granules. Substances present in α granules include platelet factor 4 which has heparin-neutralizing activity and may thus potentiate the action of thrombin, and the platelet mitogenic factors which stimulate growth of endothelial and smooth muscle cells and of skin fibroblasts.

Number and life-span

The normal range for the platelet count in peripheral blood is about $160–450 \times 10^9/l$ (see Table 1.3); slightly lower values are seen during the first three months of life. Small cyclical variations in the platelet count may be seen in some individuals of both sexes, with a periodicity of 21–35 days; in pre-menopausal women the fall usually occurs during the two weeks preceding menstruation. The platelet counts of women are slightly higher than those of men.[42, 43] There are also slight racial variations in the normal platelet count. For example, values lower than those quoted above have been reported in Australians of Mediterranean descent.[44] In addition, Nigerians have lower platelet counts than Caucasians,[45] as have Africans and West Indians living in the United Kingdom.[46]

Table 1.8 Characteristics of various types of platelet granules[40,41]

Granule	Contents	Appearance
Dense bodies (δ granules)	Serotonin, calcium, storage pool of ATP and ADP, pyrophosphate	Very dense, may have 'bull's eye' appearance
α granules	β thromboglobulin, platelet factor 4, platelet mitogenic factor, fibrinogen, fibronectin, factor-VIII-related antigen, albumin, thrombospondin	Granules of identical appearance on EM; less electron-dense than dense bodies; distinguished from each other by ultrastructural cytochemistry
Lysosomal granules (λ granules)	Acid phosphatase, β-glucuronidase, arylsulphatase	
Peroxisomes	Catalase	Smaller than α and λ granules

Functions[47]

Large quantities of energy are used during various platelet functions. This energy is mainly derived from the metabolism of glucose by the glycolytic pathway and tricarboxylic acid cycle. The energy is held as ATP within a metabolic pool which is distinct from the storage pool of adenine nucleotides situated in the dense bodies.

Platelets play an essential role in the haemostatic mechanism. When endothelial cells of vessel walls are damaged and denuded, platelets adhere to subendothelial connective tissue (basement membrane and microfibrils of elastin) via a specific receptor on the platelet membrane, glycoprotein I. This adhesion requires calcium ions and von Willebrand factor (p. 319). Platelets also adhere to collagen via other specific membrane receptors. Adhesion is followed within seconds by the transformation of the platelet from its original discoid shape to a spiny sphere (a potentially reversible process) and within a few minutes by the release of the contents of some platelet granules (the release reaction). Initially, the contents of the dense bodies are released; with stronger stimulation, some α granules are also discharged. The ADP released from the dense bodies, and possibly also traces of thrombin generated by the activation of the clotting cascade, cause an interaction of other platelets with the adherent platelets and with each other (secondary platelet aggregation) with further release of ADP from the aggregating platelets. Aggregation induced by ADP (and by adrenaline and collagen) is preceded by an alteration of the cell membrane leading to calcium-dependent binding of fibrinogen to specific platelet receptors associated with membrane glycoprotein IIb-IIIa; binding of fibrinogen to platelets may provide a recognition site for platelet–platelet interaction during aggregation.[48] The process of secondary aggregation continues until a platelet plug occludes the damaged vessel. The release reaction may be mediated through thromboxane A_2 synthesized in the platelet from arachidonic acid released from membrane phospholipids (the conversion of arachidonic acid to thromboxane A_2 requires the enzymes cyclo-oxygenase and thromboxane synthetase). The formation of a fibrin clot around the platelet plug is initiated by the activation of factor XII by contact with subendothelial structures (see p. 320). The exposure of certain membrane phospholipids (platelet factor 3) in aggregated platelets plays a role in the formation of this fibrin clot. These platelet phospholipids participate in: (a) the formation of factor Xa through a reaction involving factors IXa, VIII, X and calcium; and (b) in the reaction between factors II, V, Xa and calcium (see p. 319).

In addition to their primary role in haemostasis, platelets have several other functions. They participate in the generation of the inflammatory response by releasing factors which increase vascular permeability and attract granulocytes. The α granules of the platelet contain mitogenic factors which promote the regeneration of damaged endothelial cells. These mitogenic factors also stimulate fibroblast proliferation and may therefore promote the healing of wounds. Furthermore, platelets remove the pharmacologically active substance 5HT from their microenvironment by taking it up and concentrating it in the dense granules; they thus serve as 'detoxifying' cells. Platelets also have a limited capacity for phagocytosis. Finally, platelets play a role in pathological processes such as thrombosis and the rejection of transplants and have also been implicated by some workers in the pathogenesis of atherosclerosis.

Platelet function may be tested *in vivo* or *in vitro*. The bleeding time is the most useful *in vivo* measure of platelet function and may be determined according to the method of Ivy or Duke. The Ivy test, which is performed on the forearm, is more sensitive in detecting an abnormality than the Duke test, which is performed on the ear lobe. In the Ivy test, a sphygmomanometer cuff is applied and inflated to a pressure of 40 mm to raise the venous pressure. A set number of punctures of a defined depth are made in the skin with a lancet and the time till bleeding stops is measured.[49] In a variation of the Ivy test an incision through a template is used rather than a puncture.[50] The bleeding time is predominantly a measure of platelet number and function though some prolongation is caused by severe defects of coagulation factors, including overdose of oral anticoagulants. If platelet numbers are known to be normal, then a prolonged bleeding time usually indicates an intrinsic platelet defect (e.g. an inherited or an aspirin-induced defect) or an extrinsic defect (e.g. inhibition by uraemic toxins, or failure to interact with an abnormal surface due to a lack of high-molecular-weight von Willebrand's factor). The Hess test is also an *in vivo* test of platelet function, but is not very useful because a positive result is often consequent on capillary fragility rather than a platelet defect.

Platelet functions which may be investigated *in vitro* include adhesion, aggregation, clot retraction and contribution to the intrinsic coagulation pathway. Adhesion can best be tested by passing whole blood through rabbit aorta stripped of its endothelium and quantitating the number of adherent platelets.[51] Both adhesion and aggregation are tested by passing blood through a glass bead column and determining the percentage of retained platelets; this test is difficult to standardize. Aggregation is most readily tested by the use of an aggregometer which measures optical density of platelet-rich plasma; as aggregation is induced (e.g. by ADP, adrenaline [epinephrine], collagen or the antibiotic ristocetin) the optical density falls; if platelets disaggregate the optical density rises again. It is also possible to measure adenosine triphosphate (ATP) release during platelet aggregation. Clot retraction is assessed by measuring the volume of serum expressed by whole blood which is allowed to clot in a glass tube at 37°C for 1h; a high haematocrit may interfere with clot retraction. The contribution of the platelet to the intrinsic pathway of blood coagulation (see p. 319) may be tested by the prothrombin consumption test (which shows defective conversion of prothrombin to thrombin when there is a deficiency of platelet number or function) or the platelet factor 3 availability test or the thromboplastin generation test (which test for the ability of the platelet to accelerate the intrinsic pathway of coagulation).

ALTERATIONS IN THE BLOOD IN PREGNANCY

In most women, the haemoglobin level begins to fall at about the sixth to eighth week of a normal pregnancy, reaches its lowest level at about the thirty-second week and increases slightly thereafter. The extent of fall varies markedly from woman to woman but haemoglobin levels less than 10 g/dl are probably abnormal. The average fall is about 1.5–2 g/dl. This physiological 'anaemia' occurs despite an average increase in the red cell mass of about 300 ml and results from an average increase in the plasma volume of about a litre.[52] The reticulocyte percentage is increased, plateauing at about 6% between 25 and 35 weeks. The mean corpuscular volume and MCH rise during pregnancy in the absence of any deficiency of vitamin B_{12} or folic acid. Serum iron falls. Transferrin synthesis increases due to a direct hormonal effect (similar changes are seen in subjects taking oral contraceptives); the transferrin concentration and total iron binding capacity increase. The serum vitamin B_{12} level falls steadily throughout pregnancy reaching its lowest level at term; this is a physiological change and is not indicative of deficiency. About 10% of normal women have serum vitamin B_{12} levels below 100 ng/l during the last trimester. There is a return to non-pregnant levels by six weeks postpartum.[53] Red cell and serum folate levels also fall[53] and 20–30% of women have subnormal red-cell folate levels at term. Physiological needs for iron and folic acid are increased, and in subjects with reduced stores and/or poor intake (see pp. 159 and 179) deficiency may occur. The haemoglobin F level increases slightly. The percentage of F-cells (p. 124) is increased at mid-term but returns to non-pregnant levels by term. The ESR rises early in pregnancy and is highest in the third trimester. The white-cell count increases, due to an increase of neutrophils and monocytes. Total WBCs of 10–15 x 10^9/l are common during pregnancy and postpartum levels may reach 20–40 x 10^9/l. Metamyelocytes and myelocytes are seen in the blood in about a quarter of subjects and promyelocytes may also be present. 'Toxic' granulation and Döhle bodies[54] (see p. 210) are common and are a physiological change. The neutrophil alkaline phosphatase rises early in pregnancy and remains elevated; a further rise occurs during labour, with a return to non-pregnant levels by six weeks postpartum. The bactericidal capacity of neutrophils is increased and in 40–60% of subjects in the second and third trimester, an increased proportion of neutrophils are positive in the nitro-blue tetrazolium test (see p. 207). Lymphocyte and eosinophil counts are decreased. The basophil count may rise. Consistent changes in the platelet count have not been reported, but some fall may occur.[55] In pregnancy, several coagulation factors, including factor VIII and fibrinogen increase and fibrinolytic activity decreases.

Fetal cells, for example fetal red cells and fetal lymphocytes,[56] enter the maternal circulation during pregnancy as well as at delivery. This phenomenon is common enough to be regarded as physiological, although it may have adverse effects when the mother becomes sensitized to fetal antigens (see Chapter 2).

REFERENCES

1. Meites S, ed. Pediatric clinical chemistry, a survey of reference (normal) values, methods, and instrumentation, with commentary. 2nd ed. Washington: American Association for Clinical Chemistry, 1981: 381.
2. Bain BJ. Clin Lab Haematol 1983; 5: 45.
3. Dacie JV, Lewis SM, eds. Practical haematology. 6th ed. Edinburgh: Churchill Livingstone, 1984.
4. Guest GM, Brown EW. Am J Dis Child 1957; 93: 486.
5. Saarinen UM, Siimes MA. J Pediatr 1978; 92: 412.
6. Serjeant GR, Grandison Y, Mason K, Serjeant B, Sewell A, Vaidya S. Clin Lab Haematol 1980; 2: 169.
7. Koerper MA, Mentzer WC, Grecher G, Dallman PR. J Pediatr 1976; 89: 580.
8. Schmaier BA, Maurer HM, Johnston CL, Scott RB, Stewart LM. J Pediatr 1974; 84: 559.
9. Giorno R, Clifford JH, Beverly S, Rossing RG. Am J Clin Pathol 1980; 74: 765.
10. Hows J, Hussein S, Hoffbrand AV, Wickramasinghe SN. J Clin Pathol 1977; 30: 181.
11. Mollison PL, Veal N. Br J Haematol 1955; 1: 62.
12. Donohue DM, Motulsky AG, Giblett ER, Pirzio-Biroli G, Viranuvatti V, Finch CA. Br J Haematol 1955; 1: 249.
13. Mollison PL. Blood transfusion in clinical medicine. 7th ed. Oxford: Blackwell Scientific Publications, 1983.
14. Alderman EM, Fudenberg HH, Lovins RE. Blood 1981; 58: 341.
15. Grimes AJ. Human red cell metabolism. Oxford: Blackwell Scientific Publications, 1980.
16. Harris JW, Kellermeyer RW. The red cell. Production, metabolism, destruction: normal and abnormal. Cambridge, Mass: Harvard University Press, 1970.
17. Barcroft J. The respiratory function of the blood. Cambridge University Press, 1928.
18. Marchesi VT. Blood 1983; 61: 1.
19. Bessis M. Living blood cells and their ultrastructure. Berlin: Springer, 1973.
20. Deiss A, Kurth D. Am J Clin Pathol 1970; 53: 481.
21. Hillman RS, Finch CA. Br J Haematol 1969; 17: 313.
22. Wintrobe MM, Lee GR, Boggs DR, et al. Clinical hematology. 8th ed. Philadelphia: Lea and Febiger, 1981: 1885.
23. Cartwright GE, Athens JW, Wintrobe MM. Blood 1964; 24: 780.
24. Bain BJ, England JM. Br Med J 1975; 1: 306.
25. Bain BJ, Seed M, Godsland I. J Clin Pathol 1984; 37: 188.
26. Orfanakis NG, Ostlund RE, Bishop CR, Athens JW. Am J Clin Pathol 1970; 53: 647.
27. Dittmer DS. Blood and other body fluids. Washington: Federation of American Societies for Experimental Biology, 1961: 125.
28. Shaper AG, Lewis P. Lancet 1971; ii: 1021.
29. Ezeilo GC. Lancet 1972; ii: 1003.
30. Soothill JF, Segal AW. In: Hardisty RM, Weatherall DJ, eds. Blood and its disorders. 2nd ed. Oxford: Blackwell Scientific Publications, 1983: 629.
31. Beeson PB, Bass DA. The eosinophil. Philadelphia: Saunders, 1977.
32. Anwar ARE, Kay AB. J Immunol 1977; 119: 976.
33. Kay AB. Br J Haematol 1976; 33: 313.
34. Butterworth PE, David JR. N Engl J Med 1981; 304: 154.
35. Dvorak AM, Dvorak HF. Arch Pathol Lab Med 1979; 103: 551.
36. Zucker-Franklin D. Blood 1980; 56: 534.
37. Furth R van, Raeburn JA, Zwet TL van. Blood 1979; 54: 485.
38. Chapman EH, Kurec AS, Davey FR. J Clin Pathol 1981; 34: 1083.
39. Goodman JW, Goodman DR. In: Dunn CDR, ed. Current concepts in erythropoiesis, Chichester: Wiley, 1983: 59.
40. White JG. Am J Clin Pathol 1979; 71: 363.
41. Berndt MC, Castaldi PA, Gordon S, Halley H, McPherson VJ. Aust NZ J Med 1983; 13: 387.
42. Stevens RF, Alexander MK. Br J Haematol 1977; 37: 295.
43. Bain BJ. Scand J Haematol 1985; 35: 77.
44. Behrens WE von. Blood 1975; 46: 199.
45. Essien EM, Usanga EA, Ayeni O. Scand J Haematol 1973; 10: 378.
46. Bain BJ. (in preparation.)
47. Packham MA. Thromb Haemost 1983; 50: 610.
48. Agam G, Livne A. Blood 1983; 61: 186.
49. Bain B, Forster T. Thromb Haemost 1980; 43: 131.
50. Mielke CH, Kaneshiro MM, Maker IA, Weiner JM, Rapaport SI. Blood 1969; 34: 204.
51. Tschopp TP, Weiss HJ, Baumgartner HR. J Lab Clin Med 1974; 83: 296.
52. Lange RD, Dynesius R. Clin Haematol 1973; 2: 433.
53. Cooper BA. Clin Haematol 1973; 2: 461.
54. Abernathy MR. Blood 1966; 27: 380.
55. Sejeny SA, Eastham RD, Baker SR. J Clin Pathol 1975; 28: 812.
56. Schröder J, Chapelle A de la. Blood 1972; 39: 153.

Antibodies, complement and blood group antigens

SOME CHARACTERISTICS OF ANTIGENS

An antigen is a substance which elicits an immune response; an immune response is a specifically altered reaction of an organism to a substance it has previously come in contact with. Most naturally occurring antigens are structurally-complex macromolecules such as proteins, carbohydrates, lipids and nucleic acids; blood group antigens are macromolecules present on the surfaces of blood cells. The immune responses which may be elicited by an antigen could be positive or negative and include 1) the production of cells which react with and 'destroy' the antigen (cellular immunity), 2) the production of antibody which reacts with the antigen and, frequently, leads to its subsequent destruction (humoral immunity) and 3) the acquisition of a specific unresponsiveness to an antigen (immunological tolerance). Although antigens are complex molecules, a single molecular species of antibody reacts only with a very small part of the antigen (the antigenic determinant).

A blood cell antigen is an inherited characteristic and its inheritance is determined by a particular gene present at a specific locus on a chromosome. If an individual is homozygous for the gene in question, the same gene will also be present at the identical locus on the homologous chromosome. The pair of loci on the homologous chromosomes may, however, have different genes; two or more genes which could occupy the same locus are termed alleles.

SOME CHARACTERISTICS OF ANTIBODIES[1, 2, 3, 4]

An antigen stimulates B-lymphocytes, capable of responding to it, to proliferate and subsequently differentiate into plasma cells. Antibodies or immunoglobulins are proteins synthesized by plasma cells in response to an antigen; they are capable of specifically combining with that antigen. The progeny of a single B-lymphocyte, responding to one antigen and secreting identical antibody, are designated a clone. A primary immune response is one that occurs after first exposure to a foreign antigen. The response that occurs after an adequately spaced second exposure is called a secondary immune response. The latter is more brisk and associated with the production of larger quantities of antibody than a primary response. An important difference between a primary and secondary response lies in a considerably larger number of cells responding to antigen in the latter.

An immunoglobulin molecule has a basic structure of two pairs of covalently linked chains, the longer pair being designated heavy chains and the shorter pair light chains (Fig. 2.1). This basic

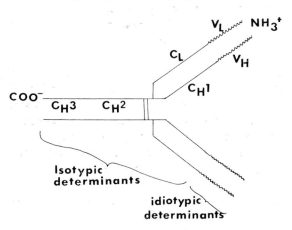

Fig. 2.1 Basic structure of an immunoglobulin molecule.

structure may occur in a monomeric form or as a dimer or a larger polymer. The heavy chain can be divided into at least five regions: three regions showing little heterogeneity in structure and thus designated the constant regions (C_H1, C_H2 and C_H3), one region showing great heterogeneity and thus designated the variable region (V_H), and

a joining region (J) between C_H1 and V_H. The pair of heavy chains in each antibody molecule may be of one of five types. The type of heavy chain divides immunoglobulins into five classes, IgG (γ heavy chains), IgM (μ heavy chains), IgA (α heavy chains), IgD (δ heavy chains) and IgE (ε heavy chains) (Table 2.1). There are, in addition, four subclasses of IgG (IgG$_1$, IgG$_2$, IgG$_3$ and IgG$_4$) and two subclasses of IgA. The class and subclass of an immunoglobulin molecule are determined by the structure of the constant region of the heavy chain. Each immunoglobulin molecule has identical light chains which are of one of two types, κ or λ. The light chains can be divided into three regions, a constant region (C_L), a variable region (V_L) and a joining region (J).

The structure of immunoglobulin molecules is determined by three sets of genes. The genes coding for the synthesis of the heavy chain are on chromosome 14 and are grouped into variable region genes (V), joining region genes (J), constant region genes (C) and diversity genes (D). The genes for the κ chain are on chromosome 2, and those for the λ chain on chromosome 22. Each set of genes for a light chain includes genes for the variable region (V), genes for the joining region (J), and genes for the constant region (C).

In germ cells and cells not committed to the B-cell lineage, genes for the variable region of the heavy chain are separated from the diversity, joining and constant region genes. At some critical point in commitment to the B-cell lineage distant genes are brought into juxtaposition (by translocation or somatic rearrangement) in the order $V_H - D - J_H - C_H$ to form a transcription unit producing a precursor of messenger RNA which, after removal of introns, becomes the messenger RNA for one of the heavy chains. Similarly, sets of genes for each of the light chains are brought into juxtaposition in the order $V_L - J_L - C_L$ and can then code for messenger RNA for the light chain. Gene rearrangement proceeds until one set of light chain genes is effectively rearranged and can be expressed: κ gene rearrangement occurs first and λ genes are rearranged only if neither of the κ genes is effectively rearranged. Heavy and light chains are synthesized separately on ribosomes, in close to

Table 2.1 Some characteristics of the various classes of immunoglobulins

	IgG	IgA	IgM	IgD	IgE
Serum concentration (g/l)	8–16	1.4–4.0	0.5–2.0	<0.4	0.02–0.04
% intravascular distribution	45	42	75	75	50
$T_\frac{1}{2}$(d)	21	6	5	2.8	2.2
Sedimentation constant (Svedberg)	7	7	19	7–8	8
Molecular weight	140 000	140 000	900 000	180 000	190 000

equimolecular amounts. Assembly of immuno-globulin molecules occurs mainly in the cisternae of the smooth endoplasmic reticulum. Re-arrangement of heavy chain genes precedes re-arrangement of light chain genes and indicates that a cell is committed to the B-cell lineage; a cell showing rearrangement of heavy chain genes only may be designated an early pre-B-cell.

Antibody specificity of an immunoglobulin molecule is conveyed by certain hypervariable re-gions within the V_H and V_L regions of the amino-terminal ends of the molecule, which form a specific antigen-combining site. The unique amino acid sequences of the variable region de-termine the idiotype of a molecule. The idiotypic determinants are themselves antigenic and anti-idiotypic antisera may be raised against them. T-cells and B-cells carry idiotypic determinants which are important in antigen recognition. Each individual is capable of producing $10^6 - 10^8$ dif-ferent species of antibody molecules, each with its unique idiotype. The constant regions of the heavy and light chains show only limited varia-tion which leads to the formation of some twenty variants which are designated isotypes; for ex-ample $IgG_1\kappa$, $IgG_2\kappa$ and $IgM\lambda$ are different iso-types. A single plasma cell or a single clone of plasma cells produces only one idiotype but, in some circumstances, may produce more than one isotype; for example, $IgD\kappa$ and $IgM\kappa$ of the same idiotype may occur together on single cells or clones of cells. Immunoglobulin molecules also show inherited differences which are known as allotypes. Allotypic determinants include the Gm markers of the γ chain and the Inv (or Km) mar-kers of the κ chain. Some characteristics of the

various classes of immunoglobulin including their concentration in normal serum are shown in Table 2.1.

IgG molecules usually exist as monomers. They have two antibody combining sites and are therefore said to be divalent. They account for most of the antibodies formed in a secondary im-mune response. IgA molecules may be present as monomers, dimers or larger polymers. IgA anti-bodies are present in secretions and are important in immune responses at mucosal surfaces. IgM molecules are usually pentamers and therefore have 10 potential antigen-binding sites. IgA di-mers and IgM in pentameric form have an addi-tional chain, the J chain, which is secreted by plasma cells. In addition a 'secretory piece' of epithelial origin is added to IgM and IgA secreted at mucosal surfaces. IgM is generally the first and predominant class of antibody to be pro-duced in a primary immune response. IgM mole-cules are important in clearing intravascular par-ticulate antigens. Because of their pentameric structure the distance between two of the antigen-binding sites on a single IgM molecule is long enough for one molecule to join together antigens on adjacent red cells and thus cause agglutination of red cells suspended in normal saline. By contrast, the smaller IgG molecules have a shorter distance between their two binding sites and do not usually cause agglutination of red cells in saline. IgD and IgE immunoglobulin molecules are both present as monomers. The function of IgD is unknown. IgE is concerned with the release of histamine and other sub-stances from basophils and mast cells in response to antigenic stimulation (see p. 15). Specific structural arrangements towards the carboxy-terminal end of the two heavy chains (Fc piece, see Fig. 2.1) determine whether an immunoglobulin molecule combines with the first component of complement and activates the complement cascade, crosses the placenta, or combines with receptors on macrophages, eosinophils, basophils or mast cells. Only IgG molecules cross the placenta. Molecules of the IgG_1 and IgG_3 subclasses of IgG can activate complement and combine with specific receptors on macrophages; IgM also activates complement and IgG_2 molecules may do so to a lesser extent. Structures in the Fc piece of IgG and IgM molecules combine respectively with receptors on two specific subsets of T-lymphocytes, $T\gamma$ and $T\mu$. Aggregated IgG molecules combine with receptors on B-lymphocytes.

Blood group antibodies

Antibodies are designated heteroantibodies if they recognize antigens of other species, alloantibodies (or isoantibodies) if they recognize antigens of other individuals of the same species and autoantibodies if they recognize self-antigens. A heterophil antibody is one produced following exposure to an antigen from one species which recognizes similar or identical antigens in another species.

Blood group alloantibodies are formed following exposure to blood cells bearing antigens not present in the recipient. Such exposure may follow blood transfusion or feto-maternal haemorrhage.

Antibodies which react with red cell antigens may also be evoked by exposure to non-erythroid antigens whose structure closely resembles that of blood group antigens. Red cell antibodies which occur in subjects who have not been exposed to the appropriate red cell antigens are designated 'naturally-occurring antibodies'. All normal A, B or O subjects have naturally-occurring antibodies to antigens of the ABO system (Table 2.2). These antibodies are probably evoked by antigens of gut bacteria and, if so, are heteroantibodies. Naturally-occurring antibodies are usually IgM and thus agglutinating. They have maximal activity at low temperature (0–4°C) and are therefore designated cold antibodies.

Antibodies developed in response to exposure to red cell antigens are designated 'immune' antibodies (although there is no reason to think that naturally-occurring antibodies are not also the result of an immune response). Immune antibodies may be IgG, IgM or IgA. In comparison with naturally-occurring antibodies, immune antibodies are less likely to agglutinate red cells, and are more likely to have optimal activity at higher temperatures (37°C), therefore being designated warm antibodies. Red cell antigens differ in their degree of antigenicity and individuals vary in the likelihood of response to a given antigen: normal individuals may fail to respond even to repeated exposure to a given antigen.

Table 2.2 Distribution of ABO and Lewis antigens and antibodies on red cells and in secretions and serum

Blood group	Genotype	Secretor (SeSe or Sese)			Non-secretor (sese)		
		Antigens on erythrocytes	Antigens in secretions	Antibodies in serum	Antigens on erythrocytes	Antigens in secretions	Antibodies in serum
A	AA or AO	A, H	A, H	anti-B★	A, H	Nil	anti-B★
B	BB or BO	B, H	B, H	anti-A	B, H	Nil	anti-A
AB	AB	A, B, H	A, B, H	Nil★	A, B, H	Nil	Nil★
O	OO	H	H	anti-A anti-B	H	Nil	anti-A anti-B
Lewis positive†	LeLe or Lele	Le^b [Le(a−b+)]	$Le^a\ Le^b$	Nil	Le^a [Le(a+b−)]	Le^a	Nil
Lewis negative†	lele	Nil [Le(a−b−)]	Nil	anti-Le^a in 20 per cent	Nil [Le(a−b−)]	Nil	anti-Le^{bL}

★ Subjects who are group A_2 or A_2B may produce anti A_1.
† With regard to Lewis groups this table is a simplification; for further details see Mollison.[12]

The majority of normal sera contains naturally-occurring antibodies of the ABO system, and also a low-titre cold autoantibody of anti-I specificity. Subjects who have been exposed to blood cells may also have alloantibodies. Pathological autoantibodies may also occur and may lead to autoimmune haemolytic anaemia. It is often harder to demonstrate the specificity of autoantibodies than of alloantibodies, but specificity may be demonstrated within the Rhesus system (warm autoimmune haemolytic anaemia) or within the Ii or P systems (cold haemagglutinin disease and paroxysmal cold haemoglobinuria, respectively) (see pp. 145–148).

Antibodies may lead to intravascular or extravascular destruction of red cells. IgG_1, IgG_3 and IgM antibodies which fix complement and activate the complement cascade may cause intravascular lysis of red cells. If complement is fixed but activation proceeds only to C3 then intravascular lysis does not occur, but the red cells may be removed by the mononuclear phagocyte system, the macrophages thereof having receptors for activated C3. Macrophages also have Fc receptors which recognize the carboxy-terminal end of IgG_1 and IgG_3 molecules and may thereby clear antibody-coated cells even if complement is not bound. The mononuclear phagocyte system may phagocytose part of the membrane of an antibody-coated cell and release the remainder of the cell as a spherocyte. Antibody-coated cells may also be destroyed by K (killer) cells, a subclass of lymphocytes with Fc receptors (ADCC, antibody-dependent cellular cytotoxicity). Platelets also have Fc receptors which bind IgG_1 and IgG_3 preferentially, and IgG_2 and IgG_4 to a lesser extent; by this mechanism immune complexes may induce platelet aggregation and the release reaction (see pp. 278 and 279).[5]

COMPLEMENT

The term complement (C) describes a group of plasma proteins which are sequentially activated by events such as antigen-antibody interactions; activation leads to the production of potent biological mediators including substances promoting chemotaxis and phagocytosis, and causing anaphylaxis. Complement may be activated through two interacting pathways, the classical pathway (activated by antigen-antibody complexes containing IgG_1, IgG_2, IgG_3 or IgM) and the alternative pathway (activated by aggregates of IgG or IgA, as well as by various foreign substances). Activation of the entire complement cascade leads to lysis of cells, for example, erythrocytes coated with antibody. The classical and alternative pathways of complement activation and the membrane attack mechanism are shown in Figure 2.2. A prerequisite for activation of the classical pathway is the binding of an antibody of appropriate class or subclass to a cellular antigen. The first component of complement, C1, then binds to the Fc portion of the antibody molecule. C1 is a complex of C1q with a tetramer $C1r_2 - Ca^{++} - C1s_2$. Binding of the C1q component to the Fc portion of the Ig leads to autoactivation of C1r which then activates C1s. C1s in turn activates both C4 and C2 with subsequent formation of the bimolecular complex C42. C42 can attach to other sites on the cell membrane thus amplifying the reaction. C42 activates C3 to C3 (C3b) which also attaches to new sites on the cell membrane with further amplification of the process. C423 cleaves C5 to form C5b which again attaches to the membrane at distant sites, subsequently binding C6, C7 and C8 to the membrane. When the C5-8 complex has attached to the membrane it acts as as a receptor for C9 which enters the membrane; C9 polymers form a 'doughnut' in the membrane, allowing cellular constituents to leave the cell through the central hole. C3b is cleaved to inactive forms. It is initially converted to C3c and C3d,g; subsequently C3d,g is cleaved to C3d and C3g. The cleavage of C3 and C5 produces chemotaxins and anaphylatoxins. Certain activated complement components also promote phagocytosis. Monocytes, macrophages and neutrophils bind to C4b (C4), C3b (C3) and C5b.

The alternative pathway of complement activation provides an alternative mechanism for activation of C3 and C5, which is independent of C1, C4, and C2; it requires C3 (C3b) which may be provided by the classical pathway but is also slowly generated spontaneously. C3b complexes with factor B in the presence of Mg^{++}

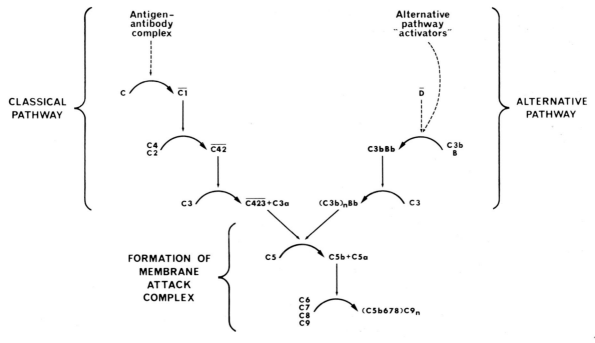

Fig. 2.2 Classical and alternative pathways of complement activation, and the membrane attack mechanism.

and the complex is then activated by factor D to form C3b,Bb which has C3-convertase activity (analogous to $\overline{C42}$ in the classical pathway). C3b, Bb activates C3 and combines with it to form $(C3b)_n Bb$ which has C5-convertase activity. Properdin (factor P) is not essential for the alternative pathway but enhances it by binding to C3b, Bb and increasing its stability.

Not only does the alternative pathway augment the activation of C3 by antigen-antibody triggering of the classical pathway but it also provides a mechanism for activation by IgA, and by non-immunological activators such as bacterial endotoxin, particulate polysaccharides (such as zymosan, agarose and inulin), most metazoan and protozoan parasites and some tumour cells[6] and various foreign surfaces. Such 'activators' of the alternative pathway are actually protectors rather than activators. They require generation of small amounts of C3b in the fluid phase. They then provide a surface for adsorption of C3b, protect it from plasma inhibitors, and allow increased generation of C3b (Fig. 2.2). During cardiopulmonary bypass, haemodialysis, and exposure of blood to nylon filters there is activation of com-

plement via the alternative pathway. The cells of patients with paroxysmal nocturnal haemoglobinuria can be damaged through both the classical and alternative pathways.

The complement system interacts with the coagulation, fibrinolytic and kinin pathways (Fig. 9.2).

The complement cascade requires Ca^{++} and Mg^{++}, Ca^{++} being part of the C1 molecular complex. Citrate, EDTA and other chelating agents thus render complement inactive. As heparin also has anticomplementary activity, serological tests dependent on complement are performed on serum rather than plasma. Complement activation may be detected by the presence of certain complement components attached to the cell membrane or by the occurrence of cell lysis. The former can be detected by the antiglobulin test using antiglobulin reagents with anticomplement activity. Such reagents must be active against C3d as only inactive C components may remain on the cell surface (anti-C3c activity is commonly also present in antiglobulin reagents). If serological tests depend on the presence of complement for antibody detection, then serum must be fresh, or stored appropriately (at 4°C for up to 24 hours or at −20°C for longer periods); if these circumstances are not met complement may be added in the form of fresh AB serum.

Subjects with inherited deficiencies of various complement components may suffer from susceptibility to infection and syndromes resembling systemic lupus erythematosus which are probably due to failure to solubilize and clear immune complexes.[7] Acquired complement deficiency is seen in diseases characterized by antigen-antibody interaction.

RED CELL ANTIGENS

The blood group antigens of the red blood cells may be shared with other body cells (e.g. ABO antigens), restricted to red blood cells (e.g. Rhesus antigens), or be primarily tissue antigens which can be absorbed on to and readily eluted from red blood cells (e.g. Lewis antigens). Although red cell antigens are inherited characteristics, they may be modified by disease. For example, bacterial enzymes may convert A_1 antigen to B-like-antigen during bacterial infection, there may be weakening of expression of A, B, Lewis[b] and I antigens in acute myeloid leukaemia, and Rhesus antigens may be lost in myeloproliferative disorders.[8, 9] The antigens are membrane proteins or glycoproteins, antigenic specificity being conveyed by terminal sugars or by amino acid sequences. A blood group system is a group of antigens, produced by allelic genes or gene complexes, whose inheritance is independent of other blood group antigens; when a blood group system is produced by a gene complex, as in the rhesus system, the group of antigens is determined by a DNA sequence so short that cross-over within it is very uncommon.

Red cell antigens are recognized by antibodies directed against them, and conversely the specificity of antibodies against red cells is determined by studying their interaction with panels of red blood cells bearing known antigens. The interaction of antigen and antibody may cause agglutination of red cells which is recognized macroscopically or microscopically; this is charac-

teristic of IgM antibodies if sufficiently potent. Non-agglutinating antibodies (e.g. most IgG antibodies) may be detected by an antiglobulin test (Coombs test) in which red cells which have been exposed to the antibody are then exposed to an anti-human-globulin with a specificity against both immunoglobulin G (IgG) and complement (often bound to red cells by the action of antibodies). Anti-human-globulin causes agglutination of red cells which are coated with IgG or complement. Some antibodies which bind complement and activate the entire complement sequence may also be detected by their ability to cause red cell lysis. An antiglobulin test in which the patient's serum is first incubated with normal red cells is termed an indirect antiglobulin test (IAGT; indirect Coombs test) whereas a test in which the patient's cells are examined is termed a direct antiglobulin test (DAGT; direct Coombs test). Special techniques which increase the ease of detection of a reaction between a red cell antigen and antibody include the suspension of cells in albumin, the suspension of cells in low ionic strength saline (LISS) rather than in normal saline, and the pretreatment of cells with various enzymes (e.g. papain). Red cell antigens may also be detected by the use of proteins or glycoproteins of non-immune origin (usually lectins of plant origin) which cause agglutination of red cells bearing specific antigens. The detection of red cell antigens in secretions and dried blood stains requires special techniques (see p. 38).

Red cells carry dozens of antigenic markers; only the ones of major importance will be discussed in detail. Table 2.3 shows the frequency of blood group antigens in a Caucasian (predominantly UK) population together with representative figures for Blacks and Chinese.[10, 11] In general, West Indian and American Blacks have an antigen frequency intermediate between Caucasian and African Black frequencies.

ABO, Lewis, Ii and P antigens

The antigens of the ABO (ABH), Lewis, Ii and P blood group systems (Tables 2.2 and 2.3)[12] are formed by the addition of specific sugar residues to a common precursor. The A and B antigens on red blood cells are either glycoproteins or glycolipids and in secretions are glycoproteins. A and B antigens are formed from H substance whose formation requires the presence of the *H* gene. The product of this gene is an enzyme (a glycosyltransferase), which adds a specific sugar to the common precursor thereby converting it into H substance (the allelic gene *h* has no recognized gene product). The products of the *A* and *B* genes are also transferases which add a further sugar to H substance. The *O* gene is an amorph (no recognized gene product). The Lewis antigens, Le^a (Lewis^a) and Le^b (Lewis^b) are structurally related to the A and B antigens. Le^a is formed by addition of a sugar to the precursor of H under the influence of the *Le* gene. The formation of Le^b requires the addition of two sugars to the precursor of H and requires the presence of the *H*, *Le* and *Se* (*secretor*) genes. The I and i antigens are structurally related to the ABO system, both being stages in the synthesis of H, A and B. I and i are not determined by allelomorphic genes, the I antigen being a further modification of i; rare subjects lacking the *I* gene have only i antigen. The antigens of the P system are also formed from the common precursor.

Secretor status

Approximately 80% of Caucasian subjects have the secretor gene *Se* (genotype *SeSe* or *Sese*) and secrete H and other ABO blood group antigens in saliva and in other body fluids, e.g. plasma, semen, tears, sweat and urine. Subjects having the *Se* and *Le* genes will have Le^a and Le^b in secretions whereas those having *Le* and *se* will have Le^a only. The antigens usually present on the red cells and in the secretions of subjects of various ABH and Lewis groups who are secretors or non-secretors are shown in Table 2.2.

The Rhesus blood group system

The Rhesus gene complex on each of a pair of homologous chromosomes codes for three Rhesus antigens, or two antigens and d, which designates a lack of the D antigen. C and c behave as alleles, as do E and e. Other less common alleles occur. The terms Rhesus positive and Rhesus

negative are most often used to indicate the presence or absence of the D antigen.

Kell blood group system

The Kell system includes five sets of antigens, three of which (Table 2.3) are clinically important. Subjects lacking Kx, the precursor of Kell antigens, may have acanthocytosis and haemolytic anaemia and may also have chronic granulomatous disease as a closely-linked genetic disorder.

Duffy blood group

The Duffy blood group system has at least three allelic genes. Only two antigens (Fy^a, Fy^b) are common in Caucasians. Black subjects of phenotype Fy (a−b−) (genotype *Fy^{c}Fy^c*) have red cells which resist invasion by *Plasmodium vivax*.

MNSs system

M and N are allelic genes, as are S and s. M and N antigenic specificities are conveyed by differences in the terminal polypeptides of glycophorin A of the red cell membranes. The S and s antigenic determinants are carried on glycophorin B.

Other groups

Other blood groups, of lesser importance, are included in Table 2.3.

ADVERSE EFFECTS OF RED CELL ANTIBODIES

HAEMOLYTIC TRANSFUSION REACTIONS

Haemolytic transfusion reactions may be divided into immediate and delayed. Immediate transfusion reactions occur when red cells bearing an antigen are transfused into a recipient whose plasma contains antibody to that antigen; less commonly, they may occur when plasma containing an antibody at fairly high titre is transfused into a recipient whose cells bear the relevant anti-

Table 2.3 Percentage distribution of some blood group antigens in three ethnic groups

Blood group system	Phenotype		Genotype	Caucasian (UK)	US	Black African	Chinese
ABO (ABH)	A★		$AA★$ or AO	42★	26	24	24
	B		BB or OB	8	20	21	27
	AB★		$AB★$	3★	4	3	6
	O		OO	47	49	52	43
Lewis	Le(a−b+)	Lewis +ive	H | $SeSe$ or $Sese$ | $LeLe$ or $Lele$	75	55	40–60	70
	Le(a+b−)		H | $sese$ | $LeLe$ or $Lele$	20	22	20	24
	Le(a−b−)		H | $SeSe$ or $Sese$ | $lele$	4	22	20–40	6
			H | $sese$ | $lele$	1			
P	P_1		P_1P_1 or P_1P_2	75	98		20–30
	P_2		P_2P_2	25	2		70–80
Rhesus	D(Rhesus +ive)		DD or Dd	83	90	95	100
	d(Rhesus −ive)		dd	17	10	5	0
	CcDee		$CDe/cde(R^1r)$	31.7	20	$\simeq 5$	$\simeq 0$
			$CDe/cDe(R^1R^0)$	2.1		$\simeq 11$	8
	CCDee		$CDe/CDe(R^1R^1)$	16.6	3	< 1	57
	CcDEe		$CDe/cDE(R^1R^2)$	11.5		3	26
	ccDEe		$cDE/cde(R^2r)$	11.0	15	$\simeq 2$	2
			$cDe/cDE(R^0R^2)$			$\simeq 15$	$1\frac{1}{2}$
	ccDEE		$cDE/cDE(R^2R^2)$	2.2		1	4
	ccDee		$cDe/cde(R^0r)$	2	25	24	
			$cDe/cDe(R^0R^0)$		25	34	
	cD^{u}e		various genotypes (R^{ou})	very rare	1–6	$\geqslant 6$–7	
	ccddee		cde/cde (rr)	15.1	5–6	4	<0.1
	ce^s(V)		various genotypes	<0.5	27	40	<0.5
	C^w		various genotypes	1–2	$\simeq 0$	$\simeq 0$	$\simeq 0$
Kell	K	Kell +ive	KK	.2	$\frac{1}{2}$–2	< 1	$\simeq 0$
	Kk		Kk	8.7			
	k	Kell −ive	kk	91.1		>99	100
	Kp(a+b−)		Kp^aKp^a	very rare			
	Kp(a+b+)		Kp^aKp^b	$\simeq 2$			
	Kp(a−b+)		Kp^bKp^b	$\simeq 98$			
	Js(a+b−)		Js^aJs^a	very	$\simeq 1$	$\simeq 1$	$\simeq 0$
	Js(a+b+)		Js^aJs^b	rare	$\simeq 19$	$\simeq 19$	$\simeq 0$
	Js(a−b+)		Js^bJs^b	100	$\simeq 80$	$\simeq 80$	
Duffy	Fy(a+b−)	Duffy +ive	Fy^aFy^a	20	13		99
	Fy(a+b+)		Fy^aFy^b	47	21		
	Fy(a−b+)	Duffy −ive	Fy^bFy^b	33			
	Fy(a−b−)		Fy^cFy^c	rare	50–60	75–100	
MNSs	M		MM	28	similar to Caucasian (M somewhat less common)		similar to Caucasian
	MN		MN	50			
	N		NN	22			
	S		SS(or SS^u in Blacks)	11	4	5	2
	Ss		Ss	44	23	30	
	ss		ss(or sS^u in Blacks)	45	72	63	98
	S−, s−		S^uS^u		$\simeq 1$	1–2	

Blood group system	Phenotype		Genotype	Caucasian (UK)	US	Black African	Chinese
Kidd	Jk(a+b−)	Kidd +ive	$Jk^a Jk^a$	26	} 85–90	} 90–95	} 50
	Jk(a+b+)		$Jk^a Jk^b$	50			
	Jk(a−b+)		$Jk^b Jk^b$	24			
Lutheran	Lu(a+b−)	Lutheran +ive	$Lu^a Lu^a$	0.1		similar to Caucasian	not known
	Lu(a+b+)		$Lu^a Lu^b$	7.5			
	Lu(a−b+)		$Lu^b Lu^b$	92.4			
Diego	Di(a+b−)	Diego +ive	$Di^a Di^a$	} very rare		≃0	} 2½–5
	Di(a+b+)		$Di^a Di^b$				
	Di(a−b+)		$Di^b Di^b$	≃100		≃100	

* Among Caucasians, subgroups of A are divided between A_1 and A_2 in the ratio of 4:1. A_2 is also frequent in Blacks; it is very rare in Chinese.

gen. A delayed transfusion reaction occurs when a patient who has previously been immunized has a rising titre of antibody following transfusion with destruction of red cells usually occurring at 6–8 days.

Immediate transfusion reactions

Immediate transfusion reactions are exemplified by those due to anti-A or anti-B. They are usually consequent on transfusion of incompatible red cells due to a clerical error, or transfusion of group O blood containing a high titre of anti-A or anti-B into an A or B recipient. Rapid intravascular haemolysis occurs with consequent haemoglobinaemia and haemoglobinuria and, sometimes, disseminated intravascular coagulation (DIC) and renal failure. Jaundice may follow. The DIC results from release of thromboplastic substances from lysed red blood cells; complement activation may also contribute since activated C5 causes the generation of tissue factor activity from leucocytes.[13] Renal failure is due to acute tubular necrosis and is related to shock (consequent on complement activation) and disseminated intravascular coagulation rather than to any specific toxic effect of haemoglobin. Initial clinical features include chest and lumbar pain, fever, rigors, dyspnoea, hypotension, vomiting and diarrhoea. Later clinical features are those of jaundice and renal failure. Immediate transfusion reactions may be fatal, death being due to irreversible shock, haemorrhage (secondary to DIC) and renal failure.

Delayed transfusion reactions

Delayed transfusion reactions are exemplified by those due to Rhesus antibodies. Destruction of red cells is slower and predominantly extravascular. There is anaemia, jaundice, fever, spherocytosis (Fig. 2.3), and a positive direct antiglob-

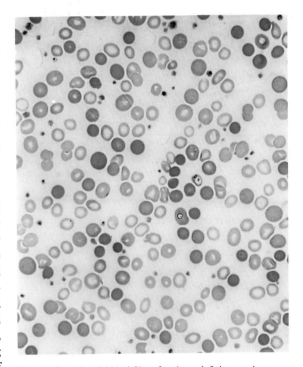

Fig. 2.3 Peripheral blood film of an iron-deficient patient who suffered a delayed transfusion reaction due to anti-D; the film shows a mixture of the patient's hypochromic microcytic red cells, and donor cells which have become spherocytic following damage by anti-D. May-Grünwald-Giemsa stain × 375.

ulin test. A small proportion of the haemolysis may be intravascular, causing haemoglobinaemia and haemoglobinuria. DIC and renal insufficiency are rare but may occur when the antibody is complement binding. It is very uncommon for delayed transfusion reactions to cause death.

HAEMOLYTIC DISEASE OF THE NEWBORN

Haemolytic disease of the newborn (HDN) occurs when maternal alloantibody (IgG) crosses into the fetal circulation and destroys incompatible fetal cells. It is now most commonly due to ABO incompatibility, with incompatibility within the Rhesus system having fallen into second place. Despite the designation 'haemolytic disease of the newborn', HDN starts during intrauterine life.

Rhesus haemolytic disease of the newborn

Rhesus haemolytic disease of the newborn due to anti-D has dropped sharply in incidence since the introduction of prophylactic therapy with anti-D in at-risk mothers. It remains the most severe form of HDN. A small number of cases of HDN are due to other antibodies within the Rhesus system, mainly anti-C or anti-E. The severity of Rhesus HDN ranges from the intrauterine death of a severely anaemic hydropic fetus, to the delivery of an infant with a normal haemoglobin level but with a positive direct antiglobulin test and a shortened red cell survival. In the most severely affected fetus there is severe anaemia with extreme reticulocytosis and erythroblastaemia. There is ascites and severe oedema with cardiomegaly, hepatomegaly (Fig. 2.4) and splenomegaly. Complicating disseminated intravascular coagulation causes thrombocytopenia and defibrination with pulmonary and subarachnoid haemorrhage and purpura. A hydropic fetus is associated with a hydropic placenta (Fig. 2.5); hydrops appears to be related to hypoalbuminaemia as well as anaemia. Accelerated red cell destruction *in utero* is associated with increased bilirubin in the amniotic fluid. Infants with less gross hydropic features may be delivered alive

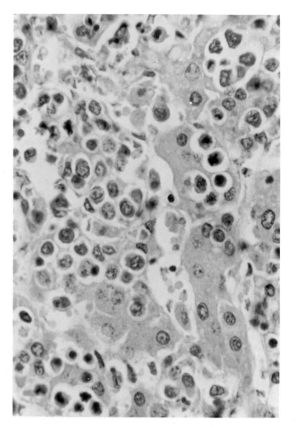

Fig. 2.4 Histology of the enlarged liver in hydrops fetalis due to Rhesus incompatibility. There is a marked increase of hepatic erythropoiesis. The erythropoietic cells are situated extravascularly between the plates of hepatocytes. Haematoxylin–eosin × 350

and may survive with treatment. Less severely affected infants may or may not be anaemic at birth but have a positive direct antiglobulin test and accelerated red cell destruction; hyperbilirubinaemia may be present at birth or develop postnatally. If hyperbilirubinaemia is not prevented, brain damage, particularly damage of the basal ganglia (kernicterus), may occur. If an infant with kernicterus survives there may be residual high-tone hearing loss, choreoathetosis and spasticity.

ABO haemolytic disease of the newborn

ABO HDN is now the commonest type of HDN but is milder than Rhesus HDN and does not cause intrauterine death. It occurs predominantly

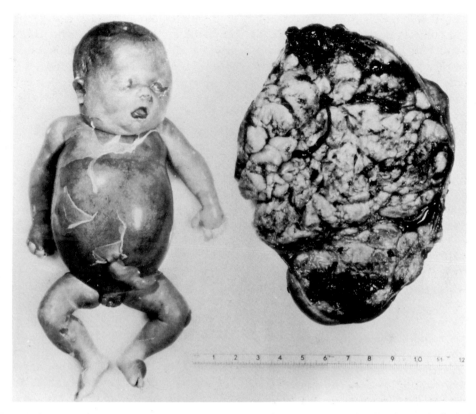

Fig. 2.5 Hydrops fetalis due to Rhesus (anti-D) haemolytic disease of the newborn; note that the placenta is also hydropic.
Courtesy of Professor P.L. Mollison

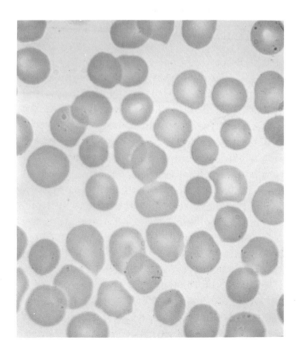

Fig. 2.6 Peripheral blood film from a baby with ABO haemolytic disease of the newborn; some spherocytes are present.
May-Grünwald-Giemsa stain. × 940.

in group A or B infants of group O mothers, since group O subjects develop higher titres of IgG anti-A and anti-B than do group B or A subjects. The relative mildness of ABO HDN is probably due to the late development of A and B antigens on fetal red cells and the presence of antigen sites capable of absorbing antibody on non-erythroid cells. ABO HDN causes anaemia, spherocytosis (Fig. 2.6), erythroblastaemia, reticulocytosis, and hyperbilirubinaemia which is occasionally severe enough to necessitate exchange transfusion. The direct antiglobulin test may be weakly positive (with an anti-Ig anti-human-globulin reagent) or negative.

THE HLA (HUMAN LEUCOCYTE ANTIGEN) SYSTEM

Human platelets and nucleated cells (with the exception of sperm and placental trophoblast) carry antigens of the human leucocyte antigen (HLA) system. Because they are important determinants of allograft rejection, HLA antigens are also designated histocompatibility antigens. HLA antigens of wide distribution which can be serologically recognized (by leuco-agglutination or granulocyte or lymphocyte cytotoxicity) are determined by genes at three loci (A, B and C) on chromosome 6. In addition a fourth locus (D) determines antigens of restricted tissue distribution which are recognized by their ability to induce blast transformation in lymphocytes which are identical at the A, B and C loci but not at the D locus (mixed lymphocyte reaction, MLR). Genes closely related to the D locus (HLA-DR) also determine antigens of restricted distribution (monocytes, macrophages, B-lymphocytes, sperm and epidermal cells) which are recognized serologically. The Ia-like antigen is a non-polymorphic product of the DR locus. HLA antigens show marked polymorphism, i.e. there are many alleles at each locus. The HLA loci are close together so that cross-over within the HLA system is unusual. The gene complex on a single chromosome is designated the haplotype. HLA antigens determined by the A, B and C loci are surface-membrane-associated glycoproteins composed of a light chain which is probably identical to β_2 microglobulin, and a heavy chain which bears the antigenic determinant. HLA antigens may be shed from cell membranes and thus appear in plasma. HLA alloantibodies are evoked by pregnancy, and by transfusion of blood or blood products containing white cells or platelets.

Many diseases show a statistical association with particular HLA antigens. For example, ankylosing spondylitis is strongly associated with HLA-B27 and coeliac disease and dermatitis herpetiformis are associated with HLA-B8. The mechanisms underlying such associations are not yet clearly established.

LYMPHOCYTE ANTIGENS

Lymphocytes carry antigens determined by the HLA-A, HLA-B and HLA-C loci; B-lymphocytes also carry antigens determined by the HLA-D and -DR loci. Lymphocytes also carry ABH, Lewis and Ii antigens and share group 5 system antigens (5a and 5b) with granulocytes and platelets.

GRANULOCYTE ANTIGENS

Granulocytes carry antigens determined by the HLA-A, HLA-B and HLA-C loci and may also have antigens of the ABH, Lewis and Ii system and the group 5 system. In addition they have granulocyte-specific antigens (NA1, NA2, NB1, NC1, ND1, NE1 and the HGA-3 systems). Alloantibodies against granulocyte antigens may be evoked by pregnancy or blood transfusion.

ADVERSE EFFECTS OF ANTI-LEUCOCYTE ANTIBODIES

Neonatal alloimmune neutropenia

This condition is caused by transplacental passage of maternal IgG alloantibodies against granulocyte-restricted antigens (NA1, NA2, NB1) present in the fetus (see p. 213).

Autoimmune neutropenia

Neutropenia may occur as a consequence of autoantibodies against granulocyte-restricted antigens (NA2, NE1).[14]

Adverse reactions to transfusion

Non-haemolytic transfusion reactions may be a consequence either of the interaction between an antibody in the recipient and the leucocytes of the donor or between the recipient's leucocytes and a high-titre antibody in donor blood. Adverse reactions may be due to granulocyte-specific antibodies or less often to HLA antibodies. The most common is a febrile reaction which may be accompanied by rigors, headache, hypotension and leucopenia. In more severe reactions obstruction of pulmonary micro-vasculature by agglutinated leucocytes leads to non-cardiogenic pulmonary oedema with cough, dyspnoea and cyanosis.[15] Such reactions may be fatal. Chest X-ray shows pulmonary infiltration without cardiomegaly. Symptoms may remit in a matter of hours; the radiological abnormality takes several days to clear.

Reduced efficacy of granulocyte transfusions

Granulocyte transfusions have been reported to be less efficacious when there is incompatibility with the recipient's plasma. When the recipient's plasma contains granulocyte agglutinins, donor granulocytes may accumulate in the liver and fail to localize at sites of infection.[16]

PLATELET ANTIGENS

Platelets carry antigens of the HLA system and weakly-expressed absorbed ABH antigens. In addition there are several platelet-specific antigen systems. Zw^a (also designated Pl^{A1}) and Zw^b (Pl^{A2}) are alleles, and are associated with the platelet membrane glycoprotein which is lacking in Glanzmann's thrombasthenia (GpIIIa) (see p. 284). $Ko(a+)$ and $Ko(b+)$ are alleles as are Pl^{E1} and Pl^{E2}. Other platelet-specific antigens determined by non-allelic genes are Duzo and Bak^a.

ADVERSE EFFECTS OF PLATELET ANTIBODIES

Antibodies against platelets may be evoked by pregnancy or blood transfusion. They may be IgG or IgM.

Neonatal alloimmune thrombocytopenia

Neonatal thrombocytopenia may be due to transplacental passage of platelet-specific IgG alloantibodies, usually anti-Zw^a(anti-Pl^{A1}) (see p. 279). Alloantibodies to HLA antigens may similarly cause neonatal thrombocytopenia.

Autoimmune thrombocytopenia (see p. 277)

Post-transfusion purpura

Post-transfusion purpura occurs in recipients who develop a platelet alloantibody, usually anti-Zw^a (anti-Pl^{A1}). The postulated mechanism is damage to recipient platelets consequent on their interaction with an immune complex of the recipient alloantibody and donor platelet antigen (innocent bystander mechanism) (see p. 280).

Recipient platelet destruction by donor antibodies

Infusion of high-titre alloantibodies to platelet-specific antigens will cause destruction of recipient platelets and fever.

Shortened survival of donor platelets

Both HLA and platelet-specific antibodies may cause markedly accelerated destruction of incompatible donor platelets; concomitant fever, rigors, headache and leucopenia may occur.

THE USE OF BLOOD GROUP SEROLOGY IN FORENSIC PATHOLOGY[17, 18]

Blood group serology plays an important role in forensic pathology. In view of the complexity and difficulty of some of the tests involved, forensic investigations should be carried out only in specialized laboratories.

Serological techniques may be used to 1) demonstrate that blood is human, 2) determine the group of blood or of a bloodstain and thus the group of the subject from whom it was derived, 3) determine the blood group of saliva or semen and 4) phenotype individuals in order to exclude or estimate the likelihood of paternity (or maternity).

Tests based on precipitation with an anti-human-globulin, such as tube precipitin tests, will confirm that blood is of human (or higher primate) origin.

Determining the bloodgroup of semen, saliva or other secretions or of bloodstains requires special techniques. Only the secretions of secretors (see p. 31) are suitable for blood grouping. Antigens may be detected by inhibition of antisera; for example, A, B and H antigens will decrease the titre of anti-A, anti-B and anti-H, respectively. If semen from the vagina is being grouped, then the ABO group and secretor status of the woman must also be studied since vaginal secretions or blood may be mixed with semen. In dried bloodstains the cells will generally have been destroyed and here also special techniques must be used for grouping. Inhibition of anti-A, -B and -H may be used (as for secretions) but more sensitive techniques which are available include absorption and subsequent elution of the specific antibody, and mixed agglutination. The latter technique can be applied not only to bloodstained fabric fibres but also to body cells, e.g. isolated skin cells, and to dandruff and hairs. The test cells or fibres following reaction with the specific antibody will show mixed agglutination with red cells bearing the same antigen.

All the above tests require rigorous controls including tests of adjoining unstained material. Secretions are tested only for ABH groups. Bloodstains may also be tested for other groups, e.g. Rhesus groups and M. A, B and H antigens are stable for prolonged periods in dried bloodstains; M is considerably less so and N is unstable.

Paternity testing

Assuming that the mother of a child is known, it may be possible to disprove that a designated man is the father by demonstrating either that the child has a red cell antigen which could not have been inherited from either parent, or alternatively that it does not have an antigen which the putative father should have passed on. Thus, in general, an A child could not be the offspring of two O parents, and an O child could not be the child of an AB father. Extremely rare exceptions to these rules are known: for example, the lack of the H gene (hh) in a child will prevent the expression of A, B and H, in which case an O child could have an AB parent, and A and B may be inherited on the same chromosome (cis AB), in which case an AB child may be produced by an O parent and an AB parent. Blood group serology can never prove paternity but can allow the probability of paternity to be estimated, particularly if the child and the putative father share an uncommon antigen. The possible ethnic origin of the mother, child and putative father must be considered in assessing the significance of blood groups; for example, if only the presence of Duffy^a (Fy^a) could be tested for, it would be very likely that those who were Fy^a negative would be Fy^b positive if subjects were Caucasians, whereas such a deduction would be untenable in Blacks with a high incidence of Fy (a-b-), genotype Fy^cFy^c. The ABO, MNSs, Rhesus, Lutheran, Kell, Duffy and Kidd systems are most useful in the study of paternity, and if used together will exclude approximately 60% of non-fathers. The P system is less useful and the Lewis system is generally too complex to be useful. Haemoglobin electrophoresis and study of haptoglobin and serum protein (Gm and Inv) groups may also be used in paternity testing, and when used in conjunction with a suitable range of tests for red cell antigens increase the chance of excluding a non-father to greater than 80%. The use of isoelectric focusing rather than electrophoresis considerably increases the number of allotypes of haptoglobin which can be detected and therefore further increases the usefulness of this marker.[19] HLA typing may also be used in paternity testing and when added to the above seven blood group systems increases the chances of excluding a non-father to approximately 97%. The same range of tests may be used for exclusion of maternity and for other problems of disputed kinship.

REFERENCES

GENERAL REFERENCES

Mollison PL. Blood transfusion in clinical medicine. 7th ed. Oxford: Blackwell Scientific Publications, 1983.

Petz LD, Swisher SN. Clinical practice of blood transfusion. New York: Churchill Livingstone, 1981.

Pittiglio DH, Baldwin AJ, Sohmer PR. Modern blood banking and transfusion practices. Philadelphia: Davis, 1983.

1. Goodman JW, Wang A-C. In: Fudenberg HH, Stites DP, Caldwell JL, Wells JV, eds. Basic and clinical immunology. Los Altos: Lange Medical Publications, 1980: 28.
2. Kincade PW. In: Kunkel HG, Dixon FJ, eds. Advances in immunology. New York: Academic Press, 1981: vol. 31.
3. Vogler LB. Clin Haematol 1982; 11: 509.
4. Leder P. Sci Am 1982; 246: 72.
5. Karas SP, Rosse WF, Kurlander RJ. Blood 1982; 60: 1277.
6. Lachmann PJ, Voak D, Oldroyd RG, Downie DM, Bevan PC. Vox Sang 1983; 45: 367.
7. Schifferli JA, Peters DK. Lancet 1983; ii: 957.
8. Kolins J, Holland PV, McGinniss MH. Cancer 1978; 42: 2249.
9. Marsh LW. Mayo Clin Proc 1977; 52: 145.
10. Race RR, Sanger R. Blood groups in man. 6th ed. Oxford: Blackwell Scientific Publications, 1975.
11. Mourant AE, Kopec AC, Demaniewska-Sobczak K. The distribution of human blood groups and other polymorphisms. London: Oxford University Press, 1976.
12. Mollison PL. Blood transfusion in clinical medicine. 7th ed. Oxford: Blackwell Scientific Publications, 1983.
13. Muhlfelder TW, Niemetz J, Kreutzer D, Beeber D, Ward PA, Rosenfeld SI. J Clin Invest 1979; 63: 147.
14. Sabbe LJM, Claas FHJ, Langerak J, et al. Acta Haematol 1982; 68: 20.
15. Andrews AT, Zmijewski CM, Bowman HS, Reihart JK. Am J Clin Pathol 1976; 66: 483.
16. McCullough J, Weiblen BJ, Clay ME, Forstrom L. Blood 1981; 58: 164.
17. Grant A, Bradbrook ID. In: Mant AK, ed. Modern trends in forensic medicine. London: Butterworths, 1973.
18. Erskine AG, Socha WW. The principles and practice of blood grouping. 2nd ed. St Louis Missouri: Mosby, 1978.
19. Dykes DD, De Furio CM, Polesky HF. Am J Clin Pathol 1983; 79: 725.

Normal haemopoiesis: cellular composition of normal bone marrow

DEVELOPMENT OF HAEMOPOIESIS[1,2]

Erythropoiesis commences on the fourteenth to nineteenth day of development of the human embryo and continues thereafter throughout life. It begins within the blood islands of the yolk sac and persists there until the end of the 12th week of gestation. Yolk sac erythropoiesis occurs intravascularly and is megaloblastic in type. It is associated with the synthesis of three embryonic haemoglobins, Gower I ($\zeta_2\varepsilon_2$), Gower II ($\alpha_2\varepsilon_2$) and Portland I ($\zeta_2\gamma_2$), and results in the production of cells which usually remain nucleated throughout their life-span. Erythropoietic foci appear in the fetal liver in the sixth week of gestation and the liver becomes the main site of erythropoiesis from the third to the sixth month. It continues to produce red cells in decreasing numbers until the end of the first week of postnatal life. Fetal hepatic erythropoiesis occurs extravascularly within the hepatic parenchyma (Fig. 3.1) and is initially megaloblastic in type but subsequently becomes macronormoblastic. It is associated with the synthesis of fetal haemoglobin (HbF; $\alpha_2\gamma_2$) and results in the production of anucleate, macrocytic red cells. Occasional foci of erythropoietic cells can be seen in certain marrow cavities between two and a half and four months of gestation; by the sixth month the marrow is an important source of red cells. The bone marrow is the major site of fetal erythropoiesis during the last trimester of pregnancy. Erythropoiesis in fetal bone marrow occurs extravascularly, is macronormoblastic in type and results in the production of macrocytic red cells: the MCV in the cord blood of full-term babies ranges between 90 and 118 fl. Erythropoiesis in fetal bone marrow appears to be regulated by erythropoietin produced extrarenally, probably in the liver. Small foci of erythroblasts occur in many tissues and organs at various times during intrauterine life but their contribution to total

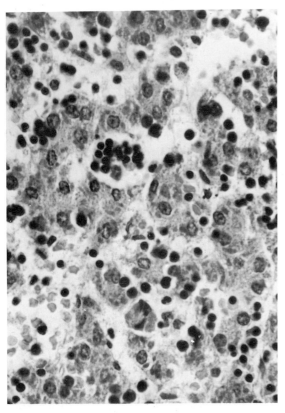

Fig. 3.1 Histological appearances of normal fetal liver during the middle trimester of pregnancy. About 40% of the area of the section consists of erythropoietic cells which are present singly or in clusters between the plates of liver cells.

Haematoxylin-eosin   × 350

erythropoietic activity is probably small. Tissues containing such foci include the lymph nodes, spleen and kidneys.

A few granulocytopoietic cells and occasional megakaryocytes can be seen in various embryonic and fetal tissues including the yolk sac, liver and lymphoid tissue. However, intra-uterine granulocytopoiesis and megakaryocytopoiesis occur largely in the fetal bone marrow.

POSTNATAL CHANGES IN THE DISTRIBUTION OF RED MARROW[1]

During the first four years of life all the marrow cavities other than those of the terminal phalanges contain red marrow consisting mainly of haemopoietic cells (by the age of 1 year, virtually all of the haemopoietic cells in the terminal phalanges have been replaced by fat cells). After the first four years an increasing number of fat cells appears amongst the haemopoietic cells of other marrow cavities. Between the ages of 10 and 14 years, the haemopoietic cells in the middle of the shafts of the long bones become virtually completely replaced by fat cells. Subsequently, these zones of non-haemopoietic yellow marrow spread both proximally and distally. Distal spread is more rapid than proximal spread and by about the twenty-fifth year the only regions of the long bones which contain red, haemopoietic marrow are the proximal quarters of the shafts of the femora and humeri. Other sites of haemopoiesis in an adult are the ribs, clavicles, scapulae, sternum, vertebrae and skull.

ORGANIZATION OF HAEMOPOIETIC MARROW[1,3]

The bone marrow contains a large number of blood vessels, some non-myelinated and myelinated nerve fibres and small amounts of reticulin. Most of the capillaries open into a network of thin-walled sinusoids which are drained by a system of collecting venules into larger venous channels. The walls of the sinusoids are lined by a single layer of flattened endothelial cells with little or no underlying basement membrane. The sinusoids are incompletely covered on the outside by a single layer of adventitial cells. In normal marrow, the reticulin is present as a scanty, incomplete network of fine branching fibres which are continuous with similar fibres in the walls of blood vessels and the endosteum (Fig. 3.2). Some thickening and concentration of fibres is seen around the walls of larger arteries and near the endosteum. The parenchymal cells of the bone marrow are situated extravascularly. About one-

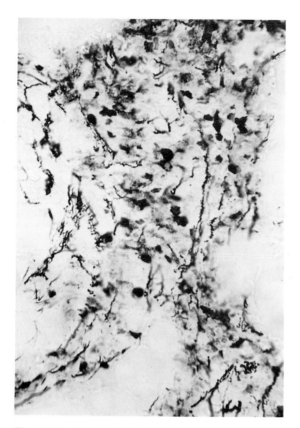

Fig. 3.2 Trephine biopsy of normal bone marrow showing fine reticulin fibres in an area of marrow close to bone.

Silver impregnation of reticulin × 375

usually lie immediately adjacent to the sinusoids. In adult bone marrow, small lymphocytes tend to occur in nodules which are 0.08-1.2 mm in their greatest diameter. Such nodules contain small numbers of reticulum cells and are held together by a reticulin network. In histological sections, about 80% of these nodules appear well-circumscribed and compact and have a follicular structure. The remainder appear as poorly-circumscribed collections of loosely arranged lymphocytes. The lymphoid follicles have blood vessels at their centre and contain some plasma cells and mast cells towards their periphery; in about 5% of the sections of lymphoid follicles, well-developed germinal centres are evident. Lymphocytes, plasma cells and mast cells also occur unassociated with lymphoid nodules. Some plasma cells occur in small clumps

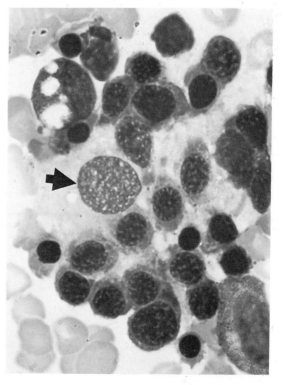

Fig. 3.3 Erythroblastic island in a smear of normal bone marrow. The island consists of several early and late polychromatic erythroblasts which are closely associated with a macrophage. The nucleus of the macrophage (arrowed) has a pale-staining lace-like chromatin structure.

May-Grünwald-Giemsa stain × 940

quarter to one-half of the volume of the red marrow of a healthy adult consists of fat cells. The remainder consists of the precursors of red cells, granulocytes, monocytes and platelets. The marrow also contains macrophages, lymphocytes, plasma cells and mast cells.

The erythropoietic and granulocytopoietic cells tend to be arranged with the more mature cells adjacent to the marrow sinusoids. The early granulocytopoietic cells are situated near bone trabeculae and small arteries. The erythroblasts are organized into erythroblastic islands composed of one or more central macrophages (reticulum cells) surrounded by one or two layers of erythroblasts[4] (Figs 3.3 and 3.4). Thin cytoplasmic processes of macrophages extend in between the erythroblasts and sometimes surround them almost completely. The megakaryocytes

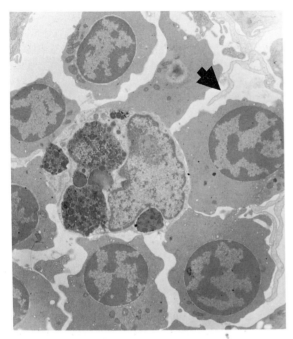

Fig. 3.4 Electron micrograph of an erythroblastic island from normal bone marrow. The central macrophage, which contains large intracytoplasmic inclusions, is surrounded by a layer of erythroblasts. Thin processes of macrophage cytoplasm (arrowed) can be seen between some of the erythroblasts.

Uranyl acetate and lead citrate   × 5500

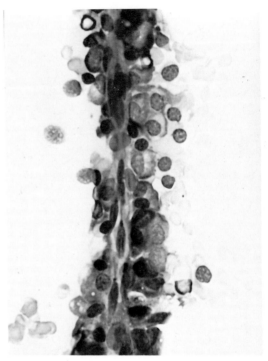

Fig. 3.5 A capillary from a smear of normal bone marrow showing plasma cells arranged along it.

May–Grünwald–Giemsa stain   × 375

grouped around a reticulum cell and others are found perivascularly (Fig 3.5).

GENERAL CHARACTERISTICS OF HAEMOPOIESIS[1]

During intra-uterine life and in the growing child, there is a progressive increase with time in the total number of haemopoietic and blood cells. By contrast, in normal adults, the total number of such cells remains more or less constant. All the haemopoietic systems of normal adults are examples of steady-state cell renewal systems in which a relatively constant rate of loss of mature cells (erythrocytes, granulocytes, monocytes and platelets) is balanced fairly precisely by the production of new cells.

The formation of blood cells of all types involves two processes: 1) the progressive development of structural and functional characteristics specific for a given cell type (i.e. cytodifferentiation); and 2) cell proliferation. The latter serves to amplify the number of mature cells produced from one precursor cell which has become committed to any particular blood cell production line.

HAEMOPOIETIC STEM CELLS AND OTHER MORPHOLOGICALLY UNRECOGNIZED PRECURSORS[5,6]

The haemopoietic cells can be divided into two categories: 1) the early precursors which have not yet been recognized morphologically with certainty but which can be studied by functional tests (described as the 'morphologically unrecognized precursors'); and 2) the morphologically recognizable precursors. The morphologically unrecognized precursors also consist of two categories: 1) haemopoietic stem cells which have both the ability to develop into at least four types of blood cells and an extensive capacity to maintain their own numbers by cell proliferation; and 2) cells which are committed to three, two or one haemopoietic differentiation pathway but which do not have a substantial capacity for self-renewal. Studies in experimental animals and in humans have clearly shown the presence of a multipotent myeloid stem cell whose progeny develop into erythrocytes, granulocytes, monocytes and megakaryocytes. Initially the myeloid stem cell was defined by its ability to form macroscopically-visible colonies composed of a mixture of cell types when injected into lethally irradiated mice; this stem cell is therefore frequently referred to as the 'colony-forming unit in spleen' or CFU-S. Subsequently, these stem cells became assayable in semi-solid culture media in which they give rise to colonies containing cells of all four myeloid lineages, i.e. granulocyte-erythrocyte – macrophage – megakaryocyte (GEMM) colonies. The myeloid stem cell is itself derived from a pluripotent haemopoietic stem cell which also gives rise to the lymphoid stem cell. Thus, cytogenetic studies have not only shown that the Philadelphia (Ph[1]) chromosome is present in the granulocytic, erythroid and megakaryocytic lineages of most patients with chronic granulocytic leukaemia (CGL), but also that this chromosome is present in the lymphoblasts of some patients with acute lymphoblastic leukaemia whose disease later evolves into CGL and in those of some patients with CGL whose disease has evolved into a lymphoblastic crisis (see p. 239). Further evidence for the existence of a pluripotent stem cell in humans comes from the demonstration that in one case of sideroblastic anaemia with glucose-6-phosphate-dehydrogenase (G6PD) mosaicism, a single G6PD isoenzyme was present in myeloid cells as well as in T- and B-lymphocytes[7] and that human GEMM colonies contain T-lymphocytes.[8]

In healthy adults most of the myeloid stem cells are in a quiescent state (i.e. in the G_0 phase) or in a prolonged G_1 phase. However, when there is an increased need for haemopoiesis, these normally quiescent stem cells become triggered into active proliferation. The morphology of the myeloid stem cell may resemble that of medium-sized lymphocytes (transitional lymphocytes). Unlike the myeloid stem cells, a high proportion of the more mature morphologically unrecognized cells which are committed to two lines, or one line, of differentiation are engaged in cell proliferation. The committed precursor cells are interposed between the stem cells and the earliest morphologically recognizable precursor cells and appear to undergo progressive restriction in their differentiation potential until they eventually become unipotent.

ERYTHROPOIESIS[1]

There are several generations of morphologically unrecognized cells which are committed to erythropoiesis. These cells have been defined and studied operationally in terms of the characteristics of the erythroid colonies they generate in appropriate semi-solid media. The most immature of such cells are referred to as the erythroid burst-forming units (BFU-E) and the most mature as the erythroid colony-forming units (CFU-E). There is a morphologically unrecognized precursor cell which is responsive to erythropoietin *in vivo* and this cell is referred to as the erythropoietin-responsive cell (ERC); the ERC may correspond to the CFU-E or a slightly earlier cell. Under the influence of erythropoietin, the ERCs develop into proerythroblasts which are the earliest morphologically recognizable red cell precursors in the marrow. The proerythroblasts then progress through several morphologically-defined cytological classes. These are, in order of increasing maturity, the basophilic erythroblasts, the early polychromatic erythroblasts, the late polychromatic erythroblasts and the marrow and blood reticulocytes. Cell division occurs in the proerythroblasts, basophilic erythroblasts and early polychromatic erythroblasts but not in more mature cells. By contrast, the results of cytodifferentiation can be seen in all classes of morphologically recognizable precursors, both proliferating and non-proliferating. There are, on average, four cell divisions in the morphologically-recognizable precursor pool so that one proerythroblast may give rise to 2^4 or 16 red cells. In normal adults,

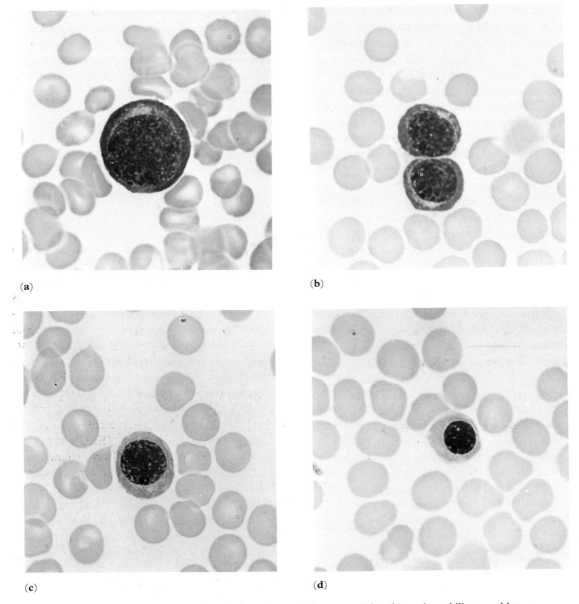

(a)   (b)

(c)   (d)

Fig. 3.6 a–d Erythroblasts from a smear of normal bone marrow. (**a**) pronormoblast (**b**) two basophilic normoblasts (**c**) early polychromatic normoblast (**d**) late polychromatic normoblast.

May–Grünwald–Giemsa stain   × 940

the time taken for a proerythroblast to mature into marrow reticulocytes and for these reticulocytes to enter the circulation is about 7 days; of this, about 2.5 days is spent in the marrow reticulocyte pool. The time taken for blood reticulocytes to mature into erythrocytes is 1–2 days. In normal individuals erythrocytes circulate for 110–120 days before they are removed and broken down by cells of the mononuclear phagocyte system.

Some of the erythropoietic cells do not develop successfully into erythrocytes but are recognized as being abnormal and phagocytosed by the bone marrow macrophages. This loss of potential erythrocytes is referred to as ineffective erythro-poiesis. The extent of ineffective erythropoiesis is small in normal marrow but is substantial in certain diseases.

Morphology of erythroblasts

Various terms have been used to describe the morphologically recognizable red cell precursors. In this book, the term *erythroblast* is used to de-scribe all nucleated red cells, normal and patho-logical; the term *normoblast* is applied only to nu-cleated red cells which resemble those seen in normal bone marrow.

In Romanowsky-stained marrow smears, the pronormoblast (Fig 3.6a) appears as a large cell with a diameter of 12–20 μm. It has a large rounded nucleus which is surrounded by a small amount of deep-blue cytoplasm; the intensity of cytoplasmic basophilia is greater than that shown by myeloblasts. The cytoplasm may show a pale perinuclear halo and frequently displays small blebs at the periphery. The nuclear chromatin

has a finely granular or finely reticular appear-ance and there are prominent nucleoli. Cells be-longing to successive cytological classes show a progressive decrease in average cell and nuclear diameter and a progressive increase in the volume of cytoplasm relative to that of the nucleus. The cytoplasm of the basophilic normoblast (Fig. 3.6b) is even more blue-staining than that of the pronormoblast. Its nuclear chromatin has a coarsely granular appearance and there are no nucleoli. The early polychromatic normoblast (Fig. 3.6c) has polychromatic cytoplasm and a nucleus containing small or moderately-large clumps of condensed chromatin. The late poly-chromatic normoblasts (Fig. 3.6d) have a dia-meter of 8–10 μm, a faintly polychromatic cyto-plasm and a small eccentric nucleus with a diameter less than 6·5 μm and containing large clumps of condensed chromatin. Eventually the nucleus becomes pyknotic and is extruded. The morphology of the resulting marrow reticulocytes is similar to that of circulating reticulocytes as described on page 7. Electron microscope

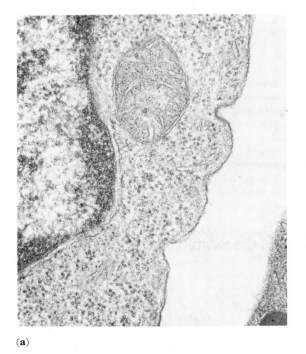

(a)

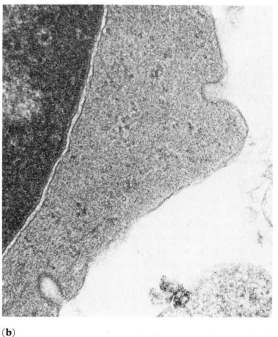

(b)

Fig. 3.7 a, b Electron micrographs of two normal erythroblasts showing characteristic surface invaginations (formation of rhopheocytotic vesicles). (**a**) Basophilic normoblast (× 45 800). (**b**) Late polychromatic normoblast (× 54 180). Clusters of polyribosomes and a mitochondrion are seen in the basophilic normoblast.

Uranyl acetate and lead citrate.

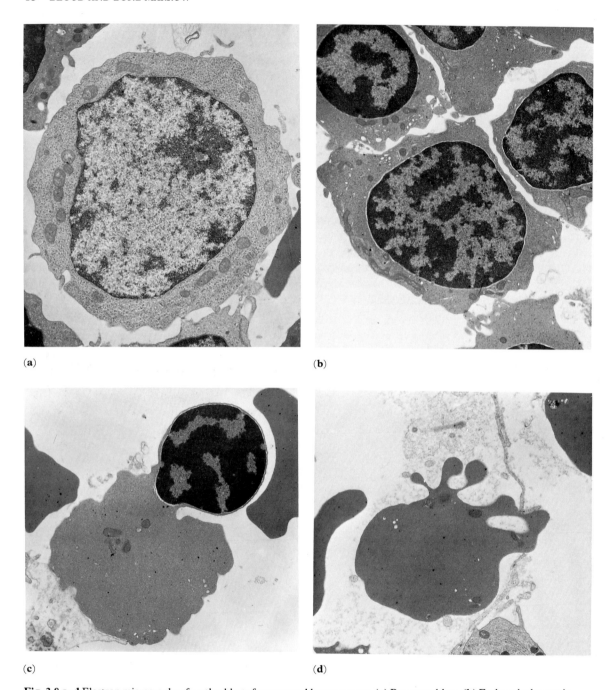

(a)

(b)

(c)

(d)

Fig. 3.8 a–d Electron micrographs of erythroblasts from normal bone marrow. (**a**) Pronormoblast. (**b**) Early polychromatic normoblast (cell in the centre). (**c**) Late polychromatic normoblast immediately prior to extruding its nucleus. (**d**) Reticulocyte in the process of entering a marrow sinusoid. Most of the cell has passed through the endothelial cell of the sinusoidal wall.

Uranyl acetate and lead citrate   × 7725

studies[4] show that all erythroblasts contain characteristic surface invaginations (Fig. 3.7) which develop into small intracytoplasmic vesicles (rhopheocytotic vesicles); the function of these vesicles is uncertain. The walls of rhopheocytotic vesicles are made up of a single membrane whose inner surface is coated with an amorphous material; the vesicles sometimes contain ferritin molecules. Pronormoblasts possess nuclei in which the chromatin is more or less totally in the form of euchromatin (expanded chromatin) with little or no nuclear-membrane-associated heterochromatin (condensed chromatin) (Fig. 3.8a). They have a fairly well-developed Golgi apparatus adjacent to a moderately-deep indentation of the nucleus, numerous polyribosomes, several mitochondria, many scattered ferritin molecules and a few lysosomal granules near the Golgi saccules. The maturation of pronormoblasts into late polychromatic normoblasts (Figs. 3.8b,c) is accompanied by 1) a progressive increase in the amount of heterochromatin both in the nucleoplasm and adjacent to the nuclear membrane; 2) a progressive decrease in the number of ribosomes; 3) a progressive increase in the electron-density of the cytoplasm due to the accumulation of haemoglobin, 4) a decrease in the number and size of the mitochondria; and 5) a tendency of intracytoplasmic ferritin molecules to aggregate into siderosomes. A Golgi apparatus persists in polychromatic erythroblasts (Fig. 3.9). The extruded nucleus of the late polychromatic erythroblast is surrounded by a very thin rim of cytoplasm and is enclosed within a cytoplasmic membrane. It is rapidly phagocytosed by adjacent macrophages. The entry of newly-formed reticulocytes into the marrow sinusoids occurs through temporary and rather narrow transendothelial channels (Fig. 3.8d).

Regulation of erythropoiesis[9]

The rate of red cell production is primarily regulated by the hormone erythropoietin whose main action is to stimulate the rate of conversion of ERC to pronormoblasts. The plasma level of this hormone is inversely related to the capacity of the blood to deliver oxygen to tissues. Thus, in most anaemic states there is an increased level of erythropoietin, which in turn causes an enhancement of the rate of erythropoiesis. The kidneys are the organs mainly concerned with erythropoietin production in adults. The secretions of various endocrine glands also influence erythropoiesis and patients with hypofunction of some endocrine glands develop a moderate anaemia (see p. 183).

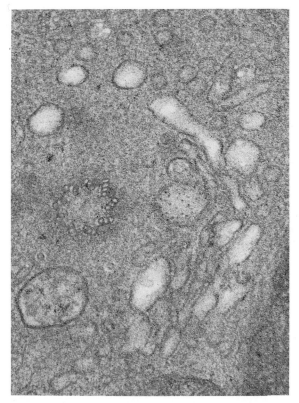

Fig. 3.9 Electron micrograph of part of a polychromatic erythroblast from normal marrow showing a centriole lying adjacent to sacs of a relatively poorly-developed Golgi apparatus.

Uranyl acetate and lead citrate   × 86 300

NEUTROPHIL GRANULOCYTOPOIESIS AND MONOCYTOPOIESIS

There are several generations of morphologically-unrecognized precursor cells concerned with the production of neutrophil granulocytes and macrophages. These have been defined on the basis of their ability to form colonies of granulocytes, macrophages or both when grown in *vitro* in semi-solid media containing appropriate colony-stimulating factors or *in vivo* within diffusion chambers implanted intraperitoneally in mice. Cells giving rise to granulocyte or macrophage colonies *in vitro* are described as colony-forming units in culture (CFU-C) or, more specifically, granulocyte-macrophage colony-forming units (CFU-GM). The available data suggest that the multipotent myeloid stem cell generates a bipotent granulocyte-macrophage progenitor cell and that the latter develops into CFU-C which are irreversibly committed to mature either into neutrophils or into macrophages. The earliest morphologically recognizable precursors in the neutrophil and monocyte-macrophage series are the myeloblasts and monoblasts respectively.

Neutrophil granulocytopoiesis[1,10]

The morphologically-recognizable cells of the neutrophil series are, in order of increasing maturity, the myeloblasts, neutrophil promyelocytes, neutrophil myelocytes, neutrophil metamyelocytes, juvenile neutrophils and the marrow neutrophil granulocytes. Cell division occurs up to and including the myelocyte stage; more mature cells are non-dividing. Cytodifferentiation occurs both in the proliferating and non-proliferating cells. The time taken for a myeloblast to mature into a marrow granulocyte and for the latter to enter the circulation is 10–12 days; about half of this time is spent in the proliferating cell pool. In normal individuals the blood neutrophils leave the circulation with a $T_{\frac{1}{2}}$ of 7.2 h (see p. 12). There is no evidence for a substantial degree of ineffective neutrophil granulocytopoiesis in normal marrow.

Morphology of neutrophil precursors (Fig. 3.10)

In Romanowsky-stained marrow smears, myeloblasts have a diameter of 10–20 μm, a large rounded or oval nucleus with finely dispersed chromatin, two to five nucleoli and a relatively small quantity of agranular, moderately deep-blue cytoplasm. They are peroxidase-negative. The neutrophil promyelocyte stage is characterized by the presence of a few to several purplish-red (azurophilic) granules, a somewhat coarser nuclear chromatin pattern and prominent nucleoli. The neutrophil myelocyte has a greater volume of cytoplasm relative to that of the nucleus, when compared with the promyelocyte. The cytoplasm is initially slightly basophilic but eventually becomes predominantly acidophilic. It contains many fine, light-pink (neutrophilic) granules in addition to some azurophilic ones. The nucleus is rounded, oval, flattened on one side or slightly indented (see Fig. 3.10d), contains coarsely-granular chromatin and usually lacks a distinct nucleolus. The neutrophil metamyelocyte has a C-shaped nucleus which displays a greater degree of condensation of nuclear chromatin than the myelocyte nucleus. Its cytoplasm stains pale pink and contains numerous neutrophilic granules. The 'band' or juvenile neutrophil (also called a 'stab form') has a U-shaped or long, relatively-narrow band-like nucleus which shows further condensation of the chromatin. The nucleus is frequently twisted into various configurations and may show one or more partial constrictions along its length. The neutrophil granulocyte differs from the 'band' neutrophil in having a segmented nucleus in which two to five nuclear masses are strung together by fine strands of chromatin; the nuclear masses contain large clumps of condensed chromatin (see Figs 1.1a and 1.5).

Ultrastructural studies[11,12] reveal that neutrophil promyelocytes contain large quantities of rough endoplasmic reticulum, many polyribosomes, a highly-developed Golgi apparatus, several large mitochondria and relatively little condensed chromatin. In successive cytological classes of increasing maturity, there is a reduction in the quantity of rough endoplasmic reticulum, ribosomes and mitochondria, a diminution of the Golgi apparatus and an increase in the amount of condensed chromatin. In addition, a large number of glycogen particles appear at the metamyelocyte and granulocyte stages. The primary (azurophilic) granules which develop at the promyelocyte stage are ellipsoidal, very electron-dense, about 0.5–1.0 μm in their long axis, and peroxidase-positive. There seem to be at least two subpopulations of specific granules, the secondary and tertiary granules, which develop

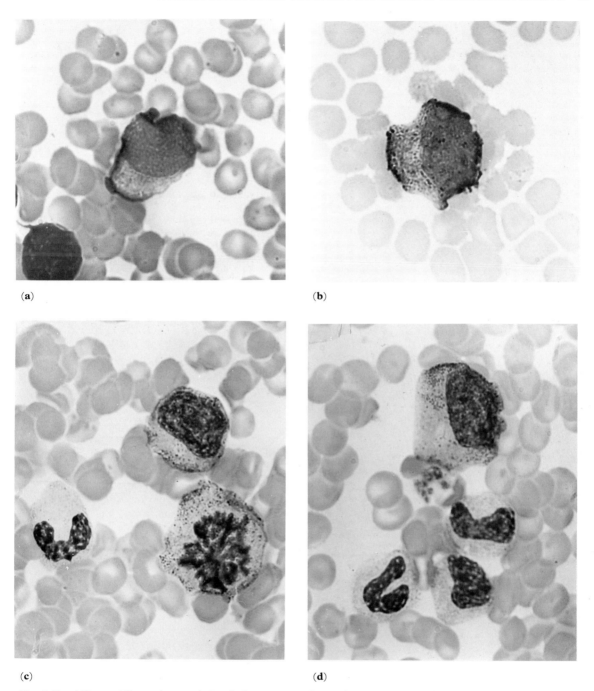

(a)   (b)

(c)   (d)

Fig. 3.10a–d Neutrophil granulocytopoietic cells from a smear of normal bone marrow. (a) Myeloblast. (b) Neutrophil promyelocyte. (c) A neutrophil myelocyte, a neutrophil myelocyte in mitosis and a late neutrophil metamyelocyte. (d) One large and two smaller neutrophil myelocytes and a band neutrophil. The two cells referred to as small myelocytes show a slight indentation in their nuclei and, for this reason, may be classified by some as early metamyelocytes rather than myelocytes. However, since a proportion of cells with slightly indented nuclei synthesise DNA, the present author includes such cells in the myelocyte compartment.

May-Grünwald-Giemsa stain   × 940

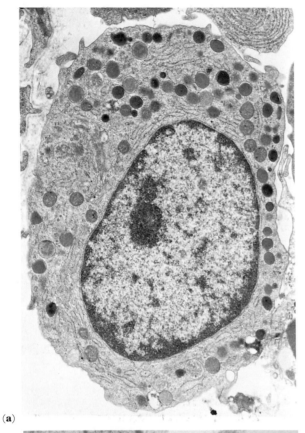

(a)

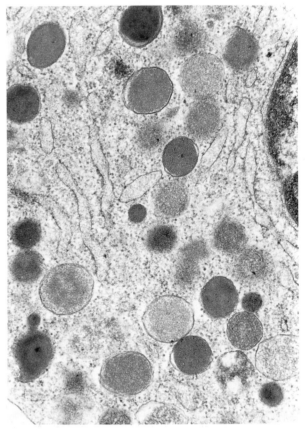

(b)

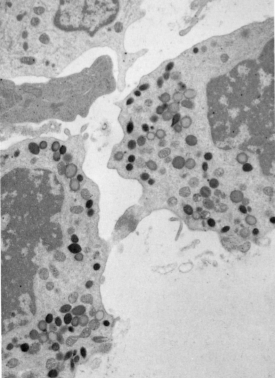

Fig. 3.11a Electron micrograph of a neutrophil myelocyte from normal bone marrow. The nucleus is rounded, contains a nucleolus and shows a small amount of nuclear-membrane-associated heterochromatin (condensed chromatin). The cytoplasm contains two morphologically distinct types of granules and many strands of rough endoplasmic reticulum.

Uranyl acetate and lead citrate   × 11 100

Fig. 3.11b The upper part of the cell in Figure 3.11a at higher magnification, showing the different appearances of the two types of granules: the very electron-dense granules are known as primary granules (and are formed at the promyelocyte stage) and the less electron-dense granules are known as secondary granules (and are formed at the myelocyte stage).

Uranyl acetate and lead citrate   × 34 200

Fig. 3.12 A neutrophil myelocyte from normal bone marrow at a late stage of cell division. The two daughter cells contain telophase nuclei and are joined together by an intercellular spindle bridge. Their cytoplasm contains a mixture of primary and secondary granules.

Uranyl acetate and lead citrate   × 10 800

at the myelocyte (Figs 3.11 and 3.12) and meta-myelocyte stages respectively. The secondary granules are large, spherical, less electron-dense than primary granules, and peroxidase-negative. The tertiary granules are small ($0.2-0.5 \mu m$ in their long axis), rounded, elongated or dumb-bell-shaped, and peroxidase-negative; their electron-density is between that of the primary granules and that of the secondary granules.

Monocytopoiesis: mononuclear phagocyte system[13]

The morphologically-recognizable precursors of the blood monocytes are, in order of increasing maturity, the monoblasts, promonocytes and marrow monocytes; only the first two of these cell types undergo division. The blood mono-cytes leave the circulation with an average $T_{\frac{1}{2}}$ of 71 h and transform into tissue macrophages. In the normal steady state there is a constant loss of tissue macrophages (e.g. by shedding of alveolar macrophages), which is balanced by the forma-tion of new macrophages from blood monocytes and to a small extent from the division of some existing macrophages. The system of cells con-cerned with macrophage production is called the mononuclear phagocyte system. At sites of in-flammation, macrophages may transform into epi-thelioid cells or develop into multinucleate giant cells. In the bone marrow, some monocyte-derived macrophages develop into osteoclasts.

Morphology of monocyte precursors

Monoblasts are agranular cells which resemble myeloblasts except for the tendency of their nu-clei to be cleft or slightly lobulated. The pro-monocytes are large cells with a rounded, oval or clearly-lobulated nucleus which consists predom-inantly of euchromatin and contains one or more prominent nucleoli. In Romanowsky-stained preparations their cytoplasm is basophilic and has a small number of azurophilic granules. The degree of basophilia is greater, the nucleus-to-cytoplasm ratio higher (>1) and the number of azurophilic granules fewer than in marrow mono-cytes. The latter resemble blood monocytes, which are described on page 15. Similar pro-portions of promonocytes, marrow monocytes and blood monocytes have IgG-Fc, IgE-Fc and C3b receptors and display non-specific esterase activity. The electron microscope shows that the cytoplasm of promonocytes contains many ribo-somes, some rough endoplasmic reticulum, a well-developed Golgi apparatus, several mito-chondria and a few granules. The latter consist of electron-dense material which is usually sur-rounded by a clear zone and contains both acid phosphatase and peroxidase. The maturation of promonocytes to marrow monocytes and blood monocytes is associated with an increase in the quantity of cytoplasmic granules and of con-densed chromatin, and a progressive decrease in the number of ribosomes. In addition, the gran-ules of monocytes do not display a peripheral clear zone. The cell membranes of promonocytes and monocytes show characteristic ruffles which appear as finger-like surface projections in thin sections.

Regulation of neutrophil granulocytopoiesis and monocytopoiesis[14]

The regulation of the production of neutrophils is closely linked to that of the production of monocytes. The colony-stimulating factors (CSF) required for the formation of neutrophil and macrophage colonies in vitro (p. 50) appear to be also involved in the formation of these cells in vivo. These factors consist of a family of glyco-proteins produced by monocytes, bone marrow macrophages and other types of cells such as fibroblasts and phytohaemagglutinin-stimulated lymphocytes. CSFs regulate the proliferation of CFU-C and promote their conversion to myelob-lasts or monoblasts. Some CSF preparations sti-mulate the production of granulocyte colonies, and others that of macrophage colonies. The available data suggest that the bone marrow macrophages play a key role in regulating the production of their own precursors as well as of granulocytes. They do this by producing both CSF as well as prostaglandin E (PGE), an inhib-itor of CFU-C.[15] Any stimulation of CSF pro-duction is followed by a CSF-mediated stimula-tion of PGE synthesis which has the effect of returning the cell system to its original steady state. Granulocytes contain inhibitors of the proliferation of granulocytopoietic cells. They also contain lactoferrin, a metal-binding glycoprotein which depresses the formation of CSF by some monocytes and macrophages.[16] These inhibitory substances may participate in the regulation of the production of monocytes and granulocytes *in vivo* by providing a negative feedback between the mass of mature granulocytes and the rate of production of new cells. Mature granulocytes in blood and tissue might also influence cell production in the marrow by removing or inactivating bacteria and their products, with the consequence that these do not reach macrophages and stimulate them to produce CSF. A reduction in the number of granulocytes in the body would lead to an increase in the bacterial antigenic load reaching the bone marrow macrophages, an increased production of CSF and, eventually, to an increased production of granulocytes.

EOSINOPHIL GRANULOCYTOPOIESIS

There is a morphologically-unrecognized precursor committed to eosinophil granulocytopoiesis which can be detected by its ability to form colonies consisting of eosinophil granulocytes when grown in a semi-solid medium containing a specific eosinophil colony-stimulating factor (produced by antigen-stimulated non-adherent spleen cells).[17] This precursor cell is described as the eosinophil colony-forming unit or CFU-Eo. The earliest morphologically recognizable eosinophil precursor is the eosinophil promyelocyte. The other more mature cells of the eosinophil series are the eosinophil myelocytes, eosinophil metamyelocytes, eosinophil band cells and marrow eosinophil granulocytes. The CFU-Eo, eosinophil promyelocytes and eosinophil myelocytes undergo cell division; the metamyelocytes, band cells and granulocytes are non-dividing cells.

Morphology

In Romanowsky-stained smears, the eosinophil promyelocyte has a large rounded nucleus with a finely-granular chromatin pattern and nucleoli. It has a moderate quantity of basophilic cytoplasm containing coarse granules, some of which are reddish-orange and others bluish in colour. The eosinophil myelocytes have a coarsely-granular chromatin pattern and polychromatic cytoplasm containing several typical eosinophil granules and few or no blue-staining granules (Fig. 3.13). The eosinophil metamyelocytes have a C-shaped nucleus, moderate quantities of condensed chromatin, a faintly polychromatic or

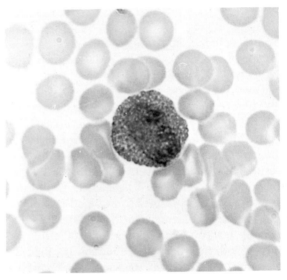

Fig. 3.13 Eosinophil myelocyte from a smear of normal bone marrow.
May–Grünwald–Giemsa stain   × 940

acidophilic cytoplasm and several eosinophilic granules. The band or juvenile eosinophils are similar to eosinophil metamyelocytes except that they have a U-shaped or long band-like nucleus. The morphology of the eosinophil granulocyte is described on page 13. Two types of eosinophil granules can be distinguished under the electron microscope,[18] homogeneous granules and crystalloid-containing granules. Eosinophil promyelocytes contain several homogeneous granules and only an occasional crystalloid-containing granule. In eosinophil myelocytes, several granules of both types are present (Fig. 3.14) and in the metamyelocytes and granulocytes crystalloid-containing granules predominate (also see p. 13).

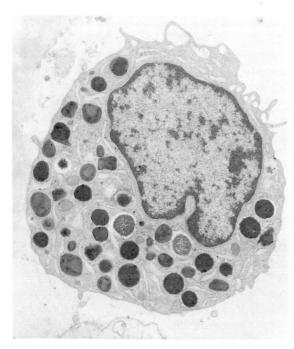

Fig. 3.14 Electron micrograph of an early eosinophil myelocyte from normal bone marrow. The nucleus shows a slight to moderate amount of condensed chromatin. The majority of the cytoplasmic granules consist of very electron-dense primary granules but there are also a few crystalloid-containing secondary granules. Two of the cytoplasmic granules contain granular material of a relatively low electron-density and display a clear halo at their periphery; these probably represent immature primary granules. The cytoplasm contains many dilated sacs of rough endoplasmic reticulum.

Uranyl acetate and lead citrate   × 8525

Regulation of eosinophil granulocytopoiesis[19]

In experimental animals, the development of an eosinophilia in response to parasitic infections occurs in two phases: an initial inductive phase which is dependent on T-lymphocytes and a subsequent phase of increased proliferation of eosinophil precursors which is dependent on a humoral factor. It appears that parasite antigens stimulate sensitized lymphocytes to release a factor which increases eosinophil granulocytopoiesis by directly or indirectly acting on CFU-Eo and the morphologically recognizable eosinophil precursors. Other studies have shown that the specific depletion of mature eosinophils by the administration of anti-eosinophil serum generates a low molecular weight substance which stimulates eosinophil granulocytopoiesis both *in vivo* and *in vitro*; this substance has been termed eosinophilopoietin.[20]

PRODUCTION OF BASOPHIL GRANULOCYTES AND MAST CELLS

The basophil granulocyte is derived from the multipotent haemopoietic stem cell. In the postnatal period, basophil granulocytopoiesis occurs in the bone marrow. The morphologically-recognizable precursors of basophil granulocytes are rounded in shape and may be subdivided into basophil myelocytes, which have round or oval nuclei, and basophil metamyelocytes, which have C-shaped, unsegmented nuclei. Characteristically, in Romanowsky-stained smears both these cell types have large basophilic cytoplasmic granules which often overlie and obscure the nucleus. However, the granules are water-soluble and so their contents may be extracted during fixation and staining. With basic dyes such as toluidine blue or methylene blue, the more mature granules stain metachromatically (i.e. a reddish-violet). The ultrastructure of the granules in basophil promyelocytes and myelocytes is similar to that of the granules of mature basophil granulocytes (see p. 15) except that the intragranular particles are finer.[21]

Recent studies have shown that the tissue mast cells are also derived from CFU-S (see p. 45) and that the latter develop within the marrow into undifferentiated precursors of mast cells.[22] These mast cell precursors circulate in the peripheral blood[23,24] and migrate into tissues where they proliferate and mature into mast cells. There are some data suggesting that both the basophil granulocyte and the mast cell might share a common bipotent morphologically unrecognized precursor cell (derived from the CFU-S). However, the exact relationship between the morphologically unrecognized precursors which are committed to the production of basophils and mast cells and those committed to the production of neutrophils, macrophages or eosinophils is still uncertain.

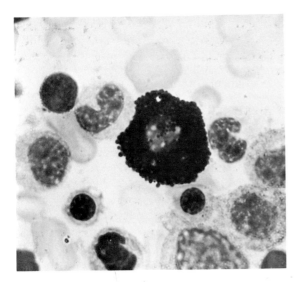

Fig. 3.15 Mast cell from a smear of normal bone marrow. The cytoplasm is packed with coarse granules only a few of which overlie the nucleus.

May-Grünwald-Giemsa stain   × 940

Mast cells vary considerably in size (diameter of 5–25 µm in smears) and can be distinguished from basophils by their generally larger size, tendency to have an elongated or ovoid shape, and the fact that the coarse, purplish-black to reddish-purple granules (Romanowsky stain) are less water-extractable and seldom overlie the nucleus (Fig. 3.15). The nucleus of the mast cell is small, round or oval, contains less condensed chromatin than that of a basophil and stains more or less uniformly. It is centrally or, occasionally, eccentrically placed. Mast cells contain histamine, heparin, hydrolytic enzymes (e.g. chloroacetate esterase) and surface receptors for IgE but, unlike basophil granulocytes (p. 15), they also contain 5-hydroxytryptamine (serotonin) and do not contain peroxidase. Mast cells (like basophils) are PAS-positive. The mast cell granules vary markedly in their ultrastructure and may be dense and amorphous, show central condensations or contain crystals or lamellar structures arranged in various ways (e.g. scrolls or whorls and parallel lamellae) (Fig. 3.16). Cells

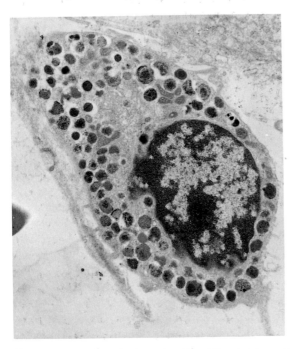

Fig. 3.16a Electron micrograph of a mast cell in normal bone marrow. The cytoplasmic granules vary considerably in their ultrastructure.

Uranyl acetate and lead citrate   × 8520

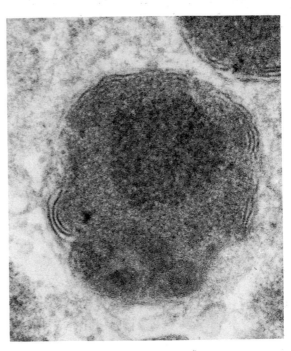

Fig. 3.16b A single granule from the cell in Figure 3.16a, at high magnification, showing central condensations and peripheral lamellae.

× 103 725

with characteristics between those of basophils and mast cells have been described.[21]

MEGAKARYOCYTOPOIESIS[1, 25]

The morphologically-unrecognized early progenitor cells committed to megakaryocytopoiesis are called the megakaryocyte colony-forming units (CFU-Meg). The latter are derived from the multipotent myeloid stem cells and develop into the earliest morphologically-recognizable member of the megakaryocytopoietic system, the megakaryoblast. The CFU-Meg is defined operationally in terms of its ability to form a small colony of megakaryocytes when grown in suitable semi-solid medium in the presence of megakaryocyte colony-stimulating factors (e.g. mitogen-stimulated spleen cell supernatants or the conditioned medium from a myelomonocytic leukaemia cell line, WEHI-3). The megakaryocytes in these colonies show more or less normal maturation and shed platelets.[26] The CFU-Meg are a diploid cell population in which DNA synthesis and nuclear division (karyokinesis) is followed by cell division (cytokinesis).

Four types of megakaryocytes can be recognized in Romanowsky-stained marrow smears. These are, in increasing order of maturity, megakaryoblasts (group I megakaryocytes), promegakaryocytes (group II megakaryocytes), granular megakaryocytes (group III megakaryocytes) and 'bare nuclei'. DNA synthesis occurs in 44% of megakaryoblasts, 18% of promegakaryocytes and in only 2% of granular megakaryocytes. This DNA synthesis is not associated with cytokinesis and results in the production of mononucleate polyploid cells. The DNA content of a megakaryoblast ranges from 4–32 c and that of a promegakaryocyte or granular megakaryocyte from 8–64 c; cells with higher DNA content are larger than those with lower content (1c = the haploid DNA content, i.e. the DNA content of a spermatozoon). The time taken for a megakaryoblast to mature into a platelet-producing granular megakaryocyte may be about six days.

Although the majority of the megakaryocytes are found in the marrow parenchyma, some whole cells enter the circulation via the marrow sinusoids. Most of the circulating megakaryocytes are trapped in the lungs and some of the pulmonary megakaryocytes appear to produce platelets.

Morphology

Megakaryoblasts and megakaryocytes are larger than other immature haemopoietic cells and this feature makes their identification relatively easy. In marrow smears, most cells with a diameter $> 20\,\mu m$ belong to the megakaryocyte series.[27] The megakaryoblasts have a very high nucleus to cytoplasm ratio, a deeply-basophilic agranular cytoplasm and a single bi-, tri- or multilobed nucleus with several nucleoli. Promegakaryocytes are usually larger than megakaryoblasts and have a lower nucleus to cytoplasm ratio and a less basophilic cytoplasm. The overlapping nuclear lobes of a promegakaryocyte are arranged in a C-shaped formation, the concavity of which sometimes contains a patch of azurophilic cytoplasmic granules. The granular megakaryocytes (Fig. 3.17) are up to $70\,\mu m$ in diameter and possess abundant pale-staining cytoplasm and numerous azurophilic cytoplasmic granules. The nucleus has multiple lobes which extend through much of the cell. Prior to the shedding of platelets, the nuclear lobes become fairly tightly packed together. The typical appearance of a megakaryocyte in a histological section of a bone marrow biopsy is illustrated in Fig. 3.18.

Ultrastructural studies[28] show that the nucleus of the megakaryoblast is lobulated and contains small quantities of condensed chromatin and several prominent nucleoli. The cytoplasm is relatively scanty and contains a well-developed Golgi apparatus within a deep indentation of the nucleus. It also contains many polyribosomes, scattered rough endoplasmic reticulum, many mitochondria, a few microtubules, a few membrane-lined vesicles representing the beginning of the demarcation membrane system, a few lysosomal vesicles containing acid phosphatase and aryl sulphatase, and a few immature α granules. The lysosomal vesicles and α granules are situated near the Golgi apparatus. The demarcation membrane system (DMS) consists of a system of cytoplasmic vesicles which seem to arise as invagin-

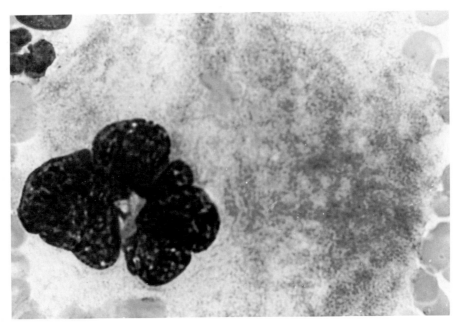

Fig. 3.17 Granular megakaryocyte from a smear of normal bone marrow.　　May–Grünwald–Giemsa stain　× 940

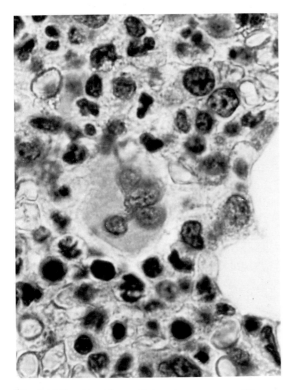

Fig. 3.18 Trephine biopsy of normal bone marrow. The very large cell with a lobed nucleus is a megakaryocyte.

Haematoxylin-eosin　× 940

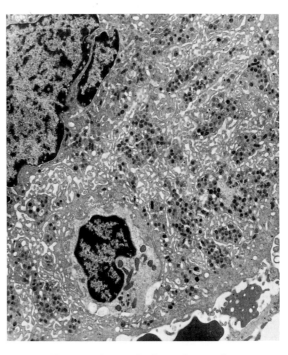

Fig. 3.19 Electron micrograph of part of a granular megakaryocyte. The extensive demarcation membrane system and numerous cytoplasmic granules can be seen in the wide intermediate zone of the cytoplasm. The cytoplasm also contains a normal-looking lymphocyte which may have been travelling through the megakaryocyte (emperipolesis).

Uranyl acetate and lead citrate　× 5300

ations of the surface membrane; the cavities of these vesicles are continuous with the exterior. The granular megakaryocytes (Fig. 3.19) have considerably more cytoplasm and a larger, more lobulated and segmented nucleus than a megakaryoblast. Three zones can often be seen in the cytoplasm: a narrow outer zone just internal to the cell membrane, a wide intermediate zone and a narrow perinuclear zone. Hardly any organelles are present in the outer zone. Many ovoid electron-dense α granules, numerous vesicles belonging to the DMS and some coated lysosomal vesicles are found in the intermediate zone, together with microtubules, ribosomes, rough endoplasmic reticulum and mitochondria. The perinuclear zone contains the Golgi apparatus, ribosomes, rough endoplasmic reticulum and mitochondria. During platelet release, the granular megakaryocytes protrude cytoplasmic processes[29] close to or directly into the marrow sinusoids; pieces of cytoplasm break away from these processes and subsequently fragment into platelets. The DMS appears to provide extra membrane for the formation of the cytoplasmic processes and to be involved in the fragmentation of these processes. The almost bare nucleus which remains after the release of platelets is surrounded by a narrow rim of cytoplasm containing a few granules and other organelles. This nucleus is phagocytosed by bone marrow macrophages.

Emperipolesis.[30, 31] This term is applied to describe the temporary presence of one cell inside the cytoplasm of another; the 'engulfed' cell can subsequently leave the engulfing cell and appears to be morphologically unaltered as a result of the interaction. If a sufficiently large number of megakaryocytes are examined, some are regularly found to display the phenomenon of emperipolesis both in normal marrow (unpublished observations) and in a wide range of clinical conditions. The cell types which may be found within megakaryocytes include granulocytes and their precursors, and lymphocytes, erythroblasts and red cells. Megakaryocytic emperipolesis may be seen in marrow smears as well as in histological sections of marrow, including thin sections used for electron microscopy; sometimes one megakaryocyte may contain several cells 'inside' it (Fig. 3.20). Although it has been claimed that

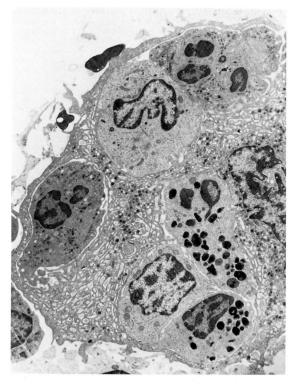

Fig. 3.20 Electron micrograph of a megakaryocyte which is apparently showing an unusual degree of emperipolesis. Although sections of six other cells (including two eosinophil granulocytes, two neutrophil granulocytes and a monocyte) are seen within the megakaryocyte profile, it is possible that at least some of these cells are not completely within the megakaryocyte but merely protruding into it.

Uranyl acetate and lead citrate   × 6 800

megakaryocytic emperipolesis may be considerably increased in patients with haemorrhage or various malignant diseases, these claims are not well-proven as they have not been made on the basis of a comparison of equal numbers of megakaryocytes from normal individuals and appropriate patients. Megakaryocytic emperipolesis is of uncertain significance but may represent a transmegakaryocytic route for the entry of blood cells into the circulation; it has been suggested that some of the intramegakaryocytic cells may enter the circulation via the processes of megakaryocytic cytoplasm which protrude into adjacent marrow sinusoids.[32] Emperipolesis is not confined to megakaryocytes. It has been described also in various non-haemopoietic cells and in malignant cells, including blast cells from patients in the acute phase of chronic granulocytic leukaemia.

Regulation of megakaryocytopoiesis

Following the induction of acute thrombocytopenia in experimental animals, there is an increase in the rate of platelet production which results in a rapid increase of the platelet count to supranormal levels. The rebound thrombocytosis is short-lived and normal platelet counts are soon re-established. Conversely, an experimentally-induced acute thrombocytosis causes a depression of the rate of platelet production which leads to a rebound thrombocytopenia prior to re-establishment of a normal platelet count. The increased rate of platelet production induced by acute thrombocytopenia results initially from an increase in the proportion of large megakaryocytes with high ploidy values and, subsequently, also from an increase in the total number of megakaryocytes in the marrow; the increase in the mean ploidy value leads to an increase in the average number of platelets produced per megakaryocyte. The depression of platelet production induced by thrombocytosis is caused by a reduction of the average size and ploidy value of megakaryocytes and a reduction in the total number of megakaryocytes in the marrow.

It is evident from the data outlined above that regulatory mechanisms operate to keep the platelet count of normal individuals within narrow limits. The details of these mechanisms are, however, uncertain. Two factors (activities) which affect megakaryocytopoiesis have been recognized: these are thrombopoietin and megakaryocyte colony-stimulating factors. Thrombopoietin regulates megakaryocyte maturation, including polyploidization, by acting both on CFU-Meg and on megakaryocytes. Its level in the plasma increases in thrombocytopenic states. Megakaryocyte colony-stimulating factors but not thrombopoietin regulate the proliferation of CFU-Meg, at least in vitro. The identity of the factor which regulates the rate of conversion of CFU-Meg to megakaryoblasts and hence the total number of megakaryocytes in the marrow is still uncertain: some workers consider this factor to be thrombopoietin.

LYMPHOPOIESIS[33]

Lymphopotent stem cells exist in fetal and postnatal haemopoietic tissues (Table 1.7) and a substantial degree of lymphopoiesis occurs in these. Much of the lymphopoiesis which occurs in normal bone marrow appears to be independent of antigenic stimulation and serves to supply the body with partially differentiated cells, some of which mature into B-lymphocytes (in the marrow) or T-lymphocytes (in the thymus) and then migrate to peripheral lymphoid tissues (spleen, lymph nodes, Peyer's patches, Waldeyer's ring). The development of bone-marrow-derived precursor cells into T-lymphocytes is dependent on an interaction of the precursor cells with the epithelial elements of the thymus and/or their products. In the case of birds, the development of the precursor cells into B-lymphocytes requires the bursa of Fabricius, an epithelial structure in the avian hind-gut. The bursa-equivalent in mammals is uncertain but is thought to be some component of the marrow. In any event, newly-formed immunologically-competent small lymphocytes with B-cell characteristics have been shown to leave the bone marrow and circulate to peripheral lymphoid tissues where they may undergo antigen-dependent proliferation and further maturation. Some B-cells undergo antigen-dependent development into plasma cells in the marrow itself. Specific antigens also stimulate T-lymphocytes present in peripheral lymphoid tissues to undergo maturation and proliferation. There appears to be a high rate of cell death during antigen-independent lymphopoiesis in both the marrow and the thymus. A hypothetical scheme of the maturation of a lymphoid stem cell into an antibody-secreting plasma cell is shown in Table 3.1. The maturation pathway for the production of memory B-cells (allowing rapid antibody production in a secondary immune response) is likely to differ from that for the production of plasma cells. A hypothetical scheme for the maturation of a lymphoid stem cell to a mature peripheral blood T-cell is shown in Table 3.2.

The distribution of lymphoid cells and plasma cells in the marrow has been described on pages 43 and 44. The light and electron microscope

Table 3.1 Hypothetical scheme of B-lymphocyte differentiation.[34,35,36] Ig, immunoglobulin; μ, heavy chain of IgM; Cμ, cytoplasmic μ chain; κ,λ, light chains of immunoglobulin; MRFC, mouse rosette-forming cell; FcR, receptor for Fc segment of Ig molecule; C3R, receptor for the third component of complement; CALLA, common ALL antigen; BA1, BA2, B1, B2, monoclonal antibodies against B-cells or their precursors; TdT, terminal deoxynucleotidyl transferase; SmIg, surface membrane immunoglobulin; CIg, cytoplasmic immunoglobulin; Ia-like, antigens related to the immune-associated antigens of the mouse.

Cell type	Immunoglobulin secretion status	Other membrane receptors	TdT	Ia-like antigen (DR locus)	CALLA	Monoclonal markers			
						BA1	BA2	B1	B2
Lymphoid stem cell	−	−	+	+	−	+/−	+	−	−
Early pre B-cell	μ gene rearranged	−	+	+	+	+/−	+	+	−
Pre B-cell	μ gene expressed; κ gene rearrangement followed by λ gene rearrangement	−	+	+	+	+/−	+	+	−
Immature B-cell	(1) Cμ Sm IgM	−	−	+	+/−	+	+	+	+
	(2) Sm IgM	MRFC +/−	−	+	−	+	−	+	+
	(3) Sm IgM Sm IgD	MRFC +/− FcR + C3R +/−	−	+	−	+	−	+	+
Mature B-cell	(1) Sm IgM Sm IgD Sm IgA or IgG	FcR + C3R +/−	−	+	−	+	−	+	+
	(2) Sm IgA or IgG	FcR + C3R +/−	−	+	−	+	−	+	−
Immunoblast									
Plasma cell	CIg	FcR +/−	−	+/−	−	−	−	−	−

Table 3.2 Maturation of T-lymphocytes.[34,37] TdT, terminal deoxynucleotidyl transferase; E rosettes, rosette formation with sheep red blood cells; Leu 1, Leu 2, Leu 3, T1, T3, T4, T5, T6, T8, T9, T10, T11, T101, and HLA DR are monoclonal antibodies (see Table 6.8 on p. 225); +, giving a positive reaction; −, giving a negative reaction; +/−, giving either a positive reaction or a negative reaction.

Cell	Site where normally found	TdT	E Rosettes, T11, Leu 5	Markers			
				Monoclonal antibodies			
				pan T, pan-thymocyte thymocyte	pan-mature T	'helper (H)' and 'suppressor (S)' markers	Others
Thymic lymphoblast (prothymocyte)	Thymic subcapsular cortex	+	−	−	−	−	−
Stage I or early thymocyte	Thymic cortex	+	+/−	T1 − or weak, T101+, Leu 1+	−	−	T9 +, T10+, HLA DR+
Stage II or common thymocyte	Thymic cortex	+/−	+/−	T1 − or weak, T101+, Leu 1+	−	T4+, Leu 3+, T5, 8+, Leu 2+	T10+, T6+, HLA DR+
Stage III or mature thymocyte	Thymic medulla	−	+	T1+, T101+, Leu 1+	T3+, Leu 4+	'H': T4+, Leu 3+ 'S': T8+, Leu 2+, T5+/−	T10+
Mature T-cell	Peripheral blood, lymph nodes	−	+	T1+, T101+, Leu 1+	T3+, Leu 4+	'H': T4+, Leu 3+ 'S': T8+, T5+/−, Leu 2+	−

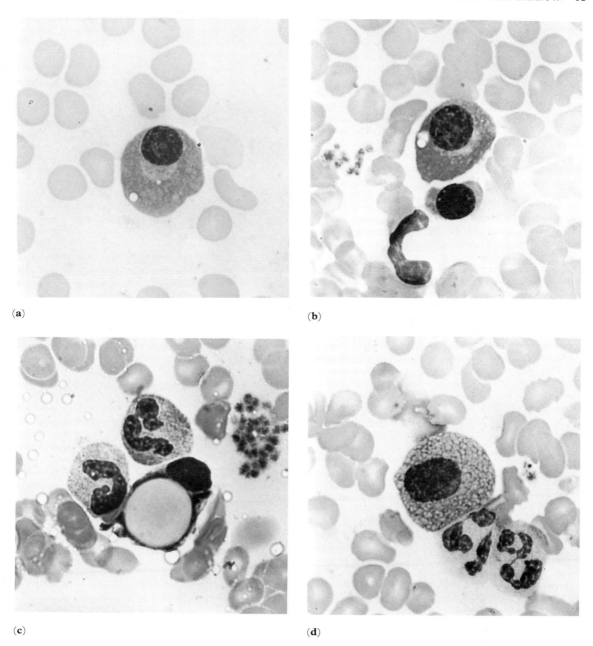

(a)

(b)

(c)

(d)

Fig. 3.21a–d Different appearances of plasma cells from smears of normal bone marrow. (**a, b**) Both plasma cells contain intracytoplasmic vacuoles and display a paler-staining crescentic zone immediately adjacent to the nucleus. This zone corresponds to the position of the Golgi apparatus. (**c**) Plasma cell containing a single Russell body. (**d**) Plasma cell with a 'reticulated' cytoplasm.

May–Grünwald–Giemsa stain   × 940

features of these cells are similar to those of the same cells in peripheral lymphoid tissue. A description of bone marrow plasma cells is given below.

PLASMA CELLS

The mature plasma cells seen in Romanowsky-stained smears of normal bone marrow may vary markedly in their morphology. The majority are 14–20 μm in diameter and have deep-blue cytoplasm with a paler paranuclear zone corresponding to the site of the Golgi apparatus; the cytoplasm may have one or more vacuoles (Fig. 3.21a,b). The nucleus is eccentric and small relative to the volume of the cytoplasm and contains moderate amounts of condensed chromatin (Fig. 3.21). The characteristic cartwheel appearance of the nucleus is only seen in histological sections, not in smears. A small proportion of normal plasma cells show a variety of additional cytological features and are then sometimes given different names. Some plasma cells contain Russell bodies (Fig. 3.21c) which are very large acidophilic cytoplasmic inclusions which stain by the periodic-acid-Schiff reaction; there is usually only one Russell body per cell. Mott cells (grape cells, or morular cells) are plasma cells containing several smaller, slightly basophilic, rounded inclusions. Some plasma cells have a reticulated appearance due to the presence of many pleomorphic inclusions (Fig. 3.21d) and others are described as 'flaming cells' as they are eosinophilic at their periphery (occasionally the entire cytoplasm may take on an eosinophilic hue). Rarely, a plasma cell may contain azurophilic rods with a crystalline ultrastructure.

When examined with the electron microscope, the cytoplasm of the mature plasma cell is seen to be packed with flattened sacs of rough endoplasmic reticulum (RER) (Figs 3.22 and 3.23a,b) which are frequently aligned parallel to each other, in a concentric arrangement or in whorls; the sacs contain an amorphous material which is thought to be immunoglobulin. The cytoplasm also contains a well-developed Golgi zone (Fig. 3.23a), some rounded primary lysosomes (which vary considerably in size) and moderate numbers

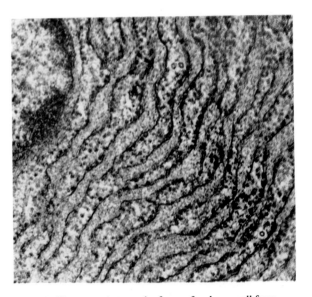

Fig. 3.22 Electron micrograph of part of a plasma cell from a normal bone marrow. There are several sacs of rough endoplasmic reticulum arranged more or less parallel to each other. The sacs contain a finely-granular material (presumably antibody) and have ribosomes attached to their outer surfaces.
Uranyl acetate and lead citrate   × 116 100

of mitochondria. Russell bodies and the inclusions within Mott cells and 'reticulated cells' consist of masses of homogeneous electron-dense material which are usually lined by RER (Fig 3.23b–d); these inclusions are thought to result from the condensation of immunoglobulin within distended cisternae of the RER. The nuclei of plasma cells contain a variable quantity of condensed chromatin (which is generally, but not always, proportional to the degree of cytoplasmic maturity) and frequently contain a well-developed nucleolus.

BONE MARROW MACROPHAGES (RETICULUM CELLS, HISTIOCYTES)

These cells are 20–30 μm in diameter, irregular in shape, and have voluminous cytoplasm with long cytoplasmic processes at their periphery (Figs 3.3 and 3.4). In Romanowsky-stained normal marrow smears, the cytoplasm appears pale-blue and contains azurophilic granules, vacuoles, lipid droplets and, often, phagocytosed

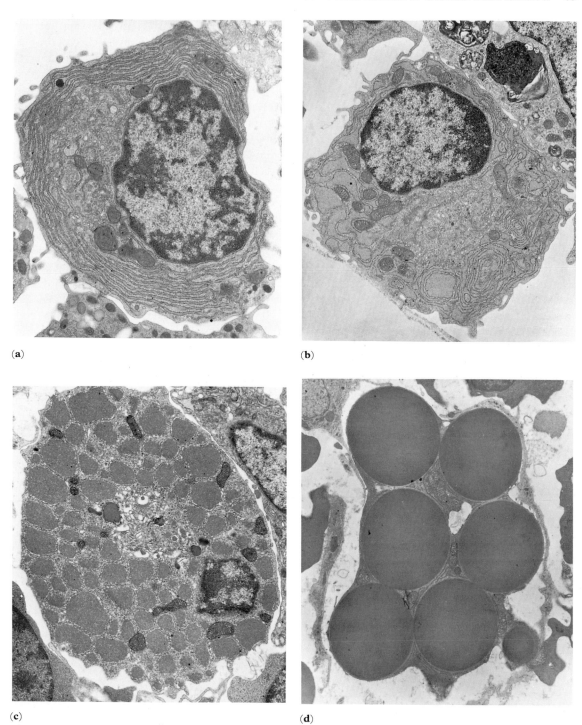

(a)

(b)

(c)

(d)

Fig. 3.23a–d Various appearances of the ultrastructure of plasma cells from normal bone marrow. (**a**) The cytoplasm is packed with rough endoplasmic reticulum aligned more or less parallel to each other. There is a large paranuclear Golgi zone, which is devoid of endoplasmic reticulum. (**b**) The endoplasmic reticulum is arranged in concentric whorls and parts of it are distended to varying extents with relatively electron-lucent material. (**c, d**) Rounded intracytoplasmic inclusions consisting of sacs of endoplasmic reticulum distended with electron-dense material.

Uranyl acetate and lead citrate   (**a**) ×9825; (**b**) ×7675; (**c**) ×7225; (**d**) ×5850

material, including extruded erythroblast nuclei and, occasionally, whole granulocytes. The nucleus of the macrophage is large, round or oval, and has a pale-staining lace-like chromatin structure and one or more large nucleoli. Macrophages are relatively fragile and their cytoplasm is frequently ruptured during the preparation of smears. Histological studies reveal that some of these cells occur within erythroblastic islands (p. 43), plasma cell islands and lymphoid nodules, and that others lie adjacent to marrow sinusoids and actually form part of the incomplete adventitial layer of the sinusoidal wall (p. 42). The cytoplasmic processes of bone marrow macrophages not only extend intimately between erythropoietic and other marrow cells but also may protrude through endothelial cells into the sinusoidal lumen. The intrasinusoidal cytoplasmic processes[38] appear to recognize and phagocytose senescent erythrocytes, abnormal or damaged cells (e.g. heat-damaged red cells, sickled red cells, red cells containing malarial parasites) and circulating particulate or colloidal material.

On electron microscopy (Fig 3.24), the eccentric nucleus often has an irregular outline and shows relatively little peripheral chromatin condensation. The cytoplasm contains numerous strands of rough endoplasmic reticulum, moderate numbers of mitochondria, scattered ferritin molecules, a moderately well-developed Golgi apparatus, centrioles and several primary lysosomes. There are also a number of membrane-bound electron-dense intracytoplasmic inclusions which vary markedly in size, shape and ultrastructure, are sometimes up to 7 μm in diameter, contain both lipid (e.g. myelin figures) and large numbers of ferritin and haemosiderin molecules, and probably represent phagocytosed cells at an advanced stage of degradation. The phagosomes of normal macrophages also occasionally contain clearly recognizable extruded erythroblast nuclei, red cells, neutrophils or eosinophils (Fig 3.25).

It is possible (but not yet proven) that bone marrow macrophages influence erythropoiesis by associating with early erythroid progenitors (one macrophage with one progenitor cell) to form an erythropoietic unit and by producing erythropoiesis-stimulating factors. As mentioned

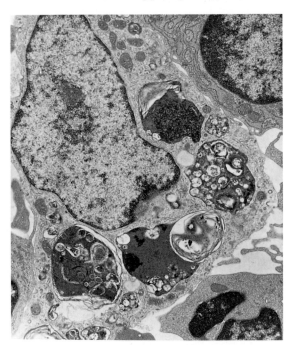

Fig. 3.24 Electron micrograph of a macrophage from normal bone marrow. The nucleus has a central nucleolus and the cytoplasm has several large pleomorphic inclusions.

Uranyl acetate and lead citrate   × 7900

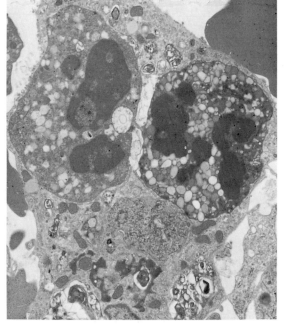

Fig. 3.25 Electron micrograph of a macrophage from normal bone marrow. The cytoplasm contains two phagocytosed granulocytes.

Uranyl acetate and lead citrate   × 7000

earlier, bone marrow macrophages are also involved in the regulation of monocytopoiesis and
granulocytopoiesis (p. 53)

OSTEOBLASTS AND OSTEOCLASTS

Groups of osteoblasts and individual osteoclasts
can occasionally be seen in Romanowsky-stained
normal marrow smears. Osteoblasts (Fig. 3.26)
appear oval or elongated and are 25–50 μm in
diameter. They have a single small eccentric nucleus with one to three nucleoli and abundant
blue-staining cytoplasm, frequently with somewhat indistinct margins. Although these cells
superficially resemble plasma cells, they are larger
and their Golgi zone is not immediately adjacent
to the nucleus. Furthermore, the nucleus of an
osteoblast does not show the heavily-stained
coarse clumps of condensed chromatin which are
characteristically seen in plasma cells. Osteoclasts

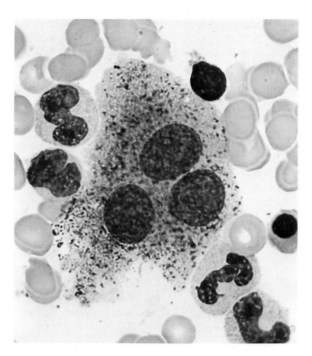

Fig. 3.27 A trinucleate osteoclast from a smear of normal
bone marrow. (Most osteoclasts have a larger number of
nuclei.)

May–Grünwald–Giemsa stain   × 940

(Fig 3.27) are giant multinucleate cells with
abundant pale-staining cytoplasm containing
many fine azurophilic granules. The individual
nuclei within a single cell are small, round or
oval, uniform in size, and have a single
prominent nucleolus. There is usually no overlap
between adjacent nuclei within the same cell. Osteoclasts must be distinguished from the other
polyploid giant cells in the marrow, the megakaryocytes. Unlike osteoclasts, the latter (when
normal) have a single large segmented and lobulated nucleus.

In histological sections, osteoblasts are found
at the surfaces of bone spicules. Osteoclasts are
also found at the surfaces of bone trabeculae
where they lie in Howship's lacunae.

CELLULAR COMPOSITION OF HAEMOPOIETIC MARROW

The bone marrow contains a mixture of fat cells
and haemopoietic cells in various proportions.

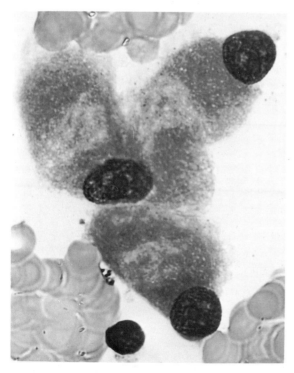

Fig. 3.26 A group of three osteoblasts from a smear of
normal bone marrow. The cytoplasm of each cell contains a
large pale-staining area (occupied by the Golgi apparatus)
which is situated at some distance from the nucleus.

May–Grünwald–Giemsa stain   × 940

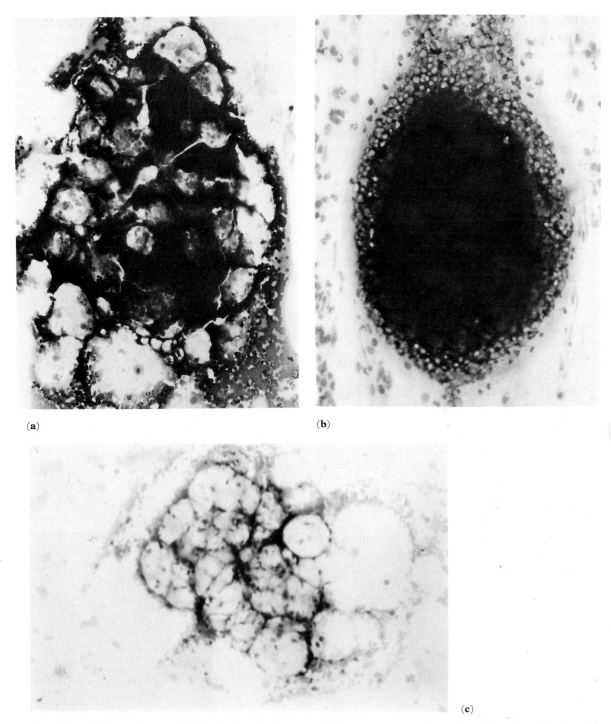

(a)

(b)

(c)

Fig. 3.28a–c Different degrees of cellularity of marrow fragments in bone marrow smears from three different individuals. (**a**) Normocellular fragments in which a little over half the volume of the fragment consists of haemopoietic cells (normal adult). (**b**) Hypercellular fragment showing virtually complete replacement of fat cells by haemopoietic cells (chronic granulocytic leukaemia). (**c**) Hypocellular fragment in which well under 25% of the volume of the fragment consists of haemopoietic cells (aplastic anaemia).

May–Grünwald–Giemsa stain   × 94

Marrow which consists predominantly of fat cells with only a very few microscopic foci of haemopoietic cells appears yellow and fatty. Marrow which contains substantial quantities of haemopoietic cells in addition to fat cells appears red.

The proportion of haemopoietic cells relative to fat cells in a sample of red marrow (i.e. the cellularity of the marrow) can be roughly assessed by examining several marrow fragments in stained marrow smears (Fig 3.28). However, cellularity is more accurately assessed from histological sections of aspirated marrow fragments, or, preferably, of specimens obtained by trephine biopsy of bone. In histological studies, cellularity is expressed as the percentage of the area of a microscopic field of marrow tissue which is occupied by haemopoietic cells. Studies of histolog-

ical sections of marrow fragments aspirated from the tibia, iliac crest and sternum of normal infants and children have shown 100% cellularity at birth, the appearance of fat cells as early as 2 weeks after birth (85% cellularity), and a cellularity of 35–80% (mean, 50%) in iliac crest and sternal aspirations from children between the ages of 18 months and 11 years.[39] In trephine biopsies from normal adults (Fig 3.29), marrow cellularity varies between 30 and 70%. Samples from adults with a cellularity of 25% or less are therefore described as hypocellular and those with a cellularity of 75% or more as hypercellular. However, in individuals aged 70 years or over, the cellularity of the marrow may normally be less than 25%, particularly in the sternum but also in the iliac crest.[40]

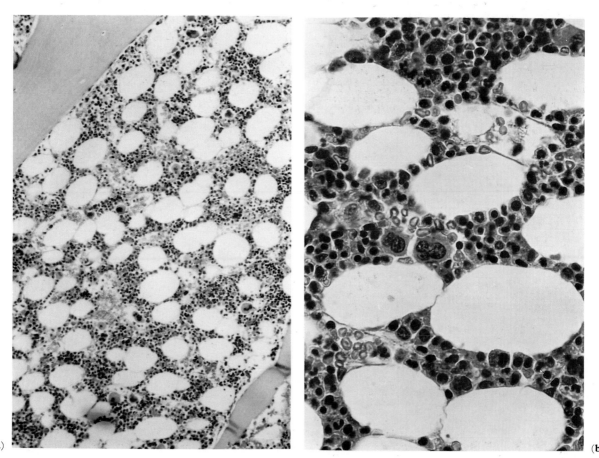

(a)　　　　　　　　　　　　　　　　　　　　　　　　　　　　　　　　　　　　　(b)

Fig. 3.29a, b Trephine biopsy of bone marrow from the posterior superior iliac spine of a normal adult. About 50% of the area between the bone trabeculae is occupied by haemopoietic cells and the remainder by fat cells.

Haematoxylin-eosin　　　(**a**) × 94; (**b**) × 375

Table 3.3 Differential counts on smears of bone marrow aspirated from healthy adults. Means, 95% confidence limits and observed ranges from 28 cases aged between 20 and 29 years and observed ranges for 63 cases aged between 20 and 93 years.[41] 2000 cells were studied in each case

Cell type	Percentages			
	Mean (20–29 years)	95% confidence limits (20–29 years)	Observed range (20–29 years)	Observed range (20–93 years)
Myeloblasts	1.21	0.75– 1.67	0.75– 1.80	0.75– 1.90
Promyelocytes	2.49	0.99– 3.99	1.00– 3.75	1.00– 4.15
Myelocytes				
neutrophil	17.36	11.54–23.18	12.25–22.65	12.00–24.35
eosinophil	1.37	0 – 2.85	0.25– 3.45	0.25– 3.45
basophil	0.08	0 – 0.21	0.00– 0.25	0.00– 0.25
Metamyelocytes				
neutrophil	16.92	11.40–22.44	11.45–23.60	8.75–27.35
eosinophil	0.63	0.07– 1.19	0.25– 1.30	0.15– 1.70
Juvenile neutrophils (stab form)	8.70	3.58–13.82	4.85–13.95	2.60–13.95
Polymorphs				
neutrophil	13.42	4.32–22.52	8.70–28.95	6.40–28.95
eosinophil	0.93	0.21– 1.65	0.45– 1.55	0.25– 2.35
basophil	0.20	0 – 0.48	0.05– 0.50	0.05– 0.65
Monocytes	1.04	0.36– 1.72	0.65– 2.10	0.50– 2.95
Plasma cells	0.46	0 – 0.96	0.10– 0.95	0.10– 2.00
Lymphocytes	14.60	6.66–22.54	9.35–25.05	6.85–25.05
Basophilic erythropoietic cells	0.92	0.40– 1.44	0.50– 1.60	0.50– 1.60
Early polychromatic erythroblasts	6.76	2.56–10.96	3.30–12.20	1.80–12.20
Late polychromatic erythroblasts	11.58	6.16–17.0	7.85–19.55	6.15–19.90
Reticulum cells	0.24	0 – 0.54	0.05– 0.65	0.05– 0.80

Table 3.4 Changes in the cellular composition of the marrow during infancy and childhood

	0–24 hours[44] ($n^\star = 19$)	2 months–1 year[45] ($n^\star = 16$)	2–20 years[45] ($n^\star = 92$)	20–29 years[41] ($n^\star = 28$)
Neutrophil series				
Mean	46.4	54.4	60.6	60.1
Range	20–73		45–77	
Lymphocytes				
Mean	12.1	25.1	16.0	14.6
Range	2–22.5		12–28	9.3–25.0
Erythroblasts				
Mean	40	19.8	23.1	19.3
Range	18.5–65		12.7–38.2	
Myeloid/erythroid ratio				
Mean	1.16	3.5	2.9	3.1
Range			1.2–5.2	2.0–8.3[46]

$\star n$ = number of marrow samples studied.

The percentage distribution of various cell types in smears of bone marrow from normal adults is given in Table 3.3. Careful quantitative histological studies of trephine biopsies of normal marrow have shown that there are, on average, about 650 megakaryocytes per 10^6 nucleated marrow cells. However, differential counts on very large numbers (e.g. 10^6) of nucleated cells in marrow smears have given lower figures, presumably because megakaryocytes tend to be firmly fixed within marrow fragments and do not readily separate and spread in conventional smears. For example, in one study of 10 normal adults, there were 99.9–266.9 (average, 183) megakaryocytes per 10^6 nucleated marrow cells.[42] When differential counts are performed on only 200–250 nucleated marrow cells, the proportion of megakaryocytes encountered varies between 0 and 6.1%.[43]

There are marked changes in the cellular composition of the marrow during the first three months of life. The percentage of erythroblasts falls progressively from 40% (range, 18.5–65%) on the first day to 8% (range, 0–20.5%) between the eighth and 10th days and remains low for a period of about three weeks. It then gradually increases again to reach a value of 16% (range, 6.5–31.5%) in the 3-month-old infant.[44] These changes appear to be secondary to an increase of arterial oxygen saturation to adult levels within three hours of birth resulting in a suppression of erythropoietin production. Erythropoietin pro-duction increases again when the infant is 6–13 weeks old. The proportion of granulocytes and their precursors increases during the first two weeks after birth and then decreases to stabilize at about 50% after the second month (Table 3.4); a slight increase is seen after the age of 4 years. The proportion of lymphocytes is relatively low in the neonate, increases markedly during the first 7–10 days and remains high throughout the first year. Adult values are reached by the age of 4 years (Table 3.5). Plasma cells are rarely seen in the marrow at birth but increase progressively to reach adult values by the age of about 12 years (Table 3.6).

Table 3.6 The prevalence of plasma cells in normal bone marrow.[49] 5000 nucleated marrow cells were assessed in each case

Age	Total number of cases	Percentage of plasma cells	
		Mean	Range
Newborn	6	0.016	0–0·04
0.5–6 months	6	0.024	0–0.06
6–12 months	5	0.068	0.02–0.16
1–2 years	7	0.118	0–0.30
2–4 years	6	0.184	0.08–0.50
4–6 years	5	0.228	0.12–0.28
6–12 years	6	0.350	0.20–0.62
12–15 years	6	0.386	0.28–0.56
21–29 years	5	0.384	0.26–0.48

Table 3.5 Changes in the prevalence of lymphocytes in the bone marrow during infancy and childhood[44,45,47,48]

Age	Total number of cases	Percentage of lymphocytes	
		Mean	Range or ±2 standard deviations
0–48 hours	24	12.3	4.0–22.0
7–10 days	28	32.7	7.5–62.0
1 month	23	46.9	12.0–73.0
3 months	12	47.0	31.0–81.0
6 months	22	47.5	±15.7
12 months	18	47.1	±22.6
1.5 years	19	43.5	±17.1
4–4.5 years	9	19.1	12.0–27.0
2–20 years	89	15.9	5.0–36.0

REFERENCES

1. Wickramasinghe SN. Human bone marrow. Oxford: Blackwell Scientific Publications, 1975.
2. Kelemen E, Calvo W, Fliedner TM. Atlas of human hemopoietic development. Berlin: Springer, 1979.
3. Bartl R, Frisch B, Burkhardt R. Bone marrow biopsies revisited. Basel: Karger, 1982: 8.
4. Bessis M. Living blood cells and their ultrastructure. Berlin: Springer, 1973.
5. Ogawa M, Porter PN, Nakahata T. Blood 1983; 61: 823.
6. Lord BI. In: Potten CS, ed. Stem cells, their identification and characterisation. Edinburgh: Churchill Livingstone, 1983: 118.
7. Prchal JT, Throckmorton DW, Carroll AJ, Fuson EW, Gams RA, Prchal JF. Nature 1978; 274: 590.
8. Messner H, Izaguirre CA, Jamal N. Blood 1981; 58: 402.
9. Erslev AJ, Caro J. In: Dunn CDR, ed. Current concepts in erythropoiesis. Chichester: Wiley, 1983: 1.

10. Athens JW. In: Gordon AS, ed. Regulation of hematopoiesis. New York: Appleton-Century-Crofts, 1970: 1143.
11. Scott RE, Horn RG. Lab Invest 1970; 23: 292.
12. Bainton DF, Ullyot JL, Farquhar MG. J Exp Med 1971; 134: 907.
13. Furth R van, Diesselhoff-den Dulk MMC, Raeburn JA, Zwet TL van, Crofton R, Oud Alblas AB van. In: Furth R van, ed. Mononuclear phagocytes. Functional aspects, part II. The Hague: Martinus Nijhoff, 1980: 279.
14. Greenberg PL. In: Fairbanks VF, ed. Current hematology. New York: Wiley, 1981: vol. 1, 219.
15. Kurland HI, Broxmeyer HE, Pelus LM, Bockman RS, Moore MAS. Blood 1978; 52: 388.
16. Broxmeyer HE, De Sousa M, Smithyman A, et al. Blood 1980; 55: 324.
17. Ruscetti FW, Cypess RH, Chervenick PA. Blood 1976; 47: 757.
18. Scott RE, Horn RG. J Ultrastruct Res 1970; 33: 16.
19. McGarry MP, Miller AM, Colley DG. In: Baum SJ, Ledney GD, eds. Experimental hematology today. New York: Springer, 1976: 63.
20. Bartelmez SH, Dodge WH, Mahmoud AAF, Bass DA. Blood 1980; 56: 706.
21. Zucker-Franklin D. Blood 1980; 56: 534.
22. Sonoda T, Kitamura Y, Haku Y, Hara H, Mori KJ. Br J Haematol 1983; 53: 611.
23. Zucker-Franklin D, Grusky G, Hirayama N, Schnipper E. Blood 1981; 58: 544.
24. Denburg JA, Richardson M, Telizyn S, Bienenstock J. Blood 1983; 61: 775.
25. Williams N, Levine RF. Br J Haematol 1982; 52: 173.
26. Vainchenker W, Bouguet J, Guichard J, Breton-Gorius J. Blood 1980; 54: 940.
27. Levine RF, Hazzard KC, Lamberg JD. Blood 1982; 60: 1122.
28. Jean G, Lambertenghi-Deliliers G, Ranzi T, Poirier-Basseti M. Haematologia 1971; 5: 253.
29. Radley JM, Haller CJ. Blood 1982; 60: 213.
30. Larsen TE. Am J Clin Pathol 1970; 53: 485.
31. Rozman C, Vives-Corrons JL. Br J Haematol 1981; 48: 510.
32. Osogoe B, Ikeda T, Ito H. Okajimas Folia Anat Jpn 1955; 27: 263.
33. Osmond DG, Miller SC, Yoshida Y. In: Wolstenholme GEW, O'Connor M, eds. Ciba Foundation Symposium 13 on haemopoietic stem cells. Amsterdam: Associated Scientific Publishers, 1973.
34. Foon KA, Schroff RW, Gale RP, et al. Blood 1982; 60: 1.
35. Mellstedt H, Holm G, Pettersson D, Peest D. Clin Haematol 1982; 11: 65.
36. Vogler LB. Clin Haematol 1982; 11: 509.
37. Thurlow PJ, McKenzie IFC. Aust NZ J Med 1983; 13: 91.
38. Marton PF. Scand J Haematol 1975; 23 (suppl).
39. Sturgeon P. Pediatrics 1951; 7: 774.
40. Harstock RJ, Smith EB, Petty CS. Am J Clin Pathol 1965; 43: 326.
41. Jacobsen KM. Acta Med Scand 1941; 106: 417.
42. Dameshek W, Miller EB. Blood 1946; 1: 27.
43. Pizzolato P. Am J Clin Pathol 1948; 18: 891.
44. Gairdner D, Marks J, Roscoe JD. Arch Dis Child 1952; 27: 128.
45. Glaser K, Limarzi LR, Poncher HG. Pediatrics 1950; 6: 789.
46. Young RH, Osgood EE. Arch Intern Med 1935; 55: 187.
47. Diwany M. Arch Dis Child 1940; 15: 159.
48. Rosse C, Kraemer MJ, Dillon TL, McFarland R, Smith NJ. J Lab Clin Med 1977; 89: 1225.
49. Steiner ML, Pearson HA. J Pediatr 1966; 68: 562.

Pathology of the marrow: general considerations

Although bone marrow function is altered in a very large number of haematological and systemic diseases, there are a limited number of types of cytological and histological change which can be detected in the marrow in disease. This chapter provides a summary of the various types of physiological or pathological change which may be seen. Details of abnormalities encountered in particular diseases are given in subsequent chapters.

EXAMINATION OF THE MARROW

The bone marrow may be examined after aspiration through a special wide-bore needle. The usual sites of aspiration are the posterior or anterior iliac crest or manubrium sterni in adults, the posterior superior iliac spine in children and infants and the medial aspect of the upper end of the tibia in infants. The aspirate, which consists of fragments of marrow tissue, individual nucleated marrow cells and a variable quantity of blood, is smeared on glass slides and examined after fixation and staining. Marrow smears should be regularly stained by a Romanowsky method and by Perls' acid ferrocyanide method for haemosiderin. In appropriate cases smears can also be stained by special methods for specific cellular constituents such as lipids, glycogen, DNA, RNA and various enzymes. Some of the special stains which may be employed are listed in Table 4.1; the diagnostic value of haematological cytochemistry has been recently reviewed.[1] Examination of marrow smears allows a detailed analysis of the morphology and

Table 4.1 Some cytochemical and histochemical stains used in haematology and their specificity. ★ = 'Non-specific esterases'

Periodic acid-Schiff (PAS) reaction (stains glycogen, glyco-proteins and other substances containing polysaccharides)

Periodic acid-silver-methenamine (stains same substances as PAS reaction)

Sudan black B (stains lipid)

Oil Red O (stains lipid)

Perls' acid ferrocyanide method (stains haemosiderin)

Alkaline phosphatase (lead methods, azo-dye methods)

Acid phosphatase (lead methods, azo-dye methods)

Tartrate-resistant acid phosphatase (see p. 260)

★α-naphthyl AS (or AS-D) acetate esterase

★α-naphthyl butyrate esterase

Leder stain (α-naphthyl AS-D chloroacetate esterase)

Peroxidase reaction (Graham-Knoll method)

Feulgen reaction (stains DNA)

Methyl green-pyronin (stains DNA and mainly RNA, res-pectively)

cytochemistry of cells but suffers from the disadvantage of not providing information on intercellular relationships and the histological organization of the marrow. In addition, differential counts performed on marrow smears do not always give accurate data on the prevalence of cell types in the marrow because some cell types (e.g. megakaryocytes and macrophages) may be relatively resistant to aspiration or may have a tendency to remain attached to the aspirated marrow fragments during the preparation of the smears. When marrow fragments are crushed between coverslips and the coverslips pulled apart, the resulting preparations sometimes show cell types which remain trapped within fragments when a smear is made in the conventional way (i.e. as one would make a blood smear).

Apart from its use for cytological studies with the light microscope, aspirated marrow can be used for biochemical and electron microscope studies.

The histology of the marrow is investigated by examining sections of aspirated marrow particles (either in clotted aspirates or after concentration of the particles in various ways) or by examining sections of a cylinder of bone obtained using a specially-constructed trephine needle. The usual site of trephine biopsy is the posterior superior iliac spine. Unlike marrow smears, histological sections of trephine biopsies permit an appreciation of intercellular relationships and particularly of the relationship between haemopoietic cells, non-haemopoietic cells, the blood vessels and bone. Such sections also allow a study of the quantity and distribution of reticulin and collagen in marrow. Histological sections are therefore useful for the detection of focal accumulations of malignant cells, granulomas and myelofibrosis. Histological sections are most usefully stained with haematoxylin and eosin (H & E), the periodic acid-Schiff stain (PAS), Giemsa stain, and stains for iron and reticulin. A Leder stain for chloroacetate esterase in the granules of cells of the neutrophil series can be applied to sections of marrow particles, but not to specimens which have required decalcification.[2] The various types of haemopoietic cells cannot be as easily distinguished in histological sections of paraffin-embedded decalcified trephine biopsies as in marrow smears. However, cytological detail is considerably improved if semi-thin (3μm) sections of plastic-embedded undecalcified trephine biopsies are studied.[3] It is useful to pick up the freshly obtained biopsy specimen gently with forceps and lightly touch a slide with the specimen before placing it in fixative. Such 'touch preparations' can be stained in various ways and may be useful in the identification of abnormal cells seen in histological preparations.

Examination post mortem

A variety of morphological changes occur fairly rapidly in marrow cells post mortem[4,5] (Fig. 4.1). This applies particularly to the neutrophil metamyelocytes and granulocytes which are rich in hydrolytic enzymes. Post-mortem marrow aspirations and trephine biopsies should therefore be performed as soon after death as possible and preferably not more than 3 h after death. Vacuolation of the cytoplasm of granulocytes may be first seen in smears of marrow aspirated 1½–7 h after death and the vacuolation increases progressively thereafter. Swelling of the nuclei of neutrophil metamyelocytes and granulocytes may be detected as early as 2 h after death; the swelling causes the affected metamyelocytes to look

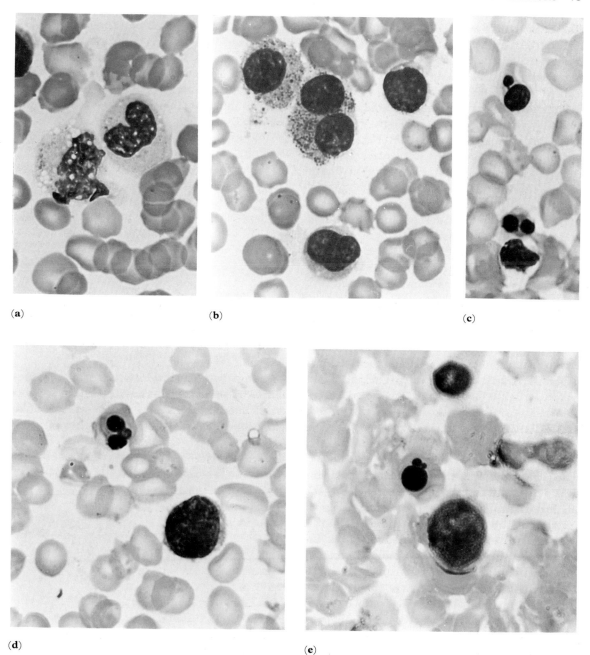

(a)

(b)

(c)

(d)

(e)

Fig. 4.1a–e Marrow smear prepared from an aspirate taken 13 hours post mortem. (**a**) Two cells of the neutrophil series showing nuclear and cytoplasmic vacuolation. (**b**) Two lymphocytes and two degenerating cells of the neutrophil series. The latter have granular cytoplasm and swollen rounded nuclear masses. (**c**) Two erythroblasts containing segmented nuclei. (**d**) Erythroblast showing lobulation of the nucleus. (**e**) Erythroblast showing nuclear budding.

May-Grünwald-Giemsa stain   × 940

Courtesy of Dr N. Francis

like myelocytes. By 8–12 h post mortem, most of the nuclei of the neutrophil metamyelocytes and granulocytes appear rounded, with a loosening of the nuclear chromatin and the appearance of structures resembling small nucleoli. The nuclear membrane is ruptured and many of the cells have indistinct cell membranes. The neutrophil myelocytes begin to lyse after 7–12 h. Karyorrhexis and budding, lobulation or segmentation of erythroblast nuclei may begin as an agonal event or during the first 2 h after death; in occasional cases, over 20% of erythroblasts may show nuclear abnormalities 25 min post mortem, but in others marked changes do not develop in less than 3 h. Reticulum cells are greatly increased in number in aspirates taken within hours of death, probably mainly because they are released into the aspirate more readily than from living marrow. The post-mortem appearances of marrow aspirated 10–20 h after death differ markedly from those obtained during life and are sufficiently confusing to have led to the incorrect diagnosis of leukaemia or malignant infiltration.

ALTERATIONS OF THE MARROW IN DISEASE

The alterations which may be seen in the marrow include changes in cellularity, alterations in the proportions or morphology of various types of marrow cells, changes in iron stores and intra-erythroblastic iron, presence of storage cells, infiltration by malignant cells, fibrosis, necrosis, the presence of specific microorganisms, haemophagocytosis, formation of granulomas, gelatinous transformation, deposition of amyloid, and vascular and embolic lesions. Marrow cells may also show various cytogenetic abnormalities.

ALTERATIONS IN CELLULARITY

The method of assessing the proportion of the marrow tissue which is composed of haemopoietic cells as opposed to fat cells (percentage cellularity), and the normal values for this parameter are discussed on page 69. Hypocellularity (i.e. cellularity $\leqslant 25\%$) is seen in Fanconi's

syndrome (p. 187), the acquired aplastic or hypoplastic anaemias (p. 188), paroxysmal nocturnal haemoglobinuria, rare cases of acute leukaemia (p. 229), and in normal adults over the age of 70 years. Hypercellularity (cellularity $\geqslant 75\%$) may be seen in a variety of conditions, including haemolytic anaemia, haemorrhage, megaloblastic (p. 169) and sideroblastic anaemias (p. 165), the congenital dyserythropoietic anaemias (p. 191), polycythaemia rubra vera (p. 196) and other chronic myeloproliferative disorders (pp. 184, 235 and 283), infections, malignant disease, myelodysplastic syndromes (p. 240), the leukaemias (p. 223) and in normal infants and young children.

ALTERATIONS IN THE FREQUENCY AND MORPHOLOGY OF VARIOUS TYPES OF MARROW CELLS

Erythroblasts and neutrophil precursors

Myeloid/erythroid ratio. Changes in the proportion of various cell types in the marrow give useful clues in the diagnosis of disease. The myeloid/erythroid ratio (M/E ratio) is commonly

Table 4.2 Causes of alterations in myeloid/erythroid (M/E) ratio

---

Reduced M/E ratio due to erythroid hyperplasia
Haemorrhagic and haemolytic states (pp. 113 and 114)
Megaloblastic anaemias (p. 169)
Sideroblastic anaemias (p. 165)
Congenital dyserythropoietic anaemias (p. 191)
Polycythaemia rubra vera (p. 196)
Secondary polycythaemia (p. 199)
Myelodysplastic syndromes (p. 240)
Erythroleukaemia (p. 234)

Reduced M/E ratio due to decreased total granulocytopoiesis
Certain drugs (p. 212)
Radiotherapy
Some cases of aplastic anaemia (p. 187)

Increased M/E ratio due to erythroid hypoplasia
Pure red cell aplasia (p. 189)
Some cases of the anaemia of chronic disorders (p. 163)

Increased M/E ratio due to increased total granulocytopoiesis
Infections
Malignant disease
Tissue necrosis
Non-infective inflammatory disease
Hypersplenism
Hereditary infantile agranulocytosis (p. 215)
During recovery from marrow suppression

used for the elucidation of disturbances in bone marrow function and is defined as the ratio between the number of cells of the neutrophil granulocyte series (including mature granulocytes) and the number of erythroblasts. The normal range for this ratio in adults is 2.0–8.3 in marrow smears[6] and 1.5–3.0 in histological sections. The M/E ratio can be used as an index of total erythropoietic activity in patients in whom there is reason to assume that the total number of marrow granulocytes and their precursors is normal (e.g. in patients with normal counts of circulating granulocytes). Conversely, the M/E ratio may be used as an index of total granulocytopoietic activity, provided that the total number of erythroblasts in the body may be assumed to be normal. Some causes of a reduced or increased M/E ratio are listed in Table 4.2.

Morphological changes in erythroblasts

Most of the erythroblasts in normal bone marrow are uninucleate, show synchrony between nuclear and cytoplasmic maturity and do not display any peculiar cytological features. In normal marrow, only 1.36 ± 0.40 ($\pm$ s.d.) per 1000 erythroblasts are binucleate.[7] Under the light microscope, 3–4% of erythroblasts show various other features such as basophilic stippling of the cytoplasm, inter-erythroblastic cytoplasmic bridges, irregularly-shaped nuclei, karyorrhexis, Howell–

Jolly bodies, asynchrony between nuclear and cytoplasmic maturation and intercellular nuclear bridges (the last three are found very infrequently). In various diseases accompanied by a disturbance of erythropoiesis, the frequency with which such cytological features are found is increased (Table 4.3); hence these cytological 'aberrations' are described as dyserythropoietic changes. Morphological abnormalities which are not encountered in normal marrow may also be found in disease states (Table 4.4). Vacuolation of the cytoplasm of erythropoietic cells has been observed during treatment with chloramphenicol and as an effect of taking excess ethanol. It has also been reported in aplastic anaemia associated with glue sniffing, in protein-energy malnutrition, riboflavine and phenylalanine deficiency, acute myeloid leukaemia and hyperosmolar

Table 4.3 Morphological abnormalities in erythroblasts which may be detected in pathological states using the light microscope

Increased proportion of cells with
1. Irregularly-shaped nuclei
2. Karyorrhexis
3. Howell–Jolly bodies
4. Binuclearity or multinuclearity
5. Intercellular cytoplasmic bridges
6. Basophilic stippling of cytoplasm
7. Orthochromatic cytoplasm
8. Vacuolation of cytoplasm
9. Internuclear chromatin bridges

Megaloblasts and macronormoblasts

Excess of coarse acid-ferrocyanide-positive siderotic granules (abnormal sideroblasts)

Ringed sideroblasts

Gigantoblasts (mononucleate or multinucleate)

Table 4.4 Ultrastructural abnormalities which may be detected in erythroblasts in pathological states

1. Long membrane-bound intranuclear clefts (> 600 nm)
2. Absence, extensive myelinization or reduplication of large parts of the nuclear membrane
*3. Separation of the nuclear membrane from the nucleus
*4. Widening of the space between the two layers of the nuclear membrane
5. Intranuclear inclusions (mitochondria, myelin figures, precipitated globin chains)
6. Deposition of electron-dense material, sometimes resembling ribosomes, on the cytoplasmic surface of the nuclear membrane
7. Different ultrastructural appearance of different nuclei within the same multinucleate cell
8. Fusion of two or more nuclei in a multinucleate cell
9. 'Swiss-cheese' appearance of the heterochromatin
*10. Mitochondrial degeneration (iron-loading, swelling, loss of cristae)
11. Abnormally large siderosomes (diameter > 300 nm)
*12. Large intracytoplasmic autophagic vacuoles (diameter ≥ 290 nm), sometimes containing degenerating mitochondria or myelin figures
*13. Intercellular spindle bridges
14. Large myelin figures lying free within the cytoplasm
15. Intracytoplasmic inclusions consisting of precipitated globin chains
16. Intracytoplasmic lipid droplets
17. Annulate lamellae
*18. Specialized regions of contact between erythroblasts
19. Presence of a double membrane 40–60 nm away from and parallel to the cell membrane
20. Reduction in electron-density of cytoplasmic matrix
21. Scarcity of ribosomes
22. Clustering of degenerating cytoplasmic organelles near the nucleus

* Found in an occasional cell in normal marrow but present with high frequency in pathological states

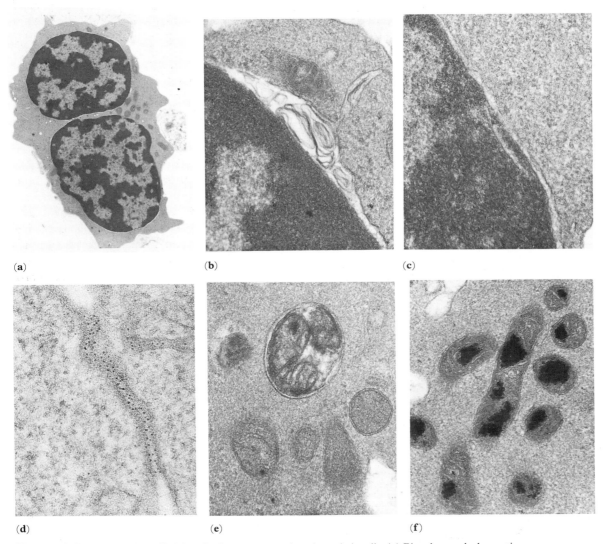

Fig. 4.2a–f Ultrastructural peculiarities affecting some normal erythropoietic cells. (**a**) Binucleate polychromatic erythroblast. (**b**) Myelinization of part of the nuclear membrane. (**c**) Intranuclear cleft. (**d**) Area of intercellular interaction with ferritin molecules between the opposing cell membranes. (**e**) Autophagic vacuole containing three mitochondria. (**f**) Iron-laden mitochondria (rare).

Uranyl acetate and lead citrate   (**a**) ×7050; (**b**) ×55 850; (**c**) ×54 450; (**d**) ×82 300; (**e**) ×45 375; (**f**) ×39 725

diabetic coma.[8] When there is asynchrony between nuclear and cytoplasmic maturation in a substantial proportion of erythroblasts, erythropoiesis is described as being megaloblastic. A detailed description and the causes of megaloblastic erythropoiesis are given on pages 169 and 172–182, respectively.

Minor ultrastructural peculiarities are seen in some of the erythroblasts of normal individuals (Fig 4.2). Thus, small autophagic vacuoles are found in 22% of erythroblast profiles, slight to substantial degrees of myelinization of the nuclear membrane in 12%, short (250–910 nm) stretches of 'duplication' of the nuclear membrane in 2%, short (260–520 nm) intranuclear clefts in 1.7% and iron-laden mitochondria in less than 0.2%.[9] Although all of the above-mentioned ultrastructural features are sometimes described as dyserythropoietic, it is likely that at least the autophagic vacuoles and the myeliniza-

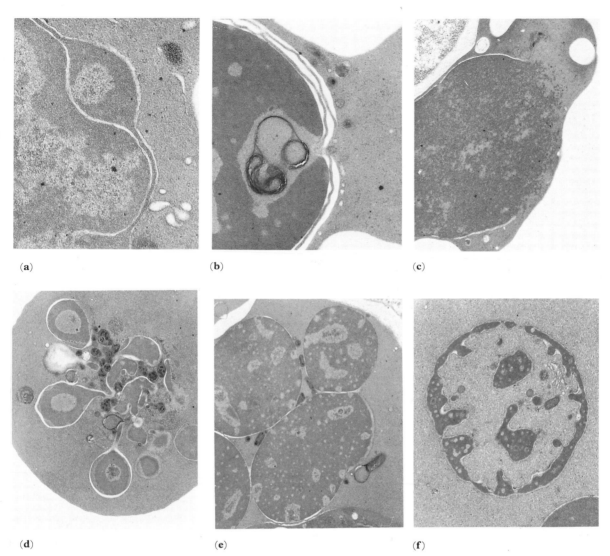

Fig. 4.3a–f Examples of ultrastructural abnormalities affecting the nuclei of erythroblasts in disorders of erythropoiesis. (a) Large intranuclear cleft (megaloblastic anaemia due to vitamin B_{12} deficiency). (b) Duplication of the nuclear membrane and an intranuclear myelin figure (HbS/β-thalassaemia). (c) Loss of part of the nuclear membrane and oozing of nuclear material into the cytoplasm (homozygous HbC disease). (d) Karyorrhexis and clumping of iron-laden mitochondria at the centre of the cell (congenital dyserythropoietic anaemia, type III). (e) Fusion of nuclei within a multinucleate erythroblast (congenital dyserythropoietic anaemia, type III). (f) 'Swiss-cheese' nucleus (congenital dyserythropoietic anaemia, type III)

Uranyl acetate and lead citrate   (a) ×36 475; (b) ×23 100; (c) ×13 325; (d) ×8 300; (e) ×8 700; (f) ×10 000

tion of membranes are the morphological manifestations of degradative processes which play an important physiological role during normal erythropoiesis.

Various ultrastructural abnormalities are seen in the erythropoietic cells of patients with disturbed erythropoiesis;[10] these are listed in Table 4·4 and illustrated in Figures 4.3 and 4.4.

Although most of these are not specific for any particular disease, certain patterns of abnormality are characteristic of specific diseases or groups of diseases. For example, although a short stretch of double membrane may be found parallel to the cell membrane in an occasional erythroblast in other diseases, the presence of a more or less complete double membrane 40–60 nm away from

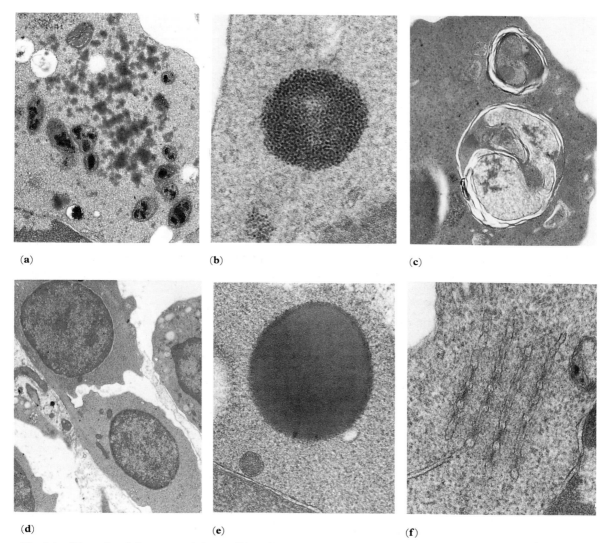

(a)

(b)

(c)

(d)

(e)

(f)

Fig. 4.4a–f Examples of ultrastructural abnormalities affecting the cytoplasm of erythroblasts in disorders of erythropoiesis. (a) Multiple small electron-dense inclusions of precipitated α chains associated with iron-laden mitochondria (HbE/β-thalassaemia). (b) Large siderosome which is not enclosed within a membrane; note that the individual ferritin molecules within the siderosome can be readily identified (HbS/β-thalassaemia). (c) Two large autophagic vacuoles containing myelin figures (homozygous HbC disease). (d) Intercellular cytoplasmic bridge containing microtubules of the mitotic spindle (homozygosity for HbE). (e) Intracytoplasmic lipid droplet (congenital dyserythropoietic anaemia, type III). (f) Annulate lamellae (thiamine-responsive anaemia)

Uranyl acetate and lead citrate   (a) ×22 750; (b) ×99 000; (c) ×24 450; (d) ×7 225; (e) ×47 500; (f) ×51 050

and parallel to the cell membrane in a high proportion of the erythroblasts is a characteristic feature of congenital dyserythropoietic anaemia type II.

Morphological changes in the neutrophil series

These include the absence of specific granules in the myelocytes and metamyelocytes in acute leukaemia and myelodysplastic syndromes (pp. 229, 242), the reduction of nuclear segmentation in the marrow granulocytes in cases of the inherited and acquired Pelger-Huët anomaly (pp. 205, 210) and the formation of giant metamyelocytes and macropolycytes in vitamin B_{12} or folate deficiency (p. 170). Giant metamyelocytes may also be found, usually in small numbers, in the absence of evidence of vitamin B_{12} or folate deficiency, in iron deficiency, infections, malignant disease and protein energy malnutrition. Macropolycytes are also not specific for vitamin B_{12} or folate deficiency, being found in infections, chronic myeloproliferative disorders, drug-induced marrow damage and protein-energy malnutrition. Increased numbers of binucleate cells of the neutrophil series occur in protein energy malnutrition and to a lesser extent in vitamin B_{12} or folate deficiency. Vacuolation of the neutrophil precursors, usually from the promyelocyte/myelocyte stage onwards may be seen in patients with acute alcoholic intoxication, severe infections, drug-induced marrow damage (e.g. chloramphenicol toxicity), protein-energy malnutrition and certain rare conditions such as the Chédiak–Higashi syndrome (p. 205), infantile genetic agranulocytosis (p. 215), hereditary transcobalamin II deficiency[11] (p. 178) and Jordans' anomaly (familial vacuolation of leucocytes)[12] (p. 208). Giant metamyelocytes, whatever the condition with which they are associated, may also be vacuolated.

Eosinophil series

An increased proportion of eosinophils and their precursors, sometimes without an associated eosinophilia in the peripheral blood, may be seen in parasitic infections, allergic disorders, certain skin diseases, Hodgkin's disease, carcinoma and collagen vascular diseases. A marrow eosinophilia is also seen in the hypereosinophilic syndrome (p. 217), chronic granulocytic leukaemia, other chronic myeloproliferative disorders and eosinophilic leukaemia.

Basophils

An increase of basophils in the marrow may be seen in chronic granulocytic leukaemia, myelofibrosis and Waldenström's macroglobulinaemia. Basophils are difficult to detect in formalin-fixed tissues, since the basophil granules are water-soluble.

Mast cells

Mast cells may be increased in the marrow in aplastic anaemia, Waldenström's macroglobulinaemia, chronic lymphocytic leukaemia, non-Hodgkin's lymphoma, myelodysplastic states, scleroderma, systemic mastocytosis and less often in a variety of other conditions.[13,14,15] Mast cells are difficult to recognize in sections stained with H & E but are detectable when stained with a Giemsa stain and, especially, with a PAS stain or Leder stain.[16]

Megakaryocytes

Conditions associated with an increased number of megakaryocytes include chronic granulocytic leukaemia, polycythaemia rubra vera, essential thrombocythaemia, myelofibrosis, infections, chronic alcoholism, malignant disease, Hodgkin's disease, other lymphomas and haemorrhage. They also include diseases such as idiopathic thrombocytopenic purpura and thrombotic thrombocytopenic purpura in which thrombocytopenia is primarily caused by a reduced platelet life-span (p. 277). A decreased number of megakaryocytes is seen in acute leukaemia, Fanconi's syndrome, the syndrome of thrombocytopenia with absent radii (p. 276), and acquired aplastic anaemia (p. 188).

The morphological abnormalities which may affect megakaryocytes are described on p. 274.

Lymphocytes

Lymphocytes are more numerous in the bone marrow in children than in adults (p. 71). An artefactual increase in the percentage of lymphocytes occurs if a bone marrow aspirate is much diluted with peripheral blood. Bone marrow lymphocytes are increased in many reactive and malignant conditions in which there is a peripheral blood lymphocytosis (e.g. infectious mononucleosis, chronic lymphocytic leukaemia). In addition, bone marrow lymphocytes may be increased in the absence of a peripheral blood lymphocytosis in Waldenström's macroglobulinaemia and non-Hodgkin's lymphoma. The majority of lymphocytes in normal bone marrow are B-cells rather than T-cells, and bone marrow infiltration is more likely to be seen in B-lymphoproliferative disorders.

A trephine biopsy will show whether a lymphocytic infiltrate is diffuse or focal and whether there is any follicle formation. In normal marrow, lymphocytes are spread diffusely through the marrow but follicles also develop, and rarely they may have germinal centres.[17, 18] The incidence of lymphoid follicles rises with age,[17] and an increased incidence is seen in pernicious anaemia,[18] chronic myeloproliferative disorders, haemolytic states, inflammatory reactions[15] and autoimmune conditions such as rheumatoid arthritis.[19] Bone marrow biopsies showing lymphoid follicles are more likely than other bone marrow biopsies to show lipid granulomas (see p. 101) and plasmacytosis.[18] A malignant lymphocytic infiltrate may be diffuse or focal and a follicular pattern may be seen. A paratrabecular pattern of infiltration is characteristic of certain non-Hodgkin's lymphomas. It may be difficult to distinguish focal lymphomatous infiltrates from benign hyperplasia of lymphoid follicles. The latter tend to be more circumscribed and smaller with some admixture of histiocytes, eosinophils and plasma cells[18,19] and, unless a germinal centre is present, consist of well-differentiated cells.[18]

Plasma cells

Normal bone marrow contains less than 1–2% of plasma cells. Plasma cells are readily detected with both H & E and PAS stains. Bone marrow plasmacytosis is very common in a wide range of pathological conditions (Table 4.5). Up to 50% of bone marrow cells may be plasma cells in benign reactive conditions.[20,22] The distinction between reactive plasmacytosis and multiple myeloma cannot always be easily made on the basis of the morphological characteristics of the plasma cells. Some features which have been found helpful are shown in Table 4.6. Russell bodies, Mott cells (see p. 64) and intranuclear inclusions resembling Russell bodies (Dutcher–Fahey bodies) may be seen in both reactive conditions and multiple myeloma. A histological section of bone marrow (either clot section or trephine biopsy) is a useful supplement to a marrow smear in the

Table 4.5 Causes of plasmacytosis in the bone marrow

Carcinoma Hodgkin's disease Iron deficiency anaemia Haemolytic anaemia Pyrexia of unknown origin Viral infection Bacterial infection Cirrhosis Collagen disorders Diabetes mellitus Cardiovascular diseases	plasma cells >2% of bone marrow cells in >20% of cases[20]
Megaloblastic anaemia Marrow hypoplasia Idiopathic thrombocytopenic purpura	plasma cells >2% of bone marrow cells in 10–20% of cases[20]
Hypersensitivity states Chronic granulocytic leukaemia Non-Hodgkin's lymphoma[21]	
Monoclonal gammopathy of uncertain significance Immunocyte-associated amyloidosis Multiple myeloma	

elucidation of the cause of plasmacytosis since it allows the distribution of plasma cells, including the presence of homogeneous nodules of these cells (which are not seen in reactive plasmacytosis), to be assessed (see Table 4.6). Haemosiderin granules may be seen in the cytoplasm of plasma cells in alcoholics and in porphyria cutanea tarda, megaloblastic anaemia, refractory normoblastic anaemia and iron overload.[25,26]

Histiocytes (macrophages); haemophagocytosis

An increase of histiocytes in the bone marrow is a common non-specific reaction to a wide variety of haematological conditions and other generalized diseases. Histiocytic proliferation may be malignant or reactive. Malignant histiocytosis is distinguishable from reactive histiocytic proliferation by the presence of pleomorphic, atypical and immature histiocytes (prominent nucleolus, distinct and thick nuclear membrane, irregular nuclear chromatin, multinuclearity).[27,28] In malignant histiocytosis, multinucleate giant cells, blast cells and promonocytes may coexist with histiocytes[29] (Fig. 4.5). Cytochemical reactions of the malignant cells are those usually seen in monocytes and histiocytes—positive reactions for

Table 4.6 Features of bone marrow plasma cells in reactive plasmacytosis and multiple myeloma[20, 22, 23]

	Reactive plasmacytosis	Multiple myeloma
Number	1–50%	1–99%
Cytology	Few cells with flaming cytoplasm; diploidy common; ⩾ four nuclei per cell rare; nucleocytoplasmic asynchrony usually not a prominent feature; nucleoli only in occasional cells	Monomorphic or pleomorphic; occasionally lymphoid;[23] substantial proportion of cells with flaming cytoplasm more likely; polyploidy common;[23] nucleocytoplasmic asynchrony common; nucleoli common; myeloma cells may be phagocytic[24]
Inclusions	Intranuclear inclusions (Dutcher–Fahey bodies) very uncommon; Russell bodies, Mott cells, azurophilic cytoplasmic spicules and unstained crystals may be seen	Intranuclear inclusions (Dutcher–Fahey bodies) more likely; Russell bodies, Mott cells, azurophilic cytoplasmic spicules and unstained crystals may be seen
Distribution	Commonly perivascular; may be aggregated around histiocytes; homogeneous nodules of plasma cells absent; broad band-like infiltrates very rare	Commonly near endosteal surface as well as perivascular;[15] homogeneous nodules of plasma cells with little intervening haemopoietic tissue and with scant supporting stroma common; broad band-like infiltrates common[22]
Associated feature	Increased lymphoid follicles and lipoid granulomas;[20] increased macrophage iron	Increased macrophage iron[20]

non-specific esterase, acid phosphatase and lyso-zyme. The cells may contain polyclonal immuno-globulin. The bone marrow infiltrate of malig-nant histiocytosis may be focal or diffuse (Fig.

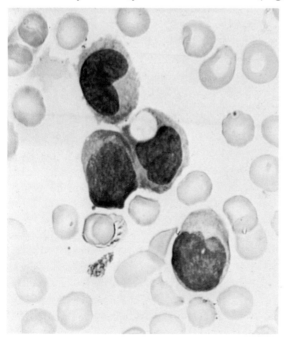

Fig. 4.5 Marrow smear from a patient with malignant histiocytosis showing promonocytes and blast cells.
May-Grünwald-Giemsa stain   × 940

4.6). In the early stages, when the percentage of malignant cells is low, the abnormality may be more readily detectable in a bone marrow aspir-ate than in a trephine biopsy. The percentage of malignant histiocytes in the bone marrow varies from 5–90.[29] The peripheral blood may show cir-culating histiocytes, monocytoid cells or blast cells. Anaemia, leucopenia, thrombocytopenia and eosinophilia may be seen. Phagocytosis by histiocytes of erythrocytes, erythroblasts and other haemopoietic cells (haemophagocytosis) is common but not universal in malignant histio-cytosis (Fig. 4.7); when erythrophagocytosis is marked the designation histiocytic medullary reticulosis is sometimes used. Haemophagocytosis may also be marked in reactive histiocytosis (Fig. 4.8) and, therefore, cannot be taken *per se* as evidence that histiocytes are malignant. Condi-tions associated with haemophagocytosis are listed in Table 4.7. Virus-associated haemo-phagocytic syndromes are particularly likely to occur in immunosuppressed patients, e.g. in patients with leukaemia or following renal transplantation.[30,34] Benign or malignant histio-cytes containing phagocytosed blood or marrow cells can be distinguished on cytological detail, and if necessary by cytochemical studies, from other malignant cells showing haemophagocytic

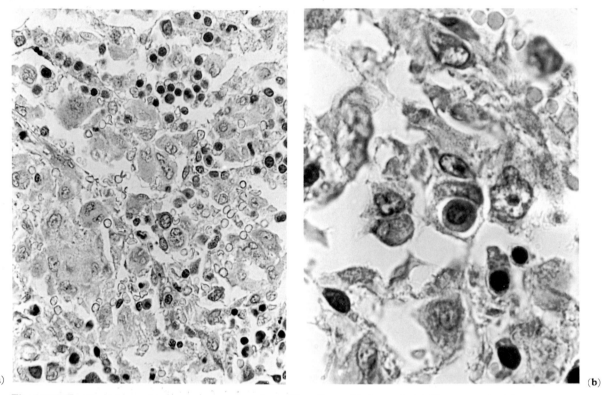

(a)

(b)

Fig. 4.6a,b Trephine biopsy of the bone marrow of a patient with malignant histiocytosis. (**a**) The marrow is diffusely infiltrated with large malignant histiocytes. (**b**) Higher-power view of the section shown in Figure 4.6a. The malignant histiocyte in the centre contains a phagocytosed haemopoietic cell.   Haematoxylin–eosin   (**a**) × 94; (**b**) × 940

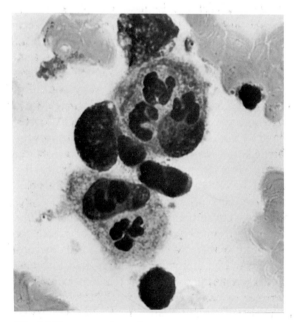

Fig. 4.7 Two macrophages from the marrow smear of a patient with malignant histiocytosis. One of the cells contains three phagocytosed granulocytes and the other contains one.

May-Grünwald-Giemsa stain   × 940

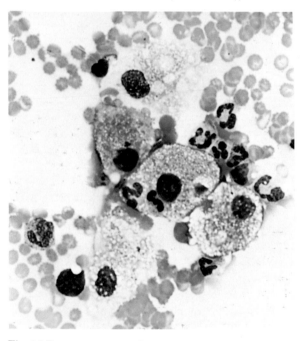

Fig. 4.8 Bone marrow smear from a patient with Gram-negative septicaemia showing reactive histiocytosis with haemophagocytosis. One of the five foamy macrophages shown in the photomicrograph contains two phagocytosed neutrophils.   May-Grünwald-Giemsa stain   × 375

Table 4.7 Conditions associated with the haemophagocytic syndrome

Malignant histiocytosis and histiocytic medullary reticulosis

Infection

    Viral infection[30,31]
        Herpes viruses e.g. herpes zoster,
            herpes simplex,[32] cytomegalovirus,
            EB virus[33]
        Adenovirus[30]
        Measles (vaccine virus)
        Parainfluenza[34]
        Vaccinia
        Congenital rubella[35]
        Kyasanur forest disease[35]

    Bacterial infection
        Salmonella typhi[36,37]
        Brucellosis[38]
        Mycobacterium tuberculosis[39]
        Legionnaires' disease[40]

    Rickettsial infection
        Rocky Mountain spotted fever[41]

    Protozoal infection
        Toxoplasmosis[42]

    Fungal infection
        Histoplasmosis[31,35]

Kawasaki's disease (mucocutaneous lymph node syndrome)[43]

Anticonvulsant lymphadenopathy

Carcinoma of the stomach[44]

T-cell lymphoma[45]

Familial erythrophagocytic lymphohistiocytosis[46]

Hodgkin's disease[47]

activity (e.g. cells of carcinomas of lung or breast,[48] medulloblastoma,[49] prolymphocytic leukaemia,[50] acute lymphoblastic leukaemia,[51] T-cell lymphoma,[52] multiple myeloma[24]). An increase of bone marrow histiocytes which do not show excessive haemophagocytic activity is commonly seen in reactive conditions, e.g. in viral infections, bacterial endocarditis,[36] mycobacterial infections[53] and histoplasmosis.[54]

Phagocytosis of cells of the granulocyte lineage only may be observed in drug-induced agranulocytosis[55] and increased erythrophagocytosis may be observed in some haemolytic states such as autoimmune haemolytic anaemia, malaria and sickle cell anaemia.

Substantial numbers of macrophages laden with lipid or mucopolysaccharide (storage cells)

are present in the marrow in a variety of disorders and these cells are discussed on page 88.

Osteoblasts and osteoclasts

An increased number of osteoblasts and osteoclasts may be seen in a bone marrow aspirate when enhanced bone remodelling is occurring. These cells are commonly increased in bone marrow aspirates containing metastatic malignant cells and they may also be increased in aspirates from bone marrows with granulomas. Vacuolated osteoblasts have been noted in Pompe's disease (type II glycogen storage disease) and have been found to be strongly PAS positive.[56]

CHANGES IN IRON STORES AND INTRAERYTHROBLASTIC IRON

Iron stores

In the bone marrow, storage iron is normally present in the form of ferritin and haemosiderin (see p. 157) and is mainly within the macrophages (see p. 64) but also in endothelial cells. The stores of haemosiderin can be assessed by examining marrow smears or histological sections of either trephine biopsies or aspirated marrow fragments. In unstained smears and sections, haemosiderin granules appear as golden-yellow or brown refractile particles. In preparations stained by Perls' acid ferrocyanide method (Prussian blue method) the haemosiderin appears as blue or bluish-black granules which may vary considerably in size. Various methods of grading haemosiderin stores semiquantitatively have been employed by different authors and one such method used in the study of both marrow smears and histological sections is given in Table 4.8. In practice, it is adequate to grade haemosiderin iron as absent (or greatly reduced), present or increased. The average size of individual haemosiderin granules increases with increasing iron stores from small (diameter 0.5–2 μm) to large (diameter > 4 μm); in subjects with normal erythropoiesis most marrow haemosiderin granules are medium-sized (2–4 μm) or small.

There have been conflicting reports regarding the relative merits of the use of smears and his-

Table 4.8 Criteria for grading iron stores in squashed marrow fragments or histological sections of marrow. The preparations are examined at high magnification ($\times 1200$). (After reference 57)

Grade	Quantity of haemosiderin	Predominant haemosiderin particle size
0	None in whole preparation	—
Trace	One or few granules in whole preparation	—
1+	Few granules in every third or fourth field	Small (0.5–2 μm)
2+	Several granules in every second or third field	Small (0.5–2 μm) and medium (2–4 μm)
3+	Granules in every field, in one or more cells	Medium (2–4 μm)
4+	Massive haemosiderin deposits	Large (>4 μm); granules often clumped

tological sections of bone marrow for the assessment of iron stores.[57,58,59] The discrepancies in the published data may have resulted from technical differences in the processing of the material for histology in the different studies because prolonged treatment of trephine biopsies in decalcifying solutions may cause leaching of haemosiderin. Another possible explanation for the discrepancies is that although a comparison between the amount of stainable iron in histological sections of trephine biopsies and the amount in marrow smears prepared from aspirates taken at the time of trephine biopsy should involve a comparison of equal volumes of marrow tissue, this criterion has not been strictly met in any of the available studies. Nevertheless, in view of the possibility that decalcification of trephine biopsies may result in the extraction of some of the haemosiderin, the best methods for the assessment of iron stores in the marrow would appear to be the study (after staining for iron) of (1) a large number of aspirated marrow fragments in smears, (2) semi-thin sections of plastic-embedded (and undecalcified) trephine biopsy specimens or (3) histological sections of adequate numbers of aspirated marrow fragments.

Marrow haemosiderin stores are either absent or virtually absent in iron deficiency anaemia from any cause (p. 158). Rarely, patients recently treated with large doses of iron dextran may develop iron deficiency anaemia in the presence of stainable iron in the marrow: in this situation the stainable iron is in a form which is unavailable for rapid mobilization.

Increased marrow haemosiderin may be found in idiopathic haemochromatosis, transfusion haemosiderosis, anaemia of chronic disorders, haemolytic anaemias with predominantly extravascular haemolysis (e.g. sickle cell anaemia, pyruvate kinase deficiency, G6PD deficiency), aplastic anaemia (p. 187) and anaemias associated with increased ineffective erythropoiesis. The latter include megaloblastic and sideroblastic anaemias, certain thalassaemia syndromes even in the absence of repeated transfusions (p. 141), congenital dyserythropoietic anaemia (p. 191) and erythraemic myelosis (p. 234). A number of mechanisms operate to increase marrow haemosiderin stores in various types of anaemia. As two-thirds of the total body iron is normally present as haemoglobin within circulating erythrocytes, it is evident that an anaemia which is not primarily due to iron deficiency and is unassociated with haemorrhage will result in a redistribution of body iron with some increase of storage iron. In addition, patients with anaemia associated with increased effective or ineffective erythropoiesis have an absolute increase in their total body iron due to increased iron absorption via the gut, there being a direct relationship between the rate of total erythropoiesis and iron absorption. The increase in iron absorption may, even in untransfused patients, eventually lead to haemosiderosis. Repeated transfusion for chronic anaemia also causes a progressive increase of iron stores as the body has no effective mechanism for getting rid of excess iron. Signs and symptoms of hepatic, cardiac and endocrine dysfunction due to haemosiderosis are usually only seen after the transfusion of about 50 litres of blood (equivalent to a total of about 25 g of iron).

There is a reasonable correlation between the cytochemical assessment of iron stores in stained preparations of marrow and biochemical determinations such as the iron content of the marrow or liver[60] or, with certain exceptions, the serum ferritin level. The causes of alterations in the serum ferritin level are given elsewhere (p. 160, Table 5.13).

Alterations in stainable non-haemoglobin iron within erythroblasts

When normal marrow smears are stained by Perls' acid ferrocyanide method and examined at high magnification (e.g. ×950) using an oil immersion lens, 20–90% of the polychromatic erythroblasts are found to contain a few (one to five) very small (usually, barely visible) blue-staining granules randomly distributed in the cytoplasm.[62,63] Such granules are termed siderotic granules and the cells containing them sideroblasts. Ultrastructural studies indicate that the siderotic granules present in normal erythroblasts correspond to intracytoplasmic aggregates of altered ferritin molecules (siderosomes or ferritin bodies) which are often membrane-bound (Fig. 4.9). In iron deficiency anaemia and, to a lesser extent, the anaemia of chronic disorders, the percentage of sideroblasts is decreased. By contrast, in a wide variety of diseases associated with an increase in the percentage saturation of transferrin (e.g. haemolytic anaemia, megaloblastic anaemia, thalassaemia, primary and secondary haemochromatosis), the number (per erythroblast) and size of siderotic granules are increased, but the granules remain randomly distributed. Erythroblasts showing this phenomenon are described as abnormal sideroblasts. Most of the siderotic granules of such erythroblasts also con-

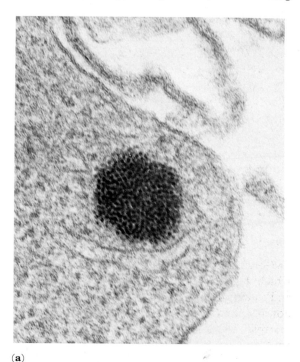
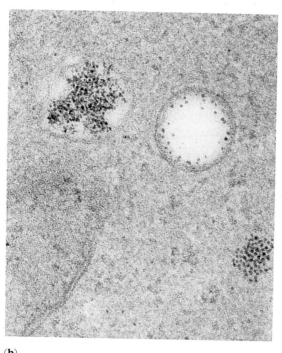

(a) (b)

Fig. 4.9a,b Different ultrastructural appearances of siderosomes in two erythroblasts from normal bone marrow. (a) Siderosome consisting of a densely-packed aggregate of haemosiderin molecules. The aggregate does not appear to be enclosed within a membrane. (b) Siderosome consisting of a membrane-bound collection of haemosiderin granules (top left). The electron micrograph also shows a smaller aggregate of ferritin molecules (bottom right) and a rhopheocytotic vesicle lined by ferritin molecules.

Uranyl acetate and lead citrate (a) ×113 300; (b) ×120 400

sist of siderosomes (albeit abnormally large ones) but a few consist of iron-laden mitochondria. In the sideroblastic anaemias, there is an increase in both the coarseness and number (per erythroblast) of siderotic granules but additionally the majority of the granules tend to be distributed in either a partial or complete perinuclear ring; cells showing such perinuclear rings are termed ringed sideroblasts; some authors require a ringed sideroblast to contain at least six perinuclear or paranuclear granules. Ultrastructural studies indicate that most of the siderotic granules within a ringed sideroblast consist of iron-laden mitochondria. The sideroblastic anaemias are discussed on page 165.

STORAGE CELLS

Gaucher cells

In Gaucher's disease (hereditary glucosyl ceramide lipidosis) typical storage cells are seen in the bone marrow (Fig. 4.10) as well as in other tissues; these cells are macrophages distended by glucocerebrosides. Gaucher's cells are large, round or oval, and have pale-blue cytoplasm with a wrinkled appearance due to the presence of many fibrillar structures (Romanowsky stain). The cytoplasm stains with Sudan black B, and the periodic acid-Schiff reaction is positive. Stains for iron give weak positive reactions. Electron microscopy reveals that the cytoplasm is packed with large elongated sacs containing characteristic tubes, 30–40 nm wide, each of which is made up of spirally arranged fibrils. Gaucher's disease is caused by an inherited deficiency of β-glucocerebrosidase. Occasionally, particularly after splenectomy, Gaucher cells may be seen in the peripheral blood. Cells resembling Gaucher cells under the light microscope (Fig. 4.11) are seen in the marrow in chronic granulocytic leukaemia, acute leukaemia,[64] thalassaemia major[65] and the congenital dyserythropoietic anaemias,[66] and have been described in two patients with Hodgkin's disease[67] and multiple myeloma,[68] respectively. However, such cells (pseudo-Gaucher cells) are ultrastructurally different from Gaucher cells.[69, 70] Pseudo-Gaucher cells are caused by an increased phagocytic load (e.g. of abnormal

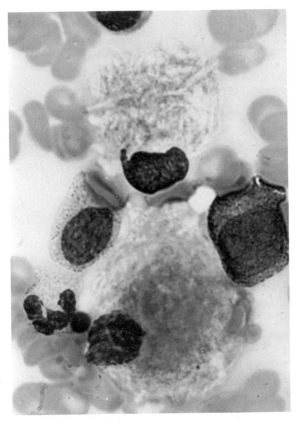

Fig. 4.10 Two Gaucher cells from the marrow smear of a patient with Gaucher's disease.
May-Grünwald-Giemsa stain   × 940

red cells or erythroblasts or leukaemic cells) on the macrophages resulting in the production of lipid in excess of that which can be metabolized, with consequent intracellular accumulation.

Sea-blue histiocytes

Sea-blue histiocytosis is an inherited condition in which large histiocytes containing excess lipid and staining sea-blue or blue-green (Romanowsky stain) are seen in the spleen, liver, bone marrow and other organs. The characteristic colour of these Romanowsky-stained histiocytes (macrophages) results from the presence of a variable number (few to numerous) of large blue-staining cytoplasmic granules. These granules contain ceroid and when unstained are yellow or brown. They stain with oil red O and Sudan black B; as the pigment ages it develops auto-

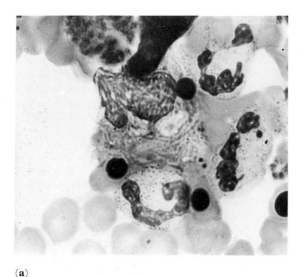

(a)

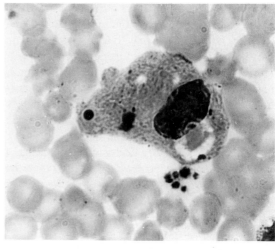

(b)

Fig. 4.11a,b Two pseudo-Gaucher cells from the marrow smear of a patient with congenital dyserythropoietic anaemia, type II.
May-Grünwald-Giemsa stain   × 940

fluorescence and, subsequently, PAS-positivity followed by acid-fast positivity.[71] Ceroid is histochemically similar to lipofuscin. Ultrastructural studies have revealed that the granules are pleomorphic and that some of them contain concentric arrangements of membrane (myelin figures).[72] Sea-blue histiocytes have also been observed in the bone marrow in chronic granulocytic leukaemia, polycythaemia rubra vera, erythraemic myelosis, multiple myeloma, Hodgkin's disease, sickle cell anaemia, thalassaemia, idiopathic thrombocytopenic purpura, lecithin-cholesterol acyltransferase deficiency, rheumatoid arthritis, Hurler's syndrome, type V hyperlipidaemia, chronic granulomatous disease, Takayasu arteritis, Hermansky-Pudlak syndrome, and a variety of other conditions.[72,73,74]

Niemann-Pick disease

Niemann-Pick disease (sphingomyelin lipidosis) is an inherited condition, due to a deficiency of sphingomyelinase, in which sphingomyelin accumulates inside the macrophages of the bone marrow and other organs. The cytoplasm of affected macrophages appears foamy, being filled with rounded lipid-containing inclusions. The inclusions stain faint blue with Romanowsky stains and variably with the periodic acid-Schiff reaction and lipid stains. These inclusions vary in their ultrastructure but often show myelin figures towards their periphery. As morphologically similar macrophages may be seen in other conditions, the Niemann-Pick cell is not pathognomonic for the disease. Peripheral-blood monocytes and lymphocytes in cases of Niemann-Pick disease have similar lipid-containing inclusions.

Other storage diseases and hyperlipidaemias[56]

Foamy histiocytes resembling those seen in Niemann-Pick disease may also be seen in the bone marrow in hypercholesterolaemia, hyperchylomicronaemia, Hand-Schüller-Christian disease, Wolman's disease, late onset cholesteryl ester storage disease and in Tangier disease (familial high-density lipoprotein deficiency). Foamy histiocytes are not pathognomonic of storage diseases, being also seen in fat necrosis, for example, as a complication of pancreatitis or following trauma.[75]

In Letterer-Siwe disease and Hand-Schüller-Christian disease, monocytes may contain amorphous lipid.

In Hurler's syndrome and other mucopolysaccharidoses, bone marrow macrophages, plasma cells and lymphocytes may have metachromatic granules which are acid mucopolysaccharides;[56] the granules stain lilac or purple with Romanowsky stains. In these conditions, the macrophages may have their cytoplasm completely filled with basophilic inclusions of varying size which are surrounded by a clear halo.

In Fabry's disease (α-galactosidase deficiency), storage of neutral glycolipids in bone marrow macrophages produces distinctive storage cells. The cytoplasm is crowded with small globular structures staining blue with Romanowsky stains and strongly with periodic acid-Schiff, Sudan black B, Luxol fast blue, oil red O, and stains for acid phosphatase.[56]

METASTATIC TUMOURS IN BONE MARROW

Metastatic carcinoma cells in bone marrow are usually distinguishable from haemopoietic cells on the basis of their larger size and their tendency to occur in clumps (Fig. 4.12). Carcinoma cells also generally show marked pleomorphism, a tendency to become multinucleate and a high mitotic-index. Some have a distinctive morphology; for example, renal carcinoma cells may have foamy cytoplasm, and mucin-secreting cells may have a 'signet-ring' appearance. Marrow aspirates from patients with metastatic carcinoma commonly have an increase of macrophages and plasma cells. Those from patients with associated osteosclerosis and bone remodelling may show

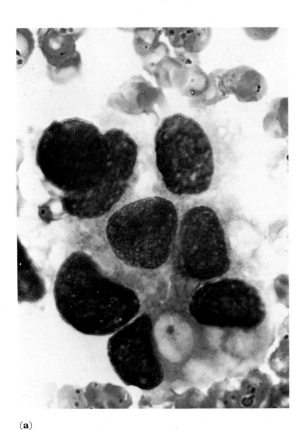

(a)

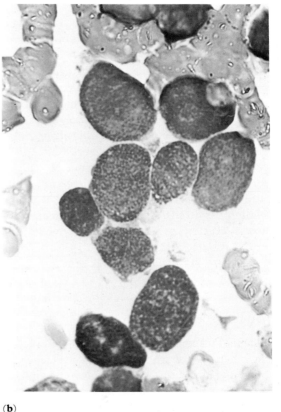

(b)

Fig. 4.12a,b Clumps of metastatic tumour cells in bone marrow smears. (a) Carcinoma of the breast. Two of the carcinoma cells contain secretory products. (b) 'Oat cell' carcinoma of the bronchus.
May-Grünwald-Giemsa stain   × 940

increased numbers of osteoblasts and osteoclasts. Necrosis of tumour cells and of bone marrow cells may occur (see p. 94). Sometimes only necrotic material is aspirated; it is important that the significance of this is appreciated and that the finding is not dismissed as an artefact due to mishandling of the specimen. Metastatic involvement of bone marrow by the small round cell tumours of childhood (neuroblastoma, medulloblastoma, retinoblastoma, rhabdomyosarcoma, Ewing's sarcoma) may be difficult to distinguish from acute lymphoblastic leukaemia (ALL) and lymphoblastic lymphoma.

In some cases of neuroblastoma, medulloblastoma and rhabdomyosarcoma, tumour cells morphologically resembling haemopoietic blasts may circulate in the peripheral blood.[76,77] In some patients the distinction between acute leukaemia and metastatic small round cell tumours can be made on the basis of morphological criteria but in others cytochemistry, electron microscopy, immunochemistry (usually with monoclonal antibodies) or other techniques are necessary. In neuroblastoma, aspirates as well as bone marrow sections may show a characteristic rosetting of tumour cells around partly fibrillar material which stains blue-grey by Romanowsky methods and eosinophilic by haematoxylin and eosin.[78] However, this diagnostic feature is lacking in the majority of patients:[79] the diagnosis may then be made by electron microscopy, which shows secretory granules, by a fluorescence assay for cellular catecholamines,[80] by tissue culture, which allows outgrowth of neurites,[80] and by immunohistochemistry for the detection of neurofilaments.[81,82] Neurofilaments may also be detected by immunohistochemistry in retinoblastoma.[81] In rhabdomyosarcoma, electron microscopy may show cross-striated myofibrils and immunohistochemistry may be used to demonstrate myosin, desmin or myoglobin.[83] In Ewing's sarcoma histological sections may show necrosis and division into irregular lobules by fibrous septa. 'Pseudorosettes' may form around blood vessels. The tumour cells usually contain glycogen, as may some neuroblastoma cells. In medulloblastoma, haemophagocytosis and autophagocytosis by tumour cells have been observed. Immunohistochemistry using monoclonal antibodies against the common leucocyte antigen and HLA-DR (Ia-like) antigen may be helpful in distinguishing acute leukaemia (in which the malignant cells are often positive) from neuroblastoma, rhabdomyosarcoma and Ewing's sarcoma, which have been demonstrated to give negative reactions.[81] The detection of terminal deoxynucleotidyl transferase (TdT) in the blasts of acute leukaemia also helps in their distinction from neuroblastoma and retinoblastoma cells, which have been demonstrated to give negative reactions.[84]

Immunohistochemistry is of use not only in demonstrating the nature of malignant cells which may be confused with leukaemic blasts, but also in detecting small numbers of malignant cells irregularly distributed between haemopoietic cells. Monoclonal antibodies against epithelial antigens have proved most useful in this regard. In one study, all carcinoma cells were positive for either milk fat globule membrane antigen (an antigen found in carcinoma of the breast but also in other carcinomas) or for simple epithelial antigen (cytokeratin filaments).[85] Immunocytochemistry using these monoclonal antibodies can be applied to cryostat sections of biopsies or to smears of bone marrow aspirates.

Cytochemical stains may help in determining the tissue of origin of malignant cells. Melanoma cells show variable degrees of cytoplasmic pigmentation, but even when pigmentation is absent a Masson-Fontana stain for melanin may still be positive.[86] Stains for mucin can be used to identify mucin-secreting carcinoma cells.

The estimation of acid phosphatase in serum obtained from aspirated bone marrow has been found to be a sensitive method of detecting metastatic involvement by prostatic carcinoma,[87] although the interpretation of an elevated level in a patient with no other evidence of metastasis is problematical.

Value of histological sections

In patients with carcinoma (and in those with lymphoma and granulomatous conditions) a bone marrow trephine biopsy is more useful in detecting lesions than either a smear or a section of aspirated bone marrow.[88,89] There is generally a

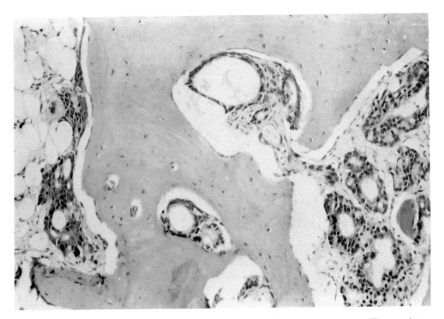

Fig. 4.13 Trephine biopsy of bone marrow showing metastases from an adenocarcinoma of the prostate. The carcinoma cells are arranged in a well-defined tubular pattern.

Haematoxylin-eosin   × 94

higher rate of detection with a section of aspirated marrow than with a smear,[90] though the reverse may be true when the marrow is infiltrated by neuroblastoma or rhabdomyosarcoma cells. The three procedures should be regarded as complementary since occasionally any one of them may detect metastases which have not been revealed by the others.[90,91,92]

Unlike smears, histological sections (either particle sections or trephine biopsies) can reveal intercellular organization such as the formation of rosettes or acini (Fig. 4.13). Metastatic lesions may be associated with dense fibrosis and an osteoblastic reaction (Fig. 4.14). There is a strong correlation between the presence of bone marrow fibrosis in response to tumour metastases and the occurrence of a leucoerythroblastic anaemia.[93]

MYELOFIBROSIS[94]

Myelofibrosis is the replacement of bone marrow tissue by collagen produced by proliferating fibroblasts. As reticulin fibres are collagen precursors and also produced by fibroblasts, increased reticulin deposition (reticulin fibrosis) may be regarded as the first stage of myelofibrosis. However, increased reticulin deposition is a common non-specific occurrence which is of little use in diagnosis. Confusion is avoided if the term myelofibrosis is restricted to increased deposition of mature collagen. Increased reticulin deposition (detected by silver stains) is seen in chronic granulocytic leukaemia, acute myeloid leukaemia, multiple myeloma, chronic lymphocytic leukaemia, acute lymphoblastic leukaemia, malignant mastocytosis, hairy cell leukaemia, Waldenström's macroglobulinaemia[95] and a variety of other conditions.

Myelofibrosis may occur as an idiopathic, apparently primary condition (see p. 184) and also in association with a number of diseases with widely differing aetiology (Table 4.9) (Fig. 4.14). Whenever extensive dense fibrosis occurs, for example in patients with metastatic carcinoma, the haematological findings may mimic those of idiopathic myelofibrosis (see p. 184). Extramedullary haemopoiesis may occur in secondary as well as in primary idiopathic myelofibrosis.[99,100] There may be no essential difference between the fibrosis seen in 'idiopathic' myelofibrosis and that associated with other chronic myeloproliferative

Table 4.9 Causes of bone marrow fibrosis (myelofibrosis)

1. *Generalized*
   Primary idiopathic myelofibrosis (agnogenic myeloid metaplasia)⋆

   In association with:
   Polycythaemic rubra vera
   Essential thrombocythaemia
   Chronic granulocytic leukaemia
   Acute myeloid leukaemia (particularly acute megakaryoblastic leukaemia[96])
   Paroxysmal nocturnal haemoglobinuria[97]
   Secondary carcinoma⋆
   Hodgkin's disease[93]
   Non-Hodgkin's lymphoma[93]
   Multiple myeloma
   Systemic mastocytosis[98]⋆
   Waldenström's macroglobulinaemia
   Nutritional and renal rickets[99,100]
   Primary hyperparathyroidism[101]
   Marble bone disease—osteopetrosis
   Osteomalacia
   Tuberculosis
   Other granulomatous disorders
   Gaucher's disease
   Grey platelet syndrome[102]
   Systemic lupus erythematosus
   Other autoimmune connective tissue disorders

2. *Focal or localized*
   Osteomyelitis
   Paget's disease
   Following bone marrow necrosis[103]
   Following irradiation of bone marrow
   Adult T-cell leukaemia/lymphoma[104]

⋆ Osteosclerosis may also occur

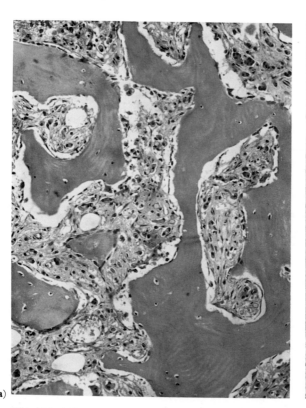
(a)

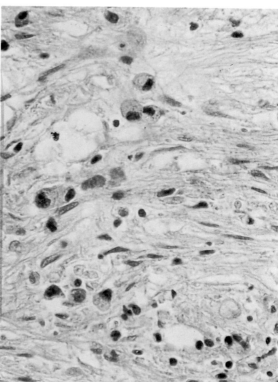
(b)

Fig. 4.14a,b Trephine biopsy of bone marrow showing myelofibrosis and osteosclerosis secondary to the presence in the marrow of scattered metastatic tumour cells from an unidentified primary tumour.

Haematoxylin-eosin   (**a**) × 94; (**b**) × 375

disorders. Thus studies employing cytogenetic and G6PD isoenzyme markers have shown that in idiopathic myelofibrosis, as in chronic granulocytic leukaemia and polycythaemia rubra vera,[105,106] the haemopoietic cells belong to a single abnormal clone whereas the fibroblasts are polyclonal. The underlying haemopoietic stem cell defect in primary idiopathic myelofibrosis is also reflected in the high incidence of a 'paroxysmal-nocturnal-haemoglobinuria-like' defect (see p. 149) in the red cells[107] which is not seen when myelofibrosis is secondary to non-haemopoietic malignancy.

The development of myelofibrosis in patients with myeloproliferative disorders may be related to secretion of platelet growth factor (which stimulates fibroblast proliferation) by megakaryocytes. Myelofibrosis is commonly found in acute megakaryoblastic leukaemia, which often presents with the clinical picture of 'acute myelofibrosis'.[96] In idiopathic myelofibrosis, necrotic megakaryocytes have been noted in fibrotic areas.[108] In chronic granulocytic leukaemia and polycythaemia rubra vera the degree of fibrosis has been related to the total number of megakaryocytes and the number of atypical megakaryocytes respectively.[108] In the congenital defect, the grey platelet syndrome, it has been hypothesized that associated myelofibrosis may be consequent on the release of granule contents (which could include platelet growth factor) from abnormal megakaryocytes. When myelofibrosis is secondary to non-haemopoietic malignancy it is likely that the tumour cells themselves promote fibrosis, since they may do so in sites other than the bone marrow. When myelofibrosis is secondary to another disorder, reversal of the fibrosis may occur when the primary condition is effectively treated.

BONE MARROW NECROSIS
(Table 4.10)[109,110]

Necrosis of bone marrow involves both the haemopoietic tissue and the non-haemopoietic tissue of the marrow. It is a common finding at autopsy[117] but is much less commonly diagnosed during life. It may be widespread and may recur

Table 4.10 Conditions associated with bone marrow necrosis[109,110]

Relatively common association
Sickle cell anaemia (particularly during pregnancy)[109]
Haemoglobin SC disease
Acute myeloid leukaemia[110,111]
Acute lymphoblastic leukaemia[103,109]
Metastatic carcinoma[109,110]
Caisson disease

Uncommon association
Chronic granulocytic leukaemia[109,112]
Megaloblastic anaemia plus infection[109]
Lymphoma[110,113]
Other haemoglobinopathies (Hb SD, HbS/β-thalassaemia, sickle trait)[110]
Embolism of bone marrow from vegetations on cardiac valve[109]
Chronic lymphocytic leukaemia[114]
Disseminated intravascular coagulation[115,116]
Multiple myeloma[117]
Malignant histiocytosis
Myelofibrosis[110]
Hyperparathyroidism[118]
Infections:
  Q fever[119]
  Mucormycosis[120]
  Typhoid fever[109]
  Gram-positive infections (e.g. streptococcus, staphylococcus)
  Gram-negative infections (e.g. *Esch. coli*)
  Diphtheria[109]
  Miliary tuberculosis[121]
  Histoplasmosis[54]

over weeks or months. Bone marrow necrosis may be due to interference with blood supply or to a failure to meet increased metabolic demands from a hyperactive marrow, or to both. Furthermore, as cancer cells have a cytolytic effect on normal bone marrow cells *in vitro*,[122] it is possible that the bone marrow necrosis which commonly accompanies malignant infiltration may be at least partly caused by cancer-cell-mediated cytotoxic effects. Bone marrow infarction may be accompanied by infarction of adjacent bone.

Necrosis of bone marrow due to interference with the blood supply is seen in sickle cell anaemia and Hb SC disease (heterozygous state for both haemoglobin S and haemoglobin C), in which the microvasculature of the bone marrow becomes intermittently obstructed by sickled cells. In these conditions pregnancy further increases the likelihood of bone marrow infarction, by inducing bone marrow hyperplasia and, thereby, also increases the likelihood of death from the embolism of necrotic marrow to the lungs. Interference with the blood supply is also the likely mechanism underlying the bone marrow necrosis which has been described in mucormycosis, since the mucorales characteristically invade vessel walls, leading to thrombosis and infarction.[120] In caisson disease (acute decompression illness) and disseminated intravascular coagulation (DIC) bone marrow infarction results from obstruction of the microvasculature respectively by bubbles of nitrogen and by thrombi. In other conditions (acute lymphoblastic leukaemia, acute myeloid leukaemia, carcinomatous infiltration of the marrow, infection coexisting with megaloblastic anaemia), the increased need of a hyperplastic marrow for oxygen and other nutrients is likely to be an important factor in the pathogenesis of the bone marrow necrosis. However, in some of these conditions the microvasculature may also be abnormal.[111] Thus, the vessels may be compressed by proliferating cells, their walls may be invaded or their lumina occluded by leukaemia[103] or carcinoma cells, or they may be thrombosed.

Bone marrow infarction causes bone pain, and when extensive a leucoerythroblastic blood picture and pancytopenia. If the patient survives the bone marrow necrosis and the underlying con-

dition, then the blood count slowly returns to normal. In the acute phase the bone marrow aspirate may appear white, pale yellowish or plum-coloured, and may be opaque. Microscopically no cellular detail is discernible (Fig. 4.15); the blurred outlines of cells are seen in a background of amorphous material which stains pink with Romanowsky stains. Trephine biopsy (Fig. 4.16) commonly shows associated bone necrosis. Osteoclasts, osteoblasts and osteocytes all appear dead. In the acute phase, skeletal radiographs are normal but bone scanning with ^{99m}Tc-sulphur-colloid shows lack of reticuloendothelial function in the infarcted area. If recovery occurs the necrotic bone marrow is replaced by fibrous tissue and new bone is laid down on the spicules of dead bone.[112] Sclerotic changes may then be seen on radiological examination. The bone scan gradually returns to normal. Extramedullary haemopoiesis has been observed in individuals with extensive bone marrow necrosis, and may be a compensatory phenomenon.[113] In patients with metastatic carcinoma, the bone marrow aspirate may show only bone marrow necrosis at one site and further aspiration at another site may be necessary to demonstrate infiltration by malignant cells. In others an aspirate may show a mix-

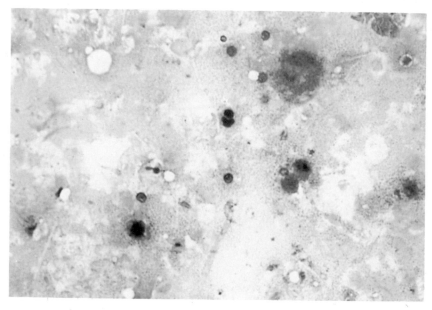

Fig. 4.15 Bone marrow smear from a patient with Ph¹-positive chronic granulocytic leukaemia showing necrosis of the marrow cells.   May-Grünwald-Giemsa stain   × 940

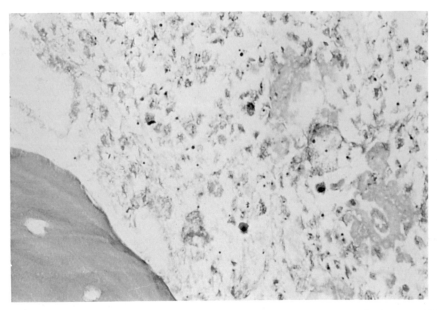

Fig. 4.16 Trephine biopsy of bone marrow showing necrosis of both the bone and the marrow. The lacunae within the bone do not contain osteocytes and appear empty.

Haematoxylin–eosin   × 375

ture of intact tumour cells with necrotic tumour and haemopoietic cells.

INFECTIONS AND THE BONE MARROW

Acute bacterial infections commonly cause a neutrophil leucocytosis, left shift and toxic granulation of neutrophils, the formation of Döhle bodies (p.210), eosinopenia and lymphopenia (see Chapter 6). The bone marrow of patients with such bacterial infections shows an increased M/E ratio due to increased neutrophil granulocytopoiesis and may, in certain circumstances (see p. 216), show a very marked reduction of the proportion of neutrophil granulocytes. The marrow may also contain occasional giant metamyelocytes. Although the cellularity of the marrow is increased (sometimes greatly), some fat cells persist.

When microbial and helminthic infections cause monocytosis or eosinophilia (see pp. 220 and 217), the marrow may show an increased proportion of cells belonging to the monocyte and eosinophil series, respectively.

A number of infections cause thrombocyto-penia by one or more mechanisms. For example, in some of the reported cases of the congenital rubella syndrome the thrombocytopenia appears to have been at least partly caused by reduced numbers of megakaryocytes in the marrow (p. 277). In other cases of the congenital rubella syndrome and in most other infections the thrombocytopenia is usually mainly caused by a decreased platelet life-span (p. 278) and is associated with normal or increased numbers of megakaryocytes in the marrow.

Suppression of erythropoiesis (with some erythroid hypoplasia) is frequent in many infections together with a sharp fall of serum iron and a slower fall of the total iron-binding capacity. Transient red cell aplasia is caused by infection by a parvovirus (see p. 190). Severe anaemia consequent on parvovirus infections has been observed in patients with an underlying haemolytic anaemia (for example, sickle cell anaemia, thalassaemia intermedia, hereditary spherocytosis and pyruvate kinase deficiency).[123]

Chronic *Plasmodium falciparum* malaria in young children is associated with a gross increase of ineffective erythropoiesis (see p. 194).

Certain infections are characterized by histiocytic proliferation, sometimes with haemophagocytosis by the histiocytes (see Table 4.7 and Fig. 4.8); others are characterized by granulomatous lesions in the bone marrow (see p. 99).

Examination of the bone marrow may be useful in the diagnosis of specific microbial infections. In patients with granulomatous lesions, acid-fast stains may show mycobacteria and periodic acid-Schiff or silver stains may show fungi within the granulomas. A Ziehl–Neelsen stain is suitable for demonstrating *Mycobacterium tuberculosis* but *Mycobacterium leprae* may fail to retain the dye, and if leprosy is suspected Fite's stain is preferred.[124] Leprosy may also be detected by the demonstration of bacilliform 'ghosts' within macrophages in marrow smears stained by a Romanowsky method.[124] *Mycobacterium tuberculosis* and atypical mycobacteria may be cultured from the bone marrow and cultures are sometimes positive in patients in whom acid-fast stains have not revealed organisms.

Brucella may also be cultured from the bone marrow and cultures are sometimes positive when simultaneous blood cultures are negative.[125]

The organism of Legionnaires' disease, *Legionella pneumophila*, may be detected in bone marrow smears by using fluorescein-labelled antiserum.[40]

Typhoid fever may cause bone marrow granulomas and the bacilli may be seen within bone marrow mononuclear cells. Culture of the bone marrow is usually positive and is a more reliable method of diagnosis than serial blood cultures or agglutinin titres.[126]

In Whipple's disease the bacterium-like inclusions, believed to be causative, may be seen within bone marrow histiocytes. They stain violet with Romanowsky stains, and black with methenamine-silver.[127]

Fungal infections, such as histoplasmosis, cryptococcosis, candidosis, blastomycosis and coccidioidomycosis, may be diagnosed by microscopy of smears or histological sections (periodic acid-Schiff and methenamine-silver stains) or by culture.[54,128,129] Morphological features often allow distinction between the different fungi.[54] Cryptococcus has a capsule which may stain with mucicarmine, and histoplasma does not.[54] In

disseminated histoplasmosis bone marrow culture is positive in 60–75% of patients;[130] culture may be positive even when organisms are not seen in bone marrow sections.

Leishmaniasis may be diagnosed by studies of bone marrow smears or sections (Figs 4.17 and 4.18) (occasionally, the organisms may also be seen in peripheral blood monocytes). A bone marrow aspirate may be helpful in the diagnosis of malaria due to *Plasmodium falciparum* when there is a strong clinical suspicion of this condition but the parasites cannot be found in the peripheral blood;[131] in these circumstances parasites may be found in marrow reticulocytes and malarial pigment may be seen in marrow macrophages.

Bone marrow aspiration is in general of little use in the diagnosis of viral infections, though cytomegalovirus infection has been diagnosed from the presence of typical giant cells with intranuclear inclusions.[132]

The bone marrow response to a microorganism depends on the immune status of an individual. The development of granulomas in response to a biologically active substance requires normal lymphocyte functions, and experimentally can be suppressed by neonatal thymectomy and antilymphocyte serum. Patients with hairy cell leukaemia and those with the acquired immunodeficiency syndrome (AIDS) may have absent or impaired granuloma formation with mycobacterial infection of the bone marrow.[133,134] In histoplasmosis, patients with normal immunity usually develop typical granulomas with scanty organisms while those with immune suppression are more likely to have marked diffuse histiocytic proliferation and bone marrow necrosis.[54]

BONE MARROW GRANULOMAS

A granuloma may be defined as a compact collection of mature cells of the mononuclear phagocyte system (p. 53).[135] Granulomas are formed by monocytes which have migrated from the blood and developed into mature macrophages and sometimes into epithelioid cells and giant cells. The giant cells may be of Langhans' type (numerous small nuclei around the periphery of

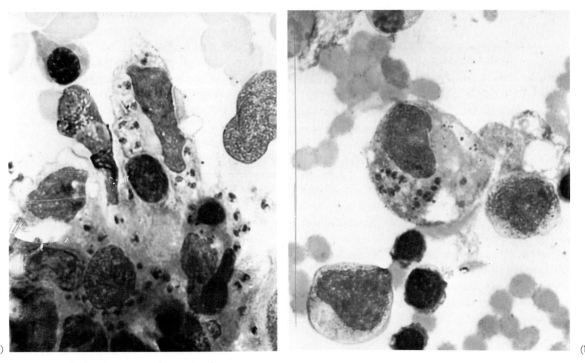

(a)   (b)

Fig. 4.17a,b Macrophages containing many Leishman-Donovan bodies, from a marrow smear of a patient with kala-azar. Each parasite contains a large ovoid or rounded nucleus and a rod-like kinetoplast situated more or less at right angles to the nucleus. Both the nucleus and kinetoplast stain reddish-violet.

May-Grünwald-Giemsa stain   × 940   *Courtesy of Dr S. Abdalla*

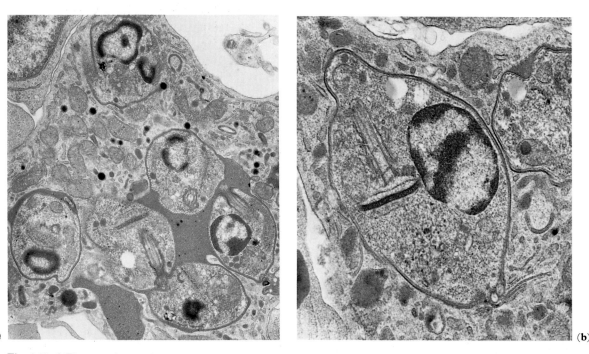

(a)   (b)

Fig. 4.18a,b Electron micrographs showing *Leishmania donovani* within the bone marrow macrophages of a patient with kala-azar. (**a**) Part of the cytoplasm of a macrophage containing six intracellular parasites. (**b**) Higher-power view of a single parasite. The periplast covering the organism, the large ovoid nucleus and the sausage-shaped kinetoplast (arranged at right angles to the nucleus) can be recognized. The kinetoplast contains an electron-dense band which runs parallel to its long axis and which contains nucleic acid.   Uranyl acetate and lead citrate   (**a**) × 13 250; (**b**) × 25 850

the cell) or foreign body type (a smaller number of nuclei of inconstant size spread irregularly through the cell). Granulomas may also contain lymphocytes, plasma cells, neutrophils and eosinophils, and necrotic or caseating areas. Suppuration may occur in granulomas caused by fungal infections. Granulomas are seen in the bone marrow in many conditions which are characterized by the presence of granulomas in other tissues (Table 4.11). They are present in about 1% of bone marrow biopsies.

Table 4.11 Causes of bone marrow granulomas

Infections
  Tuberculosis
  Brucellosis
  Leprosy[124]
  Syphilis
  Leishmaniasis
  Q fever[136]
  Toxoplasmosis[59]
  Histoplasmosis[54,137,138]
  Cryptococcosis[139]
  Infectious mononucleosis[59,137]
  Herpes zoster[137]
  Legionnaires' disease[40]
  Typhoid fever[37]

Sarcoidosis

Malignant disease
  Hodgkin's disease[137]
  Multiple myeloma[140]
  Non-Hodgkin's lymphoma[141]

Drug hypersensitivity
  Phenytoin[137,142]
  Procainamide[143]
  Oxyphenbutazone[144]
  Chlorpropamide[143]

Associated with eosinophilic interstitial nephritis[145]

Bone marrow granulomas are best detected in histological sections (Fig. 4.19), and as they may be relatively resistant to aspiration, a trephine biopsy is generally preferable to a clot section. The presence of granulomas may sometimes be suspected during the examination of marrow smears from the presence of epithelioid cells, which tend to occur in groups. These cells have abundant cytoplasm, which stains blue-grey to dark blue by a Romanowsky method, and nuclei which may be round, oval or reniform.

Patients being investigated for a suspected granulomatous condition, e.g. those with fever of unknown origin, require a marrow aspiration for culture of the aspirated material and a trephine biopsy for histological studies. If granulomas are detected, an acid-fast stain (Ziehl-Neelsen) for mycobacteria, and periodic acid-Schiff and silver stains for fungi should be carried out.

The distinction between sarcoid granulomas and those due to tuberculosis or other microbial infections is important but not always possible on histological examination alone. Caseation of granulomas is characteristic of tuberculosis but is neither invariably present nor restricted to it. In tuberculous granulomas, acid-fast bacilli may be very scanty; non-caseating granulomas with no detectable acid-fast bacilli may sometimes be due to tuberculosis rather than sarcoidosis. Both tuberculous and sarcoid granulomas may have associated eosinophils and lymphocytes and these features are not helpful in making a distinction between them. Although sarcoid granulomas do not caseate they may show eosinophilic coagulative necrosis and, in the healing stage, hyaline fibrosis.[146] Bone marrow examination is diagnostic in 15-40% of patients with miliary tuberculosis, including some patients with normal chest radiology.[130] Bone marrow examination may also be useful in the diagnosis of sarcoidosis. In one series of 30 patients granulomas were detected in 6 cases in sections of marrow aspirated from the sternum.[147] Granulomas are found in a much larger proportion at autopsy and it would be expected that trephine biopsy would yield diagnostic material more frequently than aspiration.

In granulomas due to *Mycobacterium leprae* large 'foam cells' are characteristic. Bacilli may appear as 'ghosts' within monocytes in Romanowsky-stained bone marrow smears. Foamy macrophages may also be found in the bone marrow in granulomas due to typhoid fever. Bone marrow granulomas are relatively common in brucellosis and histoplasmosis. In one series, 15 of 22 patients with serologically confirmed brucellosis had granulomas in sections of sternal marrow aspirates[147] and in another similar series, 17 of 18 iliac crest aspirates containing fragments suitable for histology showed granulomas.[125] Brucella may be cultured from infected marrow.[125] The granulomas of brucellosis tend to

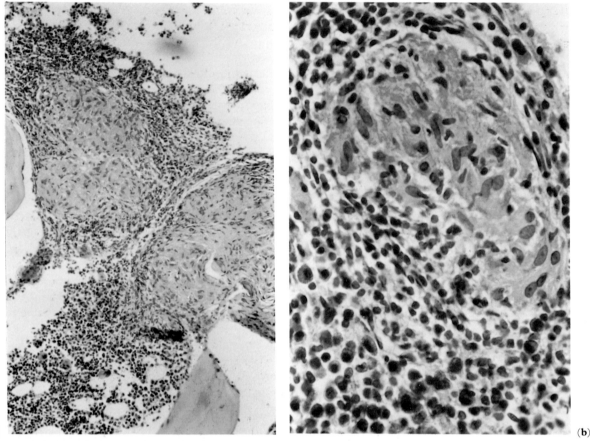

(a)   (b)

Fig. 4.19a,b Trephine biopsies of bone marrow showing sarcoid granulomas.
Haematoxylin–eosin   (**a**) ×94; (**b**) ×375

be smaller and less distinct than tuberculous or sarcoid granulomas.[147] Large granulomas, frequently with giant cells and sometimes with caseation,[130] may occur in histoplasmosis: the organisms appear blue in Romanowsky-stained films and are stained by the periodic acid-Schiff reaction and by methenamine-silver; haematoxylin and eosin staining of histological sections is less reliable than silver staining.[54] The fungi can be readily cultured from infected bone marrow.[130]

Granulomatous lesions are relatively common in infectious mononucleosis, being found, for example, in 8 of 18 cases in which particles of sternal marrow were examined by sectioning.[148] They tend to be smaller than the granulomas of tuberculosis and sarcoidosis. Caseation does not

occur but focal necrosis may.[149] Giant cells are uncommon.[148]

The granulomas described in a patient with herpes zoster were also small and non-caseating with no giant cells.[150]

Patients with Hodgkin's disease may have granuloma-like lesions associated with specific lymphomatous infiltration. They may also have bone marrow granulomas (or liver or spleen granulomas) in the absence of specific malignant infiltration of the tissue (i.e. as a non-infiltrative manifestation of the disease). It is important that failure to appreciate the nature of these lesions does not lead to misclassification of patients as having stage IV disease. In non-Hodgkin's lymphoma, lymphomatous infiltration may provoke a granulomatous response, but granulomas with benign-looking lymphocytes also occur and these are probably non-infiltrative reactive lesions analogous to those in Hodgkin's disease.[151]

Bone marrow granulomas may occur as part of a hypersensitivity reaction to drugs[143] and may coexist with other adverse reactions such as neutropenia, rash, fever and eosinophilia.

Lipogranulomas in which fat vacuoles are present both within macrophages and extracellularly do not have the same significance as other granulomas.[152] They occur more frequently in bone marrows showing plasmacytosis or lymphoid follicles than in other marrows.

Lesions which superficially resemble granulomas and need to be distinguished from them may occur in systemic mastocytosis and in angio-immunoblastic lymphadenopathy. In the former condition the lesions are composed of mast cells and collagen fibres[98] and in the latter of immunoblasts, plasma cells, lymphocytes, histiocytes and eosinophils together with arborizing capillaries,[3] and with an increase of reticulin.

GELATINOUS TRANSFORMATION[153,154]

The bone marrow of most patients with severe anorexia nervosa and some patients with cachexia secondary to chronic disorders (e.g. tuberculosis, carcinoma) contains a gelatinous material (Figs 4.20, 4.21) which appears to consist of acid mucopolysaccharide. The material is amorphous, granular or fibrillar, stains pink-purple with Romanowsky stains or haematoxylin and eosin and stains positively with Alcian blue (particularly at a high pH) and the periodic acid-Schiff stain. The haemopoietic cells are reduced in number and embedded within the gelatinous material and there is an absence or marked reduction of fat cells. A deficiency of carbohydrates and calories

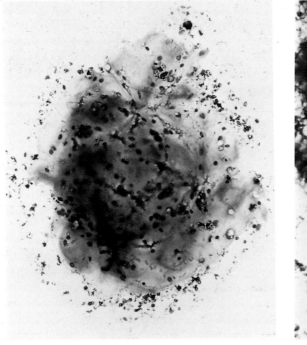

(a)

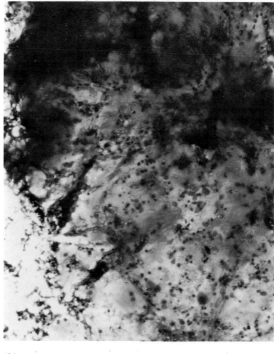

(b)

Fig. 4.20a,b Marrow fragments from a bone marrow smear of a patient with severe anorexia nervosa. (**a**) Small marrow fragment showing a few nucleated cells embedded in a pink-purple-staining gelatinous material. (**b**) Large marrow fragment, the lower part of which shows gelatinous transformation.

May-Grünwald-Giemsa stain   × 94

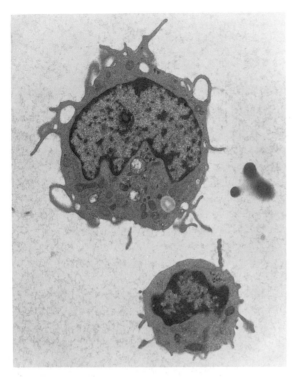

Fig. 4.21 Electron micrograph of a part of a marrow fragment from the patient with anorexia nervosa whose marrow smears are illustrated in Figure 4.20. Two nucleated cells are widely separated from each other by mucopolysaccharide which has a flocculent appearance.

Uranyl acetate and lead citrate   × 7475

may underly the gelatinous transformation and the excessive accumulation of acid mucopolysaccharide may serve to fill the marrow space normally occupied by fat cells. Interestingly, young children with protein-energy malnutrition do not show gelatinous transformation.

Marrow fragments showing gelatinous transformation do not smear properly.

AMYLOIDOSIS (see p. 301)

Amyloid deposits may be seen in the bone marrow both in smears of aspirated material and in histological sections. In Romanowsky-stained smears amyloid appears pink to purple, waxy to transparent, and has been described as resembling a cumulus cloud.[155] In histological sections of marrow, amyloid has the same appearance and staining characteristics as in other tissues (Fig. 4.22).

VASCULAR AND EMBOLIC LESIONS

Intravascular and subendothelial hyaline deposits and platelet thrombi may be seen in bone marrow vessels in thrombotic thrombocytopenic purpura.[156] Arteritis and arteriolitis may be found in the marrow in cases of any form of generalized arteritis. Giant cell arteritis has been diagnosed by bone marrow biopsy, although the vessels involved were smaller than those usually affected by this condition.[157] Granulomatous vasculitis has been seen in association with hypersensitivity reactions to drugs.[158]

Arteriosclerotic and thromboembolic lesions may be recognized. Widespread cholesterol microembolism from atherosclerotic plaques (atheroembolism) may produce a multisystem disease whose haematological manifestations include anaemia, leucocytosis, eosinophilia and elevated erythrocyte sedimentation rate. At autopsy the bone marrow shows emboli in 20% of cases; bone marrow biopsy has also allowed diagnosis during life.[159] Histologically, vessels contain acellular material with cholesterol clefts, derived from the atheromatous plaque. Intimal hyperplasia occurs. The vessel walls are initially infiltrated with granulocytes and subsequently with mononuclear cells and giant cells.

Tumour emboli are seen particularly in patients whose carcinoma is complicated by microangiopathic haemolytic anaemia.

ALUMINIUM DEPOSITION

Trephine biopsy of the iliac crest is useful for the detection of aluminium deposition in patients on haemodialysis and other patients with chronic renal failure. The aluminium is derived from oral intake and dialysis fluids and may cause dementia. Aluminium is detected by a specific aluminium stain (Irwin technique) both in bone (at the osteoid/mineralized tissue junction) and in marrow cells as coarse granules.[160] The cell which contains the aluminium is uncertain, but may be the macrophage.[160]

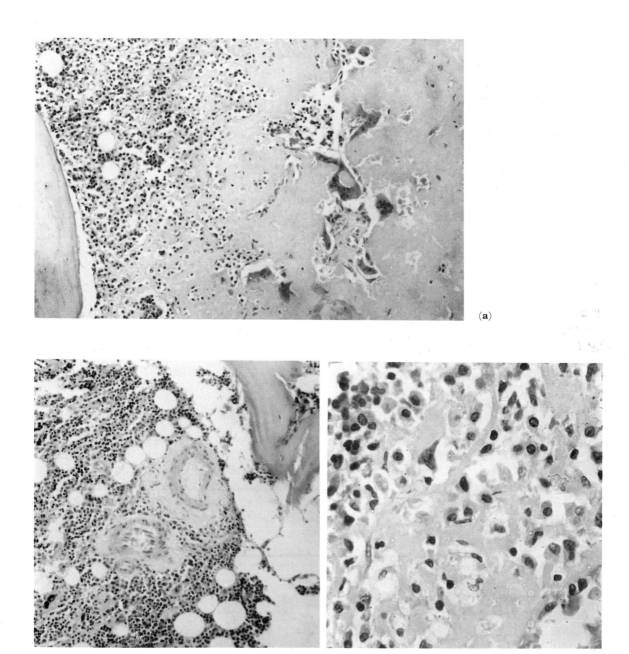

Fig. 4.22a,b,c Amyloid degeneration of the bone marrow. (a) In the right-hand half of the photomicrograph, the normal haemopoietic tissue is replaced by a nodule of amyloid which appeared faintly eosinophilic and homogeneous. (b) Two arterioles showing advanced amyloid degeneration of their walls and occlusion of their lumina with amyloid. In arterioles and small arteries, amyloid degeneration commences in the subendothelial tissues and gradually spreads outwards. (c) Higher-power view of the marrow parenchyma showing the presence of amyloid in between haemopoietic cells.

Haematoxylin-eosin   (a) ×90; (b) ×90; (c) ×350

CYTOGENETIC ABNORMALITIES IN BONE MARROW CELLS[161]

The majority of haemopoietic cells, like most other somatic cells, contain 46 chromosomes (23 pairs of homologous chromosomes) and are said to be diploid, whereas gametes have 23 chromosomes and are said to be haploid. Cells (other than diploid cells) containing a number of chromosomes which is a multiple of 23 are described as being polyploid. The only haemopoietic cells which are normally polyploid are the megakaryocytes (see p. 57). Chromosome abnormalities are common in malignant disorders of haemopoietic cells and in premalignant conditions (e.g. the myelodysplastic syndromes). Cells may be hypodiploid (having fewer than 46 chromosomes) or hyperdiploid (having more than 46 chromosomes but not a multiple of 46). The term aneuploid covers both hypodiploid and hyperdiploid cells. Pseudodiploid indicates that a cell has 46 chromosomes which are not the normal 23 pairs; loss of one or more chromosomes is balanced by gain of others. Loss of the Y chromosome from haemopoietic cells is a not uncommon age change in man. A chromosome is composed of two chromatids joined by a centromere. Chromosomes with a centrally placed centromere are termed metacentric. Those with a centromere placed closer to one end of the chromatids are termed acrocentric with the short arm being designated p and the long arm q.

In order to study the chromosomes of haemopoietic cells (i.e. the karyotype of the cell) it is necessary for the cell to be in mitosis. T-lymphocytes may be stimulated to undergo mitosis by phytohaemagglutinin and B-lymphocytes (including chronic lymphocytic leukaemia and prolymphocytic leukaemia cells) by phorbol esters or bacterial lipopolysaccharide. It is also possible to study spontaneous mitosis in bone marrow cells, or even in peripheral blood cells if there are numerous circulating immature cells, as may occur in certain leukaemias. Chromosomes may be identified to some extent by size and centromere position but more accurately by stains which show a characteristic pattern of transverse bands. Bands have been numbered to facilitate a complete description of chromosome abnormalities.

Stains which can be used for banding include quinacrine (a fluorochrome), Giemsa and acridine orange. Chromosomes of acute leukaemia cells may appear fuzzy and band poorly. The chromosomes of malignant haemopoietic cells may show abnormalities of number or structure. Aneuploidy (hypodiploidy or hyperdiploidy) is common. Monosomy (loss of one of a homologous pair) and trisomy (gain of a chromosome so that there are three homologous chromosomes) are common. For example monosomy 5 and monosomy 7 (also designated -5, -7) are common in acute myeloid leukaemias, as are deletions (del) of part of these chromosomes (designated 5-, 7- or 5q-, 7q- since these deletions are from the long arms). Trisomy 8 (also designated +8) is also common in acute myeloid leukaemia. Other abnormalities which may be seen in haemopoietic malignancies include translocation (designated t and indicating the transfer of part of one chromosome to another chromosome) (see p. 227), inversion (designated inv and indicating the inversion of a segment of a chromosome) (see p. 227), insertion (designated ins) and the formation of isochromosomes (designated i, a chromosome formed by duplication of the long or short arms of a chromosome) and marker chromosomes (designated mar, an abnormal chromosome produced by fusion of other chromosomes or parts of chromosomes). 'Double minute chromosomes' which have been seen in malignant cells of non-haemopoietic origin but not in normal cells may occur in leukaemia.[162] Studies of karyotype may be useful in demonstrating whether cells of a particular lineage belong to a malignant clone (see p. 235). Specific karyotypic abnormalities are associated with specific haemopoietic malignancies or pre-malignant states (see pp. 227, 235, 241) and also with certain causative agents. A specific translocation t (9:22) is characteristic of chronic granulocytic leukaemia (see p. 235). It is possible that the occurrence of a chromosome abnormality may actually cause a malignant proliferation, possibly by leading to activation of an oncogene (see p. 236). Chromosome abnormalities in haemopoietic malignancy are also of prognostic significance.

REFERENCES

GENERAL REFERENCE

Rywlin AM. Histopathology of the bone marrow. Boston: Little, Brown and Company, 1976.

1. Hayhoe FGJ, Quaglino D. Haematological cytochemistry. Edinburgh: Churchill Livingstone 1980.
2. Rywlin AM. Histopathology of the bone marrow. Boston: Little, Brown and Company, 1976: 10.
3. Burkhardt R, Frisch B, Bartl R. J Clin Pathol 1982; 35: 257.
4. Rohr K, Hafter E. Folia Haematol 1937; 58: 38.
5. Findlay AB. J Forensic Sci Soc 1977; 16: 213.
6. Young RH, Osgood EE. Arch Intern Med 1935; 55: 187.
7. Nemec J, Polak H. Folia Haematol 1964; 84: 24.
8. Lehane DE. Arch Intern Med 1983; 134: 763.
9. Wickramasinghe SN, Hughes M. Haematologia 1984; 17: 35.
10. Lewis SM, Verwilghen RL, eds. Dyserythropoiesis. New York: Academic Press, 1977.
11. Niebrugge DJ, Benjamin DR, Christie D, Scott CR. J Pediatr 1982; 101: 732.
12. Rozensazajn L, Klajman A, Yaffe D, Efrati P. Blood 1966; 28: 258.
13. Rywlin AM. Histopathology of the bone marrow. Boston: Little, Brown and Company, 1976: 13.
14. Yoo D, Lessin LS, Jensen WN. Ann Intern Med 1978; 88: 753.
15. Burkhardt R, Zettl K, Bartl B. Bibl Haematologica 1978; 45: 38.
16. Prokocimer M, Polliack A. Am J Clin Pathol 1980; 75: 34.
17. Rywlin AM, Ortega RS, Dominguez CJ. Blood 1974; 43: 389.
18. Maeda K, Hyun BH, Rebuck JW. Am J Clin Pathol 1977; 67: 41.
19. Dick F, Bloomfield CD, Brunning RD. Cancer 1974; 33: 1382.
20. Hyun BH, Kwa D, Gabaldon H, Ashton JK. Am J Clin Pathol 1976; 65: 921.
21. Burkhardt R, Bartl B, Sandel P, Binsack T, Bibl Haematologica 1978; 45: 55.
22. Canale DD, Collins RD. Am J Clin Pathol 1974; 61: 382.
23. Kyle RA, Bayrd ED. The monoclonal gammopathies: multiple myeloma and related plasma cell disorders. Springfield: Thomas, 1976.
24. Fitchen JH, Lee S. Am J Clin Pathol 1979; 71: 722.
25. Cook MK, Madden M. J Clin Pathol 1982; 35: 172.
26. Karcioglu GL, Hardison JE. Arch Intern Med 1978; 138: 97.
27. Lombardi L, Carbone A, Pilotti S, Rilke F. Histopathology 1978; 2: 315.
28. Carbone A, Micheau C, Caillaud J-M, Carlu C. Cancer 1981; 47: 2862.
29. Lampert ID, Catovsky D, Bergier N. Br J Haematol 1978; 40: 65.
30. Risdall RJ, McKenna RW, Nesbit ME, Krivit W, Balfour HH, Simmons RL, Brunning RD. Cancer 1979; 44: 993.
31. Daneshbod K, Kissane JM. Am J Clin Pathol 1978; 70: 381.
32. Wilson ER, Malluk A, Stagno S, Crist WM. J Pediatr 1981: 98: 260.
33. Mills MJ. JR Soc Med 1982; 75: 555.
34. Yin JAL, Kumaran TO, Marsh GW, Rossiter M, Catovsky D. Cancer 1983; 51: 200.
35. Zinkham WH, Medearis DN, Osborn JE. J Pediatr 1967; 71: 512.
36. Serck-Haussen A, Purohit GP. Br J Cancer 1968; 22: 506.
37. Macias EG. Lancet 1975; ii: 927.
38. Zuazu JP, Duran JW, Julia AF. N Engl J Med 1979; 301: 1185.
39. Chandra P, Chaudhery SA, Rosner F, Kagen M. Arch Intern Med 1975; 135: 989.
40. Weisenburgher DD, Rappaport H, Ahluwalia MS, Melvani R, Renner ED. Am J Med 1980; 69: 476.
41. Woodard BH, Farnham R, Bradford WD. Arch Pathol Lab Med 1981; 105: 452.
42. Krause JR, Kaplan SS. Scand J Haematol 1982; 28: 15.
43. Marsh WL, Bishop JW, Koenig HM. Arch Pathol Lab Med 1980; 104: 563.
44. James LP, Stass SA, Peterson V, Schumacher HR. Am J Clin Pathol 1979; 71: 600.
45. Jaffe ES, Costa J, Fauci AS. N Engl J Med 1981; 305: 103.
46. Perry MC, Harrison EG, Burgert O, Gilchrist GS. Cancer 1976; 38: 209.
47. Korman LY, Smith JR, Landaw SA, Davey FR. Ann Intern Med 1979; 91: 60.
48. Falini B, Bucciarelli E, Grignani F, Martelli MF. Cancer 1980; 46: 1140.
49. Youness E, Barlogie B, Ahearn M, Trujillo JM. Arch Pathol Lab Med 1980; 104: 651.
50. Martelli MF, Falini B, Tabilio A, Verladi A. Br J Haematol 1980; 46: 141.
51. Foadi MD, Slater AM, Pegrum GD. Scand J Haematol 1978; 20: 85.
52. Kadin ME, Kamoun M, Lamberg J. N Engl J Med 1981; 304: 648.
53. Miranda D, Vuletin JC, Kauffman SL. Arch Pathol Lab Med 1979; 103: 302.
54. Davies SF, McKenna RW, Sarosi GA. Am J Med 1979; 67: 617.
55. Tsan M-F, Mehlman DJ, Green RS, Bell WR. Ann Intern Med 1984; 84: 710.
56. Brunning RD. Hum Pathol 1970; 1: 99.
57. Lundin P, Persson E, Weinfeld A. Acta Med Scand 1964; 175: 383.
58. Fong TP, Okafor LA, Thomas W Jr, Westerman MP. Am J Haematol 1977; 2: 47.
59. Krause JR, Brubaker D, Kaplan S. Am J Clin Pathol 1979; 72: 68.
60. Gale E, Torrance J, Bothwell T. J Clin Invest 1963; 42: 1076.
61. Dacie JV, Mollin DL. Acta Med Scand 1966; 445 (suppl): 237.
62. Douglas AS, Dacie JV. J Clin Pathol 1953; 6: 307.
63. Kaplan E, Zuelzer WW, Mouriquand C. Blood 1954; 9: 203.
64. Rosner F, Dosik H, Kaiser SS, Lee SL, Morrison AN. JAMA 1969; 209: 935.

65. Zaino EC, Rossi MB, Pham TD, Azar HA. Blood 1971; 38: 457.
66. Van Dorpe A, Orshoven AB-V, Desmet V, Verwilghen RL. Br J Haematol 1973; 25: 165.
67. Lee KS, Tobin MS, Chen KTK, Ahmed F, Gomez-Leon G. Am J Med 1981; 73: 290.
68. Scullin DC, Shelburne JD, Cohen HJ. Am J Med 1979; 67: 617.
69. Lee RE, Ellis LD. Lab Invest 1971; 24: 261.
70. Wickramasinghe SN, Hughes M. Br J Haematol 1978; 38: 23.
71. Rywlin AM. Histopathology of the bone marrow. Boston: Little, Brown and Company, 1976: 145.
72. Varela-Duran J, Roholt PC, Ratliff NB. Arch Pathol Lab Med 1980; 104: 30.
73. Burns DA, Sarkany I. JR Soc Med 1979; 72: 139.
74. Tadmor R, Aghai E, Sarova-Pinhas I, Braham J. JAMA 1976; 235: 2852.
75. Rywlin AM. Histopathology of the bone marrow. Boston: Little, Brown and Company, 1976: 142.
76. Pollak ER, Miller HJ, Vye MV, Am J Clin Pathol 1981; 76: 98.
77. Nunez C, Abboud SL, Lemon NC, Kemp JA. Cancer 1983; 52: 297.
78. Head DR, Kennedy PS, Goyette RE. Am J Clin Pathol 1979; 72: 1008.
79. Franklin IM, Pritchard J. J Clin Pathol 1983; 36: 1215.
80. Reynolds CP, Smith RG, Frenkel EP. Cancer 1981; 48: 2088.
81. Andres TL, Kadin ME. Am J Clin Pathol 1983; 79: 546.
82. Kemshead JT, Goldman A, Fritschy J, Malpas JS, Pritchard J. Lancet 1983; i: 12.
83. Brooks JJ. Hum Pathol 1982; 13: 969.
84. Muehleck SD, McKenna RW, Gale PF, Brunning RD. Am J Clin Pathol 1983; 79: 277.
85. Gatter KC, Abdulaziz Z, Beverley P, et al. J Clin Pathol 1982; 35: 1253.
86. Savage RA, Lucas FV, Hoffman GC. Am J Clin Pathol 1983; 79: 268.
87. Reynolds RD, Greenberg BR, Martin ND, Lucas RN, Gaffney CN, Hawn L. Cancer 1973; 32: 181.
88. Ingle JN, Tormey DC, Tan HK. Cancer 1978; 41: 670.
89. Singh G, Krause JR, Breitfeld V. Cancer 1977; 40: 2317.
90. Anner RM, Drewinko B. Cancer 1977; 39: 1337.
91. Frey U, Senn HJ. Schweiz Med Wochenschr 1978; 108: 82.
92. Ihde DC, Simms EB, Matthews MJ, Cohen MH, Bunn PA, Minna JD. Blood 1979; 53: 677.
93. Rubins JM. Cancer 1983; 51: 308.
94. Anonymous. Lancet 1980; i: 127.
95. Lennert K. Clin Haematol 1975; 4: 331.
96. Bain BJ, Catovsky D, O'Brien M, et al. Blood 1981; 58: 206.
97. Hansen NE, Killmann SA. Blood 1970; 36: 428.
98. Sawers AH, Davson J, Braganza J, Geary CG. J Clin Pathol 1982; 35: 617.
99. Weinberg SG, Lubin A, Wiener SN, Deoras MP, Ghose MK, Kopelman RC. Am J Med 1977; 63: 125.
100. Yetgin S, Ozsoylu S. Scand J Haematol 1982; 28: 180.
101. Boxer M, Ellman L, Geller R, Wang C-A. Arch Intern Med 1977; 137: 588.
102. Breton-Gorius J, Vainchenker W, Nurden A, Levy-Toledano S, Caen J. Am J Pathol 1981; 102: 10.
103. Kundel DW, Brecher G, Bodey GP, Brittin GM. Blood 1964; 23: 526.
104. Blayney DW, Jaffe ES, Blatter WA, et al. Blood 1983; 62: 401.
105. Fialkow PJ, Jacobson RJ, Papayannopoulou T. Am J Med 1977; 63: 125.
106. Jacobson RJ, Salo A, Fialkow PJ. Blood 1978; 51: 189.
107. Kuo C, Van Voolem GA, Morrison AN. Blood 1972; 40: 875.
108. Burkhardt R. In: Catovsky D, ed. The leukaemic cell. Edinburgh: Churchill Livingstone, 1981: 49.
109. Brown CH. Bull Johns Hopkins Med Sch 1972; 131: 189.
110. Kiraly JF, Wheby MS. Am J Med 1976; 60: 361.
111. Bernard C, Sick H, Boilletot A, Oberling F. Arch Intern Med 1978; 138: 1567.
112. Bain BJ. J Clin Pathol 1980; 33: 449.
113. Carloss H, Winslow D, Kastan L, Yam LT. Arch Intern Med 1977; 137: 863.
114. Hughes RG, Islam A, Lewis SM, Catovsky D. Clin Lab Haematol 1981; 3: 173.
115. Rose MS. Lancet 1973; ii: 730.
116. Harigaya K, Watanabe S, Watanabe Y, et al. Arch Pathol Lab Med 1977; 101: 652.
117. Norgard MJ, Carpenter JT, Conrad ME. Arch Intern Med 1979; 139: 905.
118. Tavassoli M. J Miss State Med Assoc 1983; 24: 39.
119. Brada M, Bellingham AJ. Br Med J 1980; 281: 1108.
120. Caraveo J, Trowbridge AA, Amaral BW, Green JB, Cain PT, Hurley DL. Am J Med 1977; 62: 404.
121. Katzen H, Spagnolo SV. JAMA 1980; 244: 2438.
122. Lysik RM, Cornetta K, di Stefano JF, Zucker S. Cancer Res 1979; 39: 30.
123. Rao KRP, Patel AR, Anderson MJ, Hodgson J, Jones SE, Pattison JR. Ann Intern Med 1983; 98: 930.
124. Lawrence C, Schreiber AJ. N Engl J Med 1979; 300: 834.
125. Hamilton PK. Am J Clin Pathol 1954; 34: 580.
126. Guerra-Caceres JG, Gotuzzo-Herencia E, Crosby-Dagnino E, Miro-Quesada M, Carillo-Parodi C. Trans R Soc Trop Med Hyg 1979; 73: 680.
127. Rausing A. Acta Med Scand 1973; 193: 5.
128. Robert F, Durant JR, Gams RA. Arch Intern Med 1977; 137: 688.
129. Pasternak J, Bolivar R. Arch Intern Med 1983; 137: 688.
130. Ellman L. Am J Med 1976; 60: 1.
131. Cuartas F, Rothenberg J. South Med J 1972; 65: 523.
132. Penchansky L, Krause JR. South Med J 1979; 72: 500.
133. Rice L, Shenkenberg T, Lynch EC, Wheeler TM. Cancer 1982; 49: 1924.
134. Cohen RJ, Samoszuk MK, Busch D, Lagios M. N Engl J Med 1983; 308: 1476.
135. Adams DO. Am J Pathol 1976; 84: 164.
136. Desol G, Pellegrin M, Familiades J, Auvergnat JC. Blood 1978; 52: 637.
137. Pease GL. Am J Clin Pathol 1952; 22: 107.
138. Walsh TJ, Catchatourian R, Cohen H. Am J Clin Pathol 1983; 79: 509.
139. Rywlin AM. Histopathology of the bone marrow. Boston: Little, Brown and Company, 1976: 170.
140. Falini B, Tabilio A, Velardi A, Cernetti C, Aversa F, Martelli MF. Scand J Haematol 1982; 29: 211.

141. Yu NC, Rywlin AM. Hum Pathol 1982; 13: 905.
142. Wu HV, Kosmin M. Ann Intern Med 1977; 86: 663.
143. Riker J, Baker J, Swanson M. Arch Intern Med 1978; 138: 1731.
144. Andersson DEH, Langworth S, Newman HC, Ost A. Acta Med Scand 1980; 207: 131.
145. Dobrin RS, Vernier RL, Fish AJ. Am J Med 1975; 59: 325.
146. Case records of the Massachusetts General Hospital N Engl J Med 1982; 307: 1257.
147. Gormsen H. Acta Med Scand 1948; 213 (suppl): 154.
148. Hovde RF, Sundberg RD. Blood 1950; 5: 209.
149. Martin MFR. Br Med J 1977; ii: 300.
150. Schleicher EM. Am J Clin Pathol 1949; 19: 981.
151. Kadin ME, Donaldson SS, Dorfman RF. N Engl J Med 1970; 283: 859.
152. Rywlin AM, Ortega RD. Am J Clin Pathol 1972; 57: 457.
153. Mant MJ, Faragher BS. Br J Haematol 1972; 23: 737.
154. Tavassoli M, Eastlund DT, Yam LT, Neiman RS, Finkel H. Scand J Haematol 1976; 16: 311.
155. Stavem P, Larsen IF, Ly B, Rørvik TO. Acta Med Scand 1980; 208: 111.
156. Myer TJ. Semin Thromb Hemost 1981; 7: 37.
157. Enos WF, Pierre RV, Rosenblatt JE. Mayo Clin Proc 1981; 56: 381.
158. Rywlin AM. Histopathology of the bone marrow. Boston: Little, Brown and Company, 1976: 180.
159. Pierce JR, Wren MV, Cousar JB. Ann Intern Med 1978; 89: 937.
160. Kay M. J Clin Pathol 1983; 36: 1288.
161. Testa JR, Rowley JD. In: Catovsky D, ed. The leukaemic cell. London: Churchill Livingstone, 1981: 184.
162. Marinello MJ, Bloom ML, Doeblin TD, Sandberg AA. N Engl J Med 1980; 303: 704.

Disorders of the erythron

ABNORMALITIES OF RED CELL MORPHOLOGY

A number of abnormalities of red cell morphology may be seen in disease and these are described by various terms. The morphology of red cells should be examined in an area of the blood film in which only occasional red cells overlap. In such an area normal red cells (Fig. 5.1a) show some variation in diameter. They also show a central area of pallor which occupies less than a third of the diameter of the cell. The majority of normal red cells have a circular outline but occasional cells may be oval or have other shapes. The terms *anisocytosis* and *poikilocytosis* are used to describe an increased degree of variation in cell size and cell shape respectively. Poikilocytes vary considerably in their shape. They may be oval, pear or tear-drop-shaped, sickle-shaped or irregularly contracted. Red cells are described as being *normochromic* when the central area of pallor is normal in size and as being *hypochromic* when this area is larger than normal. In severely hypochromic red cells the area of pallor is very large and surrounded by a narrow rim of eosinophilic cytoplasm. Erythrocytes are described as *normocytes*, *microcytes* and *macrocytes* (Figs 5.1b and c) when their size appears to be normal, smaller than normal and larger than normal respectively. Target cells are thinner than normal and have a well-stained zone in the middle of the usual central area of pallor (Figs 5.1d and 5.2a). *Microspherocytes* are small, rounded, deeply-staining cells in which there is a loss of the central area of pallor. These cells suffer from varying degrees of loss of their central concavities and may even be completely spherical.[1] Helmet cells, triangular cells and small cells with other peculiar shapes appear to result from the fragmentation of erythrocytes by contact with fibrin strands, diseased vessel walls or foreign surfaces (e.g. cardiac valve prostheses). Such cells are collectively called *schistocytes*. There are also red cells with various types of projections (spicules) on their surface.[1, 2] On the basis of studies using the scanning electron microscope (SEM), these can be grouped into two main categories: *echinocytes* (crenated red cells) and *acanthocytes* (spur cells) (Figs 5.2a and b). When examined in the SEM,

echinocytes appear flat or spherical and have 10–30 spicules of similar length distributed evenly over the surface. In contrast, acanthocytes have 5–10 spicules of varying length irregularly distributed over the surface. Furthermore, the spicules of acanthocytes have knobby ends. In Romanowsky-stained smears, echinocytes have a serrated outline due to small projections which are more or less evenly distributed over their circumference. By contrast, acanthocytes have a few spicules of varying length and thickness projecting irregularly from the circumference. In some conditions, there is a slit-like appearance across the middle of the red cell and such cells are called *stomatocytes* (Fig. 5.2c). The term *keratocyte*[1] is used to describe a cell with two pointed projections ('horns') which appear to form as the result of the rupture of a vacuole at the cell's periphery. In several disorders, the ribosomes within reticulocytes show an abnormal tendency to form clumps of various sizes during the preparation of a Romanowsky-stained smear. Such cells show many fine or coarse basophilic dots distributed uniformly throughout the cell and are described as displaying *basophilic stippling* (Fig. 5.1c). Another type of basophilic inclusion which might be seen within erythrocytes is called a *Pappenheimer body*. These vary markedly in size from 1 μm downwards, may be single or multiple, are unevenly distributed and stain positively with the Prussian blue reaction for iron. Red cells containing Pappenheimer bodies are also called *siderocytes*. In some circumstances, one or more rounded, dark purple inclusions known as *Howell-Jolly bodies* may be found within red cells (Fig. 5.2d). These inclusions, which consist of nuclear material, are formed within erythroblasts either by karyorrhexis or from chromosome fragments which become isolated outside the nucleus when the nuclear membrane is reformed during telophase. The conditions in which the above-mentioned morphological abnormalities may be found as a prominent feature are summarized in Table 5.1.

ASSESSMENT OF ERYTHROPOIESIS

A detailed understanding of erythropoiesis in a particular patient or disease requires the assess-

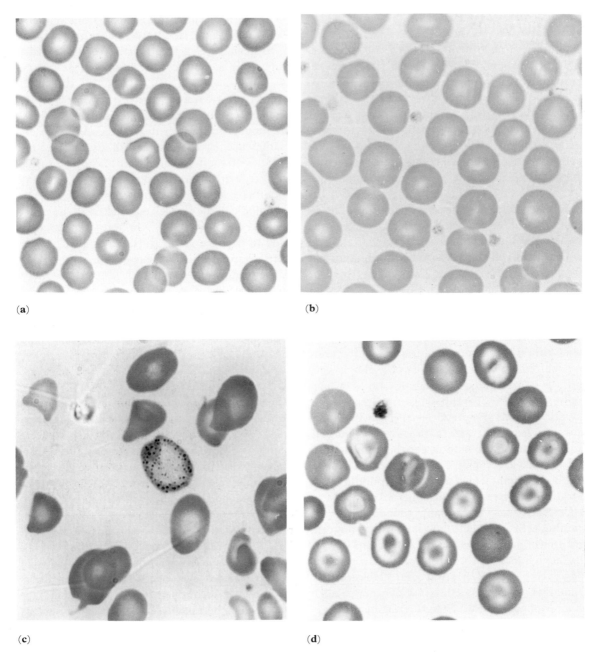

(a)

(b)

(c)

(d)

Fig. 5.1a–d Some abnormalities of red cell morphology which may be seen on examination of peripheral blood smears. (a) Normal blood film (for comparison). (b) Macrocytosis induced by chronic alcoholism. The majority of the red cells have a rounded outline, as is typical of alcohol-induced macrocytosis. (c) Oval macrocytes and other poikilocytes in severe anaemia due to vitamin B12 deficiency. One of the macrocytes displays coarse basophilic stippling. (d) High proportion of target cells in a patient with obstructive jaundice.

May–Grünwald–Giemsa stain   ×940

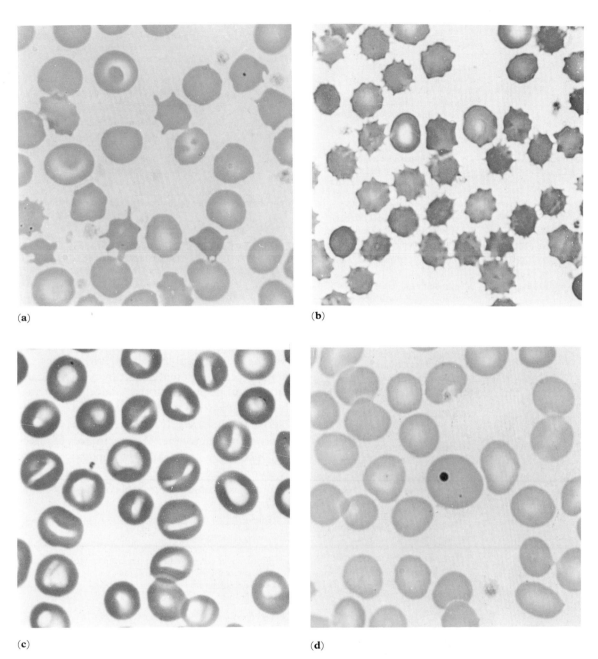

(a)

(b)

(c)

(d)

Fig. 5.2a–d Some abnormalities of red cell morphology which may be seen on examination of peripheral blood smears. (a) Acanthocytes and target cells in a haematologically normal patient subjected to splenectomy. (b) Echinocytes in blood mixed with citrate–phosphate–dextrose solution (CPD) containing adenine and stored at 4°C for 4 weeks. (c) Stomatocytes induced by acute alcoholism. (d) Howell–Jolly body within an erythrocyte of a splenectomized patient.

May–Grünwald–Giemsa stain   × 940

Table 5.1 Some causes of various abnormalities of red cell morphology

Abnormality	Significance
Hypochromia and microcytosis	Impaired synthesis of haem or globin: iron deficiency, thalassaemia syndromes, sideroblastic anaemia, congenital atransferrinaemia,[3] aluminium-induced anaemia (dialysis patients)[4]
Macrocytosis (Figs 5.1a,b)	Dyserythropoiesis or accelerated release of reticulocytes: megaloblastic erythropoiesis (e.g. vitamin B_{12} or folate deficiency, congenital dyserythropoietic anaemia types I and III, Tables 5.15, 5.16) or macronormoblastic erythropoiesis (e.g. chronic alcoholism, chronic haemolysis, Table 5.17)
Anisocytosis	Non-specific evidence of a perturbation of erythropoiesis
Target cells (Figs 5.1d, 5.2a)	Increased surface area relative to volume: thalassaemia syndromes, iron deficiency, some haemoglobinopathies (HbAC, HbCC, HbEE), liver disease, obstructive jaundice, hyposplenism, post-splenectomy, familial lecithin-cholesterol-acyltransferase deficiency[5]
Stomatocytes[6] (Fig. 5.2c)	Hereditary stomatocytosis (p. 119), the Rh null phenotype,[7] acute alcoholism, phenothiazines and other drugs
Spherocytosis	Abnormality of cell membrane: hereditary spherocytosis, membrane damage mediated by antibodies, heat, certain chemicals, hypophosphataemia
Elliptocytosis	Abnormality of cell membrane: usually hereditary; also acquired defect in various anaemias (megaloblastic anaemia, iron deficiency)
Acanthocytes (Fig. 5.2a)	Haemolytic anaemia in liver disease, hypothyroidism, anorexia nervosa, post-splenectomy, abetalipoproteinaemia,[8] haemolysis with McLeod blood type[9]
Echinocytes (Fig. 5.2b)	Neonates, recently transfused red cells, *in vitro* storage changes
Keratocytes	Uraemia
Sickle cells	Sickle cell anaemia, HbS/β-thalassaemia, HbSC disease, HbS/D-Punjab, HbS/Lepore
Schistocytes	Red cell fragmentation: cardiac valve prostheses, micro-angiopathic haemolytic anaemias including that due to malignant hypertension
Tear-drop cell	Prominent in myelofibrosis, also present in various anaemias (e.g. thalassaemia)
Basophilic stippling (Fig. 5.1c)	Lead poisoning, thalassaemia syndromes, pyrimidine 5'-nucleotidase deficiency, homozygosity for Hb Constant Spring, accelerated erythropoiesis, dyserythropoiesis
Pappenheimer bodies	Lead poisoning, sideroblastic anaemias, haemolytic anaemias, post-splenectomy
Howell–Jolly bodies (Fig. 5.2d)	Post-splenectomy, hyposplenism, megaloblastic haemopoiesis

ment of three aspects of red cell production: these are, effective erythropoiesis, ineffective erythropoiesis, and total erythropoiesis. Effective erythropoiesis is the rate of release of red cells from the marrow and ineffective erythropoiesis is the rate of loss of potential erythrocytes as a consequence of the phagocytosis of defective erythropoietic cells within the marrow. Total erythropoiesis is the overall erythropoietic activity, effective and ineffective. Various indices of effective, ineffective and total erythropoietic activity are summarized in Table 5.2. Some of these (the absolute reticulocyte count, M/E ratio and

Table 5.2 Indices of erythropoietic activity

Effective erythropoiesis
Absolute reticulocyte count (see p. 8)
Red cell turnover calculated from the mean cell life-span, red cell count and total blood volume
Red cell ^{59}Fe utilization
Red cell iron turnover

Total erythropoiesis
M/E ratio (see p. 76)
Plasma iron turnover
Total marrow iron turnover
Faecal urobilinogen excretion
Carbon monoxide production

Ineffective erythropoiesis
Discrepancy between indices of total and effective erythropoiesis
Morphological evidence of increased dyserythropoiesis (see p. 77) and erythroblast phagocytosis
Early-labelled bilirubin production after administration of labelled glycine

morphological evidence of dyserythropoiesis or of erythroblast phagocytosis) are more easily and, therefore, more frequently determined than the others. The scientific basis and the limitations of various indices of erythropoiesis have been reviewed by a number of authors.[10, 11]

ANAEMIA[12]

A person is considered to be anaemic when the haemoglobin concentration in the peripheral blood is below the normal range for the age and sex of that individual. The normal ranges at different ages are given on page 5.

The symptoms and signs of anaemia are numerous and result both from decreased tissue oxygenation leading to widespread organ dysfunction as well as from adaptive changes, particularly in the cardiovascular system. Symptoms include lassitude, easy fatiguability, dyspnoea on exertion, palpitation, angina or intermittent claudication (in older patients with degenerative arterial disease), headache, vertigo, lightheadedness, visual disturbances, drowsiness, anorexia, nausea, bowel disturbances, menstrual disturbances and loss of libido. Physical signs include pallor, signs of a hyperkinetic circulation (tachycardia, wide pulse pressure with capillary pulsation, haemic murmurs), signs of congestive cardiac failure, and haemorrhages and occasional exudates in the retina. Severe anaemia may also cause slight proteinuria, mild impairment of renal function and a low-grade fever.

Patients with a moderate degree of chronic anaemia usually have only mild symptoms attributable to the anaemia and show only slight increases in cardiac output at rest and slight decreases in mixed venous Po_2. This situation results from a substantial shift of the oxygen dissociation curve to the right (see p. 6), mainly due to an intraerythrocytic adaptation to the anaemia resulting in increased levels of 2,3-diphosphoglycerate within red cells. When the haemoglobin falls below 7–8 g/dl symptoms become more marked. The intraerythrocytic adaptation cannot by itself maintain an adequate oxygen delivery to the tissues and other compensatory mechanisms come into operation. These include: (1) an increase of stroke volume, heart rate and cardiac output at rest; (2) redistribution of blood flow with vasoconstriction in the skin and kidneys and increased perfusion of the heart, brain and muscle; and (3) reduction of the mixed venous Po_2 (which increases the arterial-venous oxygen difference).

Anaemias have been classified in various ways: two useful classifications are based on: (1) the MCV and an assessment of the size and intensity of staining of the red cells in a Romanowsky-stained blood smear (Table 5.3); and (2) the main

Table 5.3 Morphological classification of anaemia

Type	MCV
Normochromic, normocytic anaemia	Within normal range
Hypochromic, microcytic anaemia	Low
Macrocytic anaemia	High

pathogenetic mechanisms underlying the anaemia (Table 5.4). In most cases of anaemia more than one of the five mechanisms listed in Table 5.4 are involved. Various abnormalities of red cell morphology other than abnormalities of size are present in certain anaemias and may provide useful clues regarding the possible aetiology of an anaemia.

Table 5.4 Mechanisms of anaemia

1. Blood loss

2. Increased red cell destruction (haemolytic anaemia)

3. Impaired red cell formation
   (a) Decreased or inadequately increased total erythropoiesis
   (b) Greatly increased ineffective erythropoiesis

4. Splenic pooling and sequestration (see p. 156)

5. Increased plasma volume (see pp. 22 and 156)

BLOOD LOSS[13]

Acute haemorrhage results in an acute reduction of blood volume. Restoration of the blood volume occurs slowly over the next 36–72 h by an expansion of the plasma volume: the rate of recovery of the blood volume appears to be determined by the rate of addition of protein to the plasma. A gradual fall in haemoglobin level accompanies the expansion in plasma volume. Thus, the haemoglobin level is normal soon after the haemorrhage, is slightly decreased about 3 h later and gradually falls to reach its lowest value between 36 and 72 h after the bleed. The anaemia is normochromic and normocytic in type. The reticulocyte count is slightly increased 1–2 days after the haemorrhage, reaches a peak at about 7–10 days and returns to normal by about 2 weeks. The extent of the reticulocytosis is proportional to the amount of blood lost but seldom exceeds 10–15%. A few normoblasts appear in the blood after a severe haemorrhage. The leucocyte count increases within 1–2 h of acute haemorrhage, usually to the range $12–20 \times 10^9/l$ and remains elevated for several days. This leucocytosis is caused by a raised neutrophil count associated with a few neutrophil metamyelocytes and an occasional myelocyte. There is also a temporary increase in the platelet count.

The rapid loss of 500 ml of blood within a few minutes usually causes a slight fall in central venous pressure but no significant changes in the blood pressure or pulse rate. When 750 ml or more are lost rapidly, there is a substantial fall in central venous pressure, a fall in cardiac output, a fall in blood pressure and peripheral vasoconstriction. The rapid loss of 1.5–2 litres may cause unconsciousness.[14]

Chronic blood loss, such as results from chronic peptic ulcers or neoplasms of the large bowel, eventually causes the development of a hypochromic microcytic anaemia due to iron deficiency (see p. 157).

HAEMOLYTIC ANAEMIA[15, 16]

A haemolytic state is said to exist when the survival of a patient's red cells in the circulation is reduced below the normal value of 110–120 days due to lysis within the vascular tree (intravascular haemolysis), premature phagocytosis and destruction by cells of the mononuclear phagocyte system (extravascular haemolysis), or both. As normal individuals can increase the rate of red cell production to six to eight times the basal rate

in response to anaemia, patients whose mean red cell life-span is reduced to one-sixth of normal (i.e. to about 20 days) do not suffer from anaemia provided there is no impairment of bone marrow function. Such patients are said to suffer from a compensated haemolytic state. Anaemia develops when the bone marrow cannot adequately compensate for the degree of reduction of red cell life-span.

Extravascular and intravascular haemolysis[12, 17]

In the majority of haemolytic anaemias, haemolysis occurs extravascularly in the liver, spleen and bone marrow. The cells of the mononuclear phagocyte system present in these organs remove abnormal erythrocytes and red cell fragments from the circulation. The fate of these prematurely removed red cells is similar to that of normal red cells that are removed at the end of their life-span. The degradation of 1 mol of haem within these phagocytes leads to the production of 1 mol of bilirubin and 1 mol of carbon monoxide. The bilirubin enters the plasma and is transported to the liver bound to albumin. In the liver the water-insoluble bilirubin is converted to soluble glucuronides and excreted in the bile. The bilirubin is then converted by the bacterial flora of the bowel to urobilinogen and eliminated in the faeces. Some of the urobilinogen is reabsorbed from the gut and excreted in the urine. In normal adults about 1% of the circulating red cells (i.e. about 20 ml of red cells) are destroyed extravascularly per day and, provided liver function is unimpaired, this results in a serum bilirubin level of 5–17 μmol/l (0.3–1.0 mg/dl) and a daily faecal urobilinogen excretion of 50–265 mg. Patients with haemolytic anaemia usually show mild to moderate jaundice, slight hyperbilirubinaemia and an increased excretion of faecal and urinary urobilinogen. The serum bilirubin level is usually in the range 20–50 μmol/l (1–3 mg/dl). The exact level depends not only on the rate of haemolysis but also on the capacity of the liver to cope with an increased bilirubin load. In haemolytic states the body attempts to cope with the increased rate of red cell destruction both by an increase in the number of macrophages involved in erythrophagocytosis and by increasing the capacity of the liver to conjugate and excrete bilirubin. For this reason, an occasional patient with haemolytic anaemia may have a normal serum bilirubin level and may not be jaundiced.

The haemoglobin released from intravascular lysis of red cells is bound to haptoglobins, a family of haemoglobin-binding α globulins present in the plasma. The resulting haemoglobin-haptoglobin complex is rapidly cleared from the circulation by cells of the mononuclear phagocyte system. The concentration of haptoglobin is usually expressed in terms of its haemoglobin-binding capacity and in normal individuals there is sufficient to bind 0.4–2.1 g of haemoglobin per 1 of plasma. A reduction in the plasma haptoglobin level is a feature of intravascular haemolysis but is also seen in extravascular haemolysis, possibly because of a leak of some free haemoglobin into the circulation. When the amount of haemoglobin released during intravascular haemolysis exceeds the haemoglobin-binding capacity of the haptoglobins, free haemoglobin appears in the plasma. Haem is released from the free haemoglobin and binds to a specific haem-binding plasma β glycoprotein called haemopexin; the haem-haemopexin complex is removed by the liver. When the haem-binding capacity of the haemopexin is exceeded, haematin is formed and binds to albumin to produce methaemalbumin which gives the plasma a dirty brown colour. In severe intravascular haemolysis, tetrameric haemoglobin ($\alpha_2\beta_2$) and $\alpha\beta$ dimers are present in the plasma (haemoglobinaemia). The dimers pass through the glomerular filter and, when the haemoglobin level exceeds about 0.3g/l, appear in the urine (haemoglobinuria). Some of the $\alpha\beta$ dimers are metabolized in the renal tubular cells with the formation of haemosiderin granules. These granules may be seen both within shed tubular cells and extracellularly when the urine is spun and the deposit examined after staining by Perls' acid ferrocyanide method (Fig. 5.3). Thus, apart from the reduction of haptoglobin levels, the other biochemical changes of intravascular haemolysis include reduced haemopexin levels, methaemalbuminaemia (detected by Schumm's test), haemoglobinaemia (serum level >4 mg/dl), haemoglobinuria and haemosiderinuria.

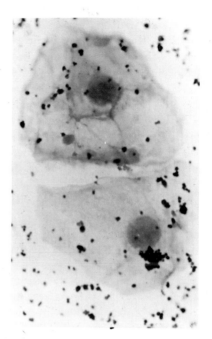

Fig. 5.3 Urinary deposit stained by Perls' acid ferrocyanide method for haemosiderin. The deposit was obtained by centrifugation of the urine of a patient with chronic intravascular haemolysis due to a malfunctioning aortic valve prosthesis and shows the presence of haemosiderin granules.

Haematological changes

These consist of morphological abnormalities in the red cells (e.g. spherocytosis, fragmentation of red cells) resulting from the disorder underlying the haemolysis and changes caused by a compensatory increase of erythropoietic activity. The latter include reticulocytosis, erythroblastaemia, macrocytosis, and erythroid hyperplasia. Most patients have a clearly increased reticulocyte percentage and absolute reticulocyte count. Reticulocyte percentages of 5–20% are usual but values as high as 50–70% may occasionally be seen. In general the extent of the increase in the reticulocyte count is proportional to the severity of the anaemia. Small numbers of erythroblasts may be present in the circulation (less than 1 per 100 leucocytes). The degree of erythroblastaemia is higher in patients with higher reticulocyte counts and may increase considerably if the haemolysis continues following splenectomy. The anaemia is generally normochromic and normocytic in type but may be macrocytic. The macrocytosis is usually associated with macronormoblastic erythropoiesis and in such cases is the result of alterations in the kinetics of erythropoiesis; the reticulocytes formed during accelerated erythropoiesis are considerably larger than normal and mature into macrocytes. Occasionally the macrocytosis may be partly or wholly due to a secondary folate deficiency and in these cases erythropoiesis is megaloblastic. The bone marrow of subjects with haemolysis shows increased cellularity due to erythroid hyperplasia, and a corresponding decrease in fat cells. The myeloid-erythroid ratio is reduced and may be as low as 0.5 (normal range, 2.0–8.3). There may be an extension of haemopoietic marrow down the long bones.

Patients with chronic haemolytic anaemias suffer from temporary aplastic crises in which morphologically recognizable erythropoietic cells virtually disappear from the marrow, the reticulocyte count falls, sometimes to zero, and the haemoglobin level falls very rapidly. Neutropenia and thrombocytopenia may also be occasionally present. Reticulocytes reappear after about 7–10 days. The aplastic crises are often associated with 'trivial' infections and may affect more than one member of a family at about the same time. Recent studies suggest that such infections are frequently caused by a parvovirus.[18, 19, 20]

There may be a substantial loss of iron in the urine of patients with chronic haemoglobinuria and haemosiderinuria and this may lead to iron deficiency.

Changes in other tissues

The increased haemolysis leads to an increased rate of production and excretion of bilirubin and, consequently, to an increased frequency of pigment gall stones. Cholecystitis or deep jaundice due to obstruction of the common bile duct may follow. The persistence of stones in the gall bladder for long periods may be associated with the subsequent development of carcinoma.

Particularly in severe congenital haemolytic anaemia, the erythroid hyperplasia may be so

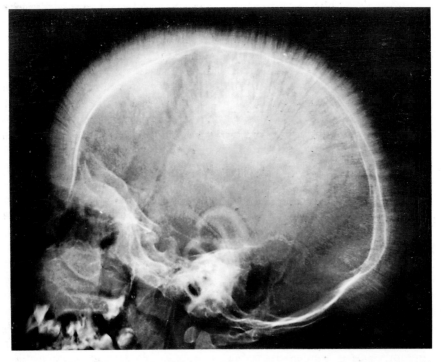

Fig. 5.4 X-ray of the skull of a patient with sickle cell anaemia. There is thickening of the parietal and frontal bones due to widening of the marrow-containing diploic space. Both tables of these bones, particularly the outer table, are abnormally thin and bony trabeculae have developed at right angles to the tables, giving a 'hair-on-end' appearance.

marked that it causes an increase in the volume of the marrow cavity, thinning of cortical bone and deformities of the bones (Fig. 5.4). Furthermore, extramedullary haemopoiesis may occur in the liver, spleen and lymph nodes.

Splenomegaly is common and is associated with an increase in phagocytic cells to cope with the high rate of destruction of abnormal red cells in this organ. In some conditions, the spleen also shows foci of extramedullary haemopoiesis. Retardation of growth may occur in children with gross splenomegaly.

Haemosiderosis may develop as a consequence of recurrent blood transfusions, an increased absorption of iron (secondary to the erythroid hyperplasia) or both.

Chronic leg ulcers over the malleoli have been occasionally observed in various types of haemolytic anaemia.

Causes of haemolytic anaemia

Haemolytic anaemia may be due to: (1) inherited abnormalities of the cell membrane, energy-generating and other metabolic pathways, or haemoglobin constitution of the red cell; or (2) various acquired abnormalities. A classification of the causes of haemolytic anaemia is given in Table 5.5.

Table 5.5 Classification of the haemolytic anaemias

Hereditary haemolytic anaemia
(a) Abnormalities of the red cell membrane
(b) Abnormalities of red cell enzymes
(c) Abnormalities of the structure or synthesis of haemoglobin

Acquired haemolytic anaemia
(a) Immune
(b) Non-immune

HEREDITARY HAEMOLYTIC ANAEMIAS

Abnormalities of the cell membrane

Hereditary spherocytosis[15, 21]

This is a familial disorder characterized by jaundice, haemolytic anaemia, the presence of microspherocytes in the blood and the disappear-

ance of the jaundice and anaemia following splenectomy. It is the commonest type of congenital haemolytic anaemia in Northern Europe, where it affects 200–300 per million of the population. Other racial groups in Europe and elsewhere are less frequently affected. The condition is inherited as an autosomal dominant and there is some evidence that the gene concerned is located on the short arm of chromosome 12. About a quarter of the cases of hereditary spherocytosis appear not to show haematological abnormalities in either parent. This is usually due to varying expression of the gene in different members of the same family and careful examination frequently shows a small population of osmotically fragile cells in one of the parents. However, there are some cases which appear, on the basis of detailed family studies, to have arisen by recent mutation.

It has been suspected for a long time that the primary defect in hereditary spherocytosis is probably some abnormality of the structure or function of the red cell membrane. The structural stability of the normal red cell membrane appears to depend on a filamentous protein meshwork (membrane skeleton) which is apposed to the inner surface of the cell membrane. The four main proteins which interact in this meshwork are spectrin, actin, protein 4.1 and ankyrin and the meshwork is tethered to the rest of the cell membrane via an attachment of ankyrin to an integral membrane protein (protein 3) which spans the lipid bilayer.[22] The interaction between spectrin and actin is enhanced by the reaction of protein 4.1 with spectrin near the spectrin-actin binding site. Recent studies have shown that in about 30% of families with hereditary spherocytosis some of the spectrin molecules are abnormal and lack the ability to bind protein 4.1.[23, 24] This abnormality would be expected to impair the interaction between spectrin and actin and thus impair the function of the membrane skeleton. The primary defect (or defects) in the membrane skeleton of the remaining 70% of cases of hereditary spherocytosis remains to be determined. The primary defects in this disorder lead to the formation of microspherocytes which have a reduced ratio of surface area to volume and are osmotically fragile. In stained blood films, micro-

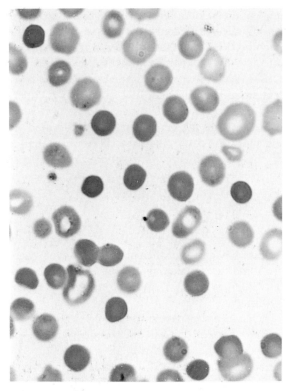

Fig. 5.5 Peripheral blood film of a patient with hereditary spherocytosis (Hb 10.9 g/dl; reticulocyte count 20%). Several microspherocytes are present; these appear as small densely-staining cells which lack a central area of pallor.

May–Grünwald–Giemsa stain   × 940

spherocytes appear as small, round, deeply-staining erythrocytes with no area of central pallor (Fig. 5.5). Careful determinations of red cell fragility curves are required for the detection of mild cases of hereditary spherocytosis in which the appearances of the blood film may be indecisive; in such cases the fragility curve may show a small 'tail' of abnormally fragile cells. Microspherocytes show an increased rate of metabolism of glucose and an increased flux of sodium into the cells which is balanced by an increased ATPase-dependent transport of sodium out of the cells.

The reticulocytes and newly-formed erythrocytes of patients with hereditary spherocytosis have a more or less normal morphology and spherocytosis develops subsequently even in the absence of the spleen; there is some increase in the degree of spherocytosis as a result of the re-peated passage of erythrocytes through the splenic circulation. Apparently, factors in the micro-environment of the splenic tissue (possibly a lack of glucose and acidosis) cause the abnormal erythrocytes to lose parts of their cell membrane and become more spherocytic. Spherocytes are less deformable than normal red cells and are therefore retarded and eventually prevented from passing from the Billroth cords to the splenic sinuses. The microspherocytes which are trapped in the splenic cords are subsequently destroyed. After splenectomy, there is only a slight reduction in the degree of spherocytosis but the red cell life-span becomes almost normal.

The age at which the diagnosis is made varies from 1–3 days to over 80 years and is governed mainly by the severity of the disorder; the disease is one of the causes of neonatal jaundice. The clinical features include mild to moderate jaundice, splenomegaly, complications resulting from gall stones and, rarely, chronic leg ulcers. Splenomegaly is almost invariably present. Gall stones may reveal themselves at an unusually young age. In a few cases biliary colic may be the first indication of the disease. The leg ulcers occur above the malleoli, are often bilateral, and usually heal following splenectomy, leaving pigmented scars. Deformities of bones secondary to erythroid hyperplasia are very uncommon. Rare cases have shown congenital skeletal abnormalities such as tower skull and deformities of the palate. Mental deficiency was associated with the disorder in one large family studied. Haemolytic and aplastic crises may occur and the latter can be life-threatening. Epidemiological evidence suggests that aplastic crises are usually due to a single transmissible agent with an incubation period of about 9 days; the agent is now known to be a human parvovirus[18, 20] (see p. 96). The blood shows all the features of a haemolytic state and, in addition, shows both spherocytosis and a high MCHC.

Hereditary elliptocytosis[15]

This disorder is characterized by the presence of many oval, elliptical or long rod-shaped red cells in the blood (Fig. 5.6). It is inherited as an autosomal dominant. In a proportion of the

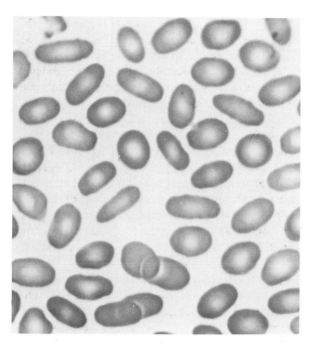

Fig. 5.6 Blood film of a case of hereditary elliptocytosis.
May–Grünwald–Giemsa stain   × 940

patients, the gene determining the elliptocytosis is situated on the same chromosome as those determining the Rh blood groups. The primary defect probably lies in an abnormality of the structure or function of the spectrin of the membrane skeleton. It also seems that more than one primary defect may cause elliptocytosis since two patients have been reported who had elliptocytosis associated with a lack of membrane band 4.1.[25, 26] The erythropoietic cells and most reticulocytes are normal in shape, the elliptocytic change usually developing after the reticulocyte stage. There is a considerable variation in the haematological changes seen in heterozygotes. The severity of the elliptical change varies from case to case and the percentage of ovalocytes or elliptocytes varies between about 25 and 90%. Most individuals show no anaemia or haemolysis, or suffer from a compensated haemolytic state, but occasional heterozygotes have a moderate haemolytic anaemia with splenomegaly. In general, anaemia usually occurs when the elliptocytosis gene is not linked with the Rh locus. Homozygotes for the elliptocytosis gene are usually diagnosed in infancy and have a severe and sometimes fatal haemolytic anaemia. They display a very abnormal blood picture with small densely-staining cells, misshapen microcytes, and red cell fragments. Both in heterozygotes and homozygotes the anaemia and jaundice are improved after splenectomy.

Hereditary macro-ovalocytosis of Melanesians[27]

This is common in Melanesia and also occurs in South-East Asia. It is inherited as an autosomal recessive trait. In addition to ovalocytosis, some macro-ovalocytes, sometimes with two areas of central pallor, and stomatocytes are present (Fig. 5.7). The red cell membrane shows a reduced expression of many red cell antigens. Anaemia does not usually occur.

Hereditary stomatocytosis

This is a newly-described type of haemolytic anaemia. There is a wide diversity in the degree of

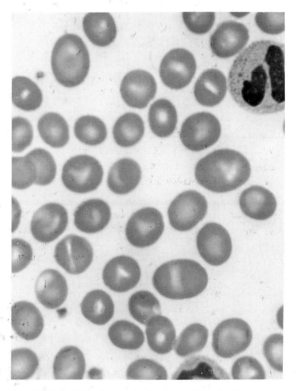

Fig. 5.7 Blood film from a Melanesian with hereditary macro-ovalocytosis. Macro-ovalocytes and stomatocytes are present.

May–Grünwald–Giemsa stain   × 940

the anaemia.[28] However, the anaemia may be severe, with reticulocyte counts up to 40%. The diagnostic feature is that 10–40% of the erythrocytes are stomatocytes: these are cells with a mouth-like slit instead of the usual circular zone of central pallor. The stomatocytes show an increased intracellular Na^+, decreased intracellular K^+, increased water content and increased osmotic fragility. The primary defect is still uncertain but appears to be an inherited abnormality in a membrane protein; affected patients may be homozygous for the abnormality.

Stomatocytosis may also be seen in the Rh null phenotype[7] and as an acquired condition[6] (see Table 5.1 and Fig. 5.2b).

Abnormalities of red cell enzymes[29, 30]

The mature red cell oxidizes most of the glucose entering it via the anaerobic glycolytic (Embden-Meyerhof) pathway (Fig. 5.8) and the remainder (less than 10%) via the pentose phosphate shunt (Fig. 5.9). The oxidation of 1 mol of glucose by the Embden–Meyerhof pathway results in the production of 2 mol of ATP and 2 mol of pyruvate and also in the generation of NADH. The ATP generated in this way plays an important role in maintaining the structural integrity of the cell: it controls the intracellular cation and water content by regulating the ATPase-dependent cation pump located in the cell membrane and also

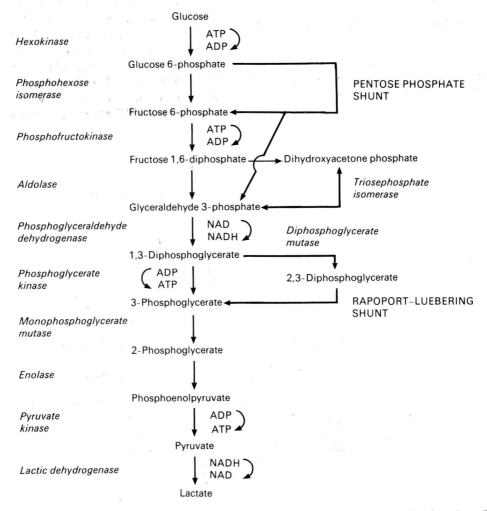

Fig. 5.8 The Embden–Meyerhof pathway of anaerobic glycolysis and its relationships to the pentose phosphate shunt (Fig. 5.9) and the Rapoport–Luebering shunt.

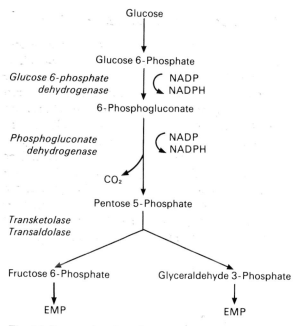

Fig. 5.9 Pentose phosphate shunt and its relationship to the Embden–Meyerhof pathway (EMP).

maintains membrane flexibility and cell shape. The NADH serves as a coenzyme for the enzyme diaphorase (NADH-dependent methaemoglobin reductase) which is concerned with reversing the constant tendency of haemoglobin to be oxidized to methaemoglobin. The special feature of the pentose phosphate shunt is that for each mol of glucose metabolized via this shunt, 2 mol of NADPH are formed. NADPH is the preferred cofactor for the enzyme glutathione reductase which maintains the tripeptide glutathione in a reduced form (Fig. 5.10). Reduced glutathione protects the -SH groups of the proteins of the red cell against oxidation and thereby maintains the normal function of membrane proteins, enzymes and haemoglobin. Reduced glutathione also inactivates small quantities of hydrogen peroxide by a reaction which is catalyzed by the enzyme glutathione peroxidase. During both these reactions the reduced glutathione becomes oxidized. A large number of enzymes are involved in the metabolic pathways concerned with the generation of ATP, reduction of methaemoglobin

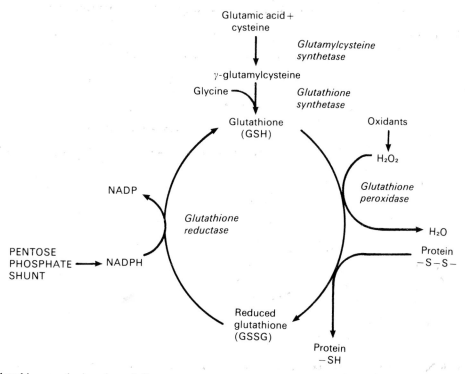

Fig. 5.10 Glutathione synthesis and metabolism.

and generation of reduced glutathione and a deficiency of any of several of these enzymes has been shown to cause haemolytic anaemia.

Glucose 6-phosphate dehydrogenase deficiency[31, 32]

Glucose 6-phosphate dehydrogenase (G6PD) catalyzes the first step of the pentose phosphate shunt and a deficiency of this enzyme constitutes the commonest metabolic defect of red cells. The usual form of the enzyme with normal activity is designated as type B. A second form with normal activity, designated type A, is present in some individuals of African ancestry and this differs from type B in one amino acid. The gene for G6PD is on the X chromosome and a deficiency of G6PD is therefore inherited as a sex-linked characteristic. Although over 250 variants of G6PD have been described, more than 95% of the cases affected by G6PD deficiency have either the A⁻ (the African type) or the Mediterranean types; not all of the remaining types cause clinical disease. It has been estimated that there are over 100 million people with a reduced red cell G6PD level in the world; for example, the deficiency affects about 10% of American Blacks and West Africans (A⁻ type), 3–35% of Sardinians (Mediterranean type) and 15–40% of Kurds (Mediterranean type). The deficiency is also found in several other countries around the Mediterranean, in the Middle East, India, Southern China, Thailand and Malaysia. G6PD deficiency is most common in hemizygous males but is also seen in homozygous females. Heterozygous females may occasionally have clinical manifestations. The G6PD activity in red cells of affected males is reduced to 8–20% of normal in the A⁻ type and to less than 5% in the Mediterranean type. This difference may account for the fact that when anaemia develops, it tends to be more severe and more persistent in those with the latter type. Reduced levels of G6PD activity lead to a failure to generate NADPH which is required to maintain the glutathione of red cells in a reduced state. Low levels of reduced gluthathione make red cell proteins susceptible to oxidation (see preceding paragraph) and under certain circumstances (mentioned below), lead to the formation within red cells of masses of denatured globin (Heinz

bodies) which become attached to the cell membrane probably by disulphide bridges. These Heinz bodies, which hinder the passage of red cells through the spleen, are pitted (together with the associated cell membrane) by splenic macrophages. The inclusion-free red cells so formed have 'damaged' membranes and are believed to undergo predominantly extravascular haemolysis. Marked oxidation of components of the cell membrane may also occur and cause intravascular haemolysis.

Most patients with G6PD deficiency have no significant haematological abnormalities except when suffering from bacterial or viral infections or following treatment with certain, presumably oxidant, drugs. A list of these drugs is given in Table 5.6. Acute intravascular and extravascular

Table 5.6 Some agents reported to cause haemolysis in some G6PD-deficient subjects[33]

Antibacterial drugs	Antimalarials
Sulphonamides	Aminoquinolines
Sulphanilamide	Primaquine
Sulphacetamide	Pamaquin
Sulphafurazole	Chloroquine★
(sulphisoxazole)	Pentaquine
Sulphasalazine	Quinine★
Sulphamethoxypyridazine	
	Analgesics
Nitrofurans	Aspirin (high dose)
Nitrofurantoin	Phenacetin
Furazolidone	Acetanilide
Nitrofurazone	
Nalidixic acid	*Others*
Chloramphenicol★	Vitamin K (water soluble
Aminosalicylates	analogues)
Sulphones (e.g. dapsone)	Naphthalene
	Probenecid
	Dimercaprol (BAL)
	Methylene blue
	Acetylphenylhydrazine
	Neoarsphenamine
	Quinidine★

★ Not shown to cause haemolysis in Blacks

haemolysis of moderate severity, sometimes causing acute renal failure or death, may develop within a few days of starting the drug. In most patients with the A⁻ variant, the haemolytic episode is self-limiting and the haemoglobin level starts to rise after about 10 days, despite continuation of the drug. This is because the cells destroyed following drug exposure are the older cells with the lowest G6PD activities and the reticulocytes and young red cells formed after a haemolytic episode have relatively high enzyme activities and are therefore resistant to the drug. Shortly after a haemolytic episode, when the reticulocyte count is high, the G6PD level may be normal. During the early stages of a haemolytic crisis, the red cells contain Heinz bodies which can be demonstrated by staining with a supravital dye such as methyl violet for about 10 min. Subsequently the only special feature in the blood may be the presence of some small, irregularly-shaped, densely-staining cells with empty spaces beneath parts of the cell membrane (Fig. 5.11).

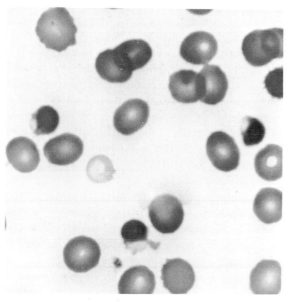

Fig. 5.11 Blood film from a patient with G6PD deficiency who developed drug-induced haemolysis. There are three irregularly-shaped, densely-staining red cells with an 'empty' area just beneath part of the cell membrane ('bite cells').

May–Grünwald–Giemsa stain   × 940

In addition to developing drug-induced haemolysis, patients with the Mediterranean type of G6PD deficiency may rapidly develop severe haemolysis after eating the broad bean, *Vicia fava*, or, rarely, after inhaling its pollen; this phenomenon is known as favism.

In Greece, Thailand and China, G6PD deficiency has been reported to be associated with and possibly responsible for many cases of severe neonatal jaundice. In these cases, kernicterus has been a common complication when exchange transfusions were not given. Curiously the blood picture returns to normal after the neonatal period. Rarely G6PD deficiency (due to an unusual enzyme variant) may cause a chronic non-spherocytic haemolytic anaemia in infancy and childhood, sometimes with splenomegaly and gall stones. The chronic haemolysis is further exacerbated by infections and oxidant drugs.

G6PD-deficient patients have some degree of protection against *Plasmodium falciparum* malaria.

Pyruvate kinase deficiency[34, 35]

Pyruvate kinase catalyses the conversion of phosphoenolpyruvate to pyruvate in the last step of the Embden–Meyerhof pathway; this conversion is associated with the generation of ATP which, as has been mentioned, is vital for the maintenance of the structural and functional integrity of the red cell. Compared with G6PD deficiency, pyruvate kinase deficiency is rare. It may present as neonatal jaundice or congenital non-spherocytic haemolytic anaemia with mild to moderate splenomegaly. The incidence of gall stones is increased; leg ulcers are rare. The clinical severity varies considerably from case to case and the diagnosis may be made any time from infancy onwards; haemoglobin levels are usually between 5 and 12 g/dl. The blood film shows no specific abnormality but if splenectomy is performed red cell morphology may become very abnormal, with numerous acanthocytes and thin macrocytes. The efficiency of tissue oxygenation may be considerably better than that suggested by the haemoglobin level as there may be a substantial decrease in the oxygen affinity of the haemoglobin as the result of an increase in the intracellular level of 2,3-diphosphoglycerate, one of the intermediary metabolites in the glycolytic pathway. The disorder is inherited as an autosomal recessive character and clinically affected patients are homozygotes for a functionally-abnormal variant of pyruvate kinase or, more commonly, double heterozygotes for two abnormal variants. Heterozygotes have levels of enzyme activity between those seen in homozygotes and normal individuals and do not usually suffer from haemolysis.

Other enzyme deficiencies[36]

A deficiency of any one of a number of red cell enzymes other than glucose 6-phosphate dehydrogenase or pyruvate kinase has been shown to account for spontaneous or drug-induced chronic haemolysis, usually in a very occasional patient. These enzymes are listed in Table 5.7. A deficiency of some of the enzymes is associated with

Table 5.7 Red cell enzyme deficiencies associated with chronic haemolysis

Embden–Meyerhof pathway
Hexokinase
Phosphohexose isomerase
Phosphofructokinase*
Aldolase*
Triosephosphate isomerase*
Phosphoglyceraldehyde dehydrogenase
Diphosphoglycerate mutase
Phosphoglycerate kinase
Pyruvate kinase

Pentose monophosphate shunt and glutathione metabolism
Glucose 6-phosphate dehydrogenase
γ-L-glutamylcysteine synthetase*
Glutathione synthetase
Glutathione reductase

Nucleotide metabolism
Adenylate kinase
Pyrimidine 5′-nucleotidase

* Associated with neurological symptoms

peculiar neurological symptoms and the deficiency of phosphofructokinase may be associated with severe muscle dysfunction. Pyrimidine 5′-nucleotidase deficiency presents as a congenital non-spherocytic haemolytic anaemia with basophilic stippling of a substantial proportion of circulating red cells and may be relatively common.

Abnormalities of the structure or synthesis of haemoglobin[37, 38]

There are three types of haemoglobin in an adult and all of them consist of four peptide (globin) chains per molecule; each globin chain is associated with a single haem group (see p. 6). Over 95% of the haemoglobin of a normal adult consists of haemoglobin A (HbA) which has two α-chains made up of 141 amino acids per chain and two β-chains made up of 146 amino acids per chain; HbA is therefore designated $\alpha_2\beta_2$. Between 1.5 and 3.4% (mean 2.5%) of the haemoglobin of an adult consists of HbA$_2$ which is composed of two α chains and two δ chains ($\alpha_2\delta_2$). The remainder (less than 1% of the total) consists of fetal haemoglobin (HbF) which consists of two α chains and two γ chains ($\alpha_2\gamma_2$). HbF molecules contain two types of γ chains which differ only in the amino acid at position 136, which may be either glycine ($^G\gamma$) or alanine ($^A\gamma$). Although very little HbF is synthesized in normal adults, HbF is the predominant type of haemoglobin synthesized during fetal life (after 8-10 weeks of gestation). The small quantity of HbF produced in most normal adults appears to be unevenly distributed within 0.5-7% of the erythrocytes (the HbF-containing cells are known as F-cells).

The information determining the order of the amino acids in the different globin chains is contained in the base sequence in the DNA of the corresponding structural genes. The structural genes coding for the synthesis of α chains are found on chromosome 16 and, in most populations, are duplicated so that there are four α genes in each diploid somatic cell. The genes coding for the non-α chains are closely linked on chromosome 11, in the order $^G\gamma-^A\gamma-\delta-\beta$. The gene coding for the γ chain is also duplicated but, unlike the duplicated α genes which are identical, the duplicated γ genes differ in one base triplet (codon). Each structural gene produces a high molecular weight precursor of its messenger RNA, known as heterogeneous nuclear RNA (HnRNA); this precursor is modified, probably within the nucleus, to produce the smaller 'mature' messenger RNA (mRNA). Globin chain synthesis occurs within the cytoplasm through an interaction of the mRNA with ribosomes, transfer RNAs and a number of cofactors.

Inherited disorders of haemoglobin can be divided into two main groups. In the first group there is an alteration in the amino acid sequence of a globin chain, usually due to a single amino acid substitution (resulting from the substitution of a single base in the genetic code). In the second group there is a depression of the rate of synthesis of one of the globin chains. In this group, which is collectively known as the thalassaemia syndromes, the amino acid sequences of the globin chains that are synthesized are usually normal. However, in some patients the thalassaemic picture results from the presence of a structurally-abnormal globin chain which is synthesized at a reduced rate (e.g. Hb Constant Spring and Hb Lepore) or of an abnormal haemoglobin which is markedly unstable (e.g. Hb Indianapolis).

Structural haemoglobin variants [37,38]

Over 250 structural variants of human haemoglobin have now been described but only a small number of these result in clinical and haematological manifestations. Most structural variants have a single amino acid substitution in the affected globin chain due to a single-point mutation affecting one base triplet (codon) in the corresponding globin gene (e.g. HbS, HbE, HbC and HbD). Occasionally the single-point mutation affects the stop codon, the base triplet which terminates the transcription of a gene into mRNA. When this happens in the α-globin gene an abnormally long α chain is produced with extra amino acids at the end of a normal α chain (e.g. in Hb Constant Spring, Hb Icaria, Hb Koya Dora, Hb Seal Rock). Other structural variants result from deletions (loss) of one or more base triplets with the consequent loss of one or more amino acids in a globin chain or from the insertion of extra base triplets leading to the presence of extra amino acids within a chain; the changes in the DNA presumably occur by abnormal crossing-over during meiosis. A few variants contain hybrid chains made of parts of δ and β chains (in Lepore and anti-Lepore haemoglobins) or γ

and β chains (in Hb Kenya). The latter are formed from δβ, βδ or γβ fusion genes which seem to originate by unequal crossing-over during meiosis. Finally, some variants (e.g. Hb Wayne, Hb Tak and Hb Cranston) are caused by 'frame shift' mutations in the region of a globin gene coding for the C-terminal residues. In this type of mutation, there is a loss of a single base in a base triplet so that the first base of the succeeding triplet is read with the affected triplet and the reading of the genetic code from that triplet onwards becomes out-of-phase and results in an amino acid sequence which is quite different from normal, with extra amino acids in the affected globin chain.

Many structural haemoglobin variants are not associated with any clinical or haematological abnormalities. The clinical and haematological disturbances which may be caused by certain structural haemoglobin variants are: (1) haemolysis and recurrent painful crises due to sickling of red cells on deoxygenation (e.g. HbS; see p. 126); (2) haemolytic anaemia due to decreased red cell deformability as a consequence of the insolubility of the deoxygenated haemoglobin variant compared with deoxy HbA (e.g. HbC; see p. 132); (3) spontaneous or drug-induced haemolytic anaemia due to the instability of the abnormal haemoglobin causing its intracellular precipitation (see p. 134); (4) congenital methaemoglobinaemia (and cyanosis) when the substitution occurs near or in the haem pocket (e.g. HbM Boston or HbM Saskatoon); (5) hereditary polycythaemia due to an increased oxygen affinity of the abnormal haemoglobin (e.g. Hb Chesapeake; see also Table 5.21); (6) anaemia and cyanosis due to a decreased oxygen affinity (e.g. Hb Kansas); (7) a thalassaemia-like syndrome due to a decreased rate of synthesis of the abnormal globin chain (e.g. Hb Constant Spring, Hb Tak, Hb Lepore and HbE), or due to marked instability of an abnormal haemoglobin (Hb Indianapolis or Hb Quong Sze); and (8) various combinations of the above (e.g. Hb Köln and Hb Brisbane not only show instability but also have a high oxygen affinity; Hb Hammersmith is unstable and has a low affinity). HbM Boston and HbM Saskatoon referred to above have low and high oxygen affinities, respectively.

Haemoglobin S

In this haemoglobin, glutamic acid at position 6 of the β-globin chain is replaced by valine. The sickle cell gene is found in most parts of tropical Africa. Its prevalence in Central and West Africa varies between about 10 and 30% and in East Africa between 0 and 40%. The gene frequency in Southern Africa is low (0–2%) except in Zambia and parts of Zimbabwe. The gene for HbS is also found in Greece (0–30%), Sicily (4%), Turkey (10–20%), Arabia (0–25%) and India (3–40%). The average prevalence of the sickle cell gene in the Caribbean and in American Blacks is about 8%. The distribution of the HbS gene corresponds to the areas of the world in which *Plasmodium falciparum* malaria is or has been endemic. The persistence of the HbS gene in high frequency in these areas has been attributed to the relative resistance of heterozygous children to severe infection with this type of malaria.

Deoxygenated HbS is about 50 times less soluble than deoxygenated HbA and, under appropriate conditions, forms long fibres (tactoids) (Fig. 5.12) which deform the red cell and give it a characteristic sickle shape (Fig. 5.13). Red cells from both heterozygotes and homozygotes for the HbS gene can be induced to sickle *in vitro* by the addition of reducing agents such as sodium metabisulphite. Sickling occurs *in vivo* in homozygotes but not usually in heterozygotes.

Sickle cell trait. Individuals with one HbA gene and one HbS gene are said to have the sickle cell trait. Their red cells contain 25–45% HbS and 55–75% HbA and do not sickle until the Po_2 is reduced to 15 mmHg or less. As this level of Po_2 is not usually achieved *in vivo*, the vast majority of cases of sickle cell trait are asymptomatic. However, cases of the trait will develop sickling crises (see section on sickle cell anaemia) if subjected to severe hypoxia such as may occur with flight in unpressurized aircraft to an altitude of approximately 3000 m. Splenic infarction has also occurred in association with marked

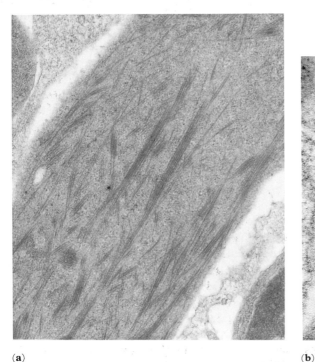

(a)

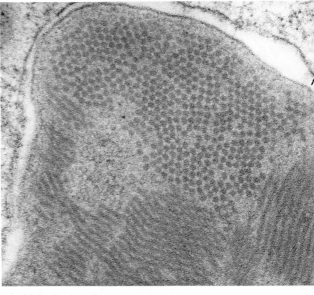

(b)

Fig. 5.12a, b Electron micrographs of two red cells from the bone marrow of a patient homozygous for haemoglobin S. The cell profiles contain fibres of polymerized deoxyhaemoglobin S, many of which have been sectioned longitudinally in (a) and transversely in (b). Uranyl acetate and lead citrate.

(a) × 29 150; (b) × 97 175

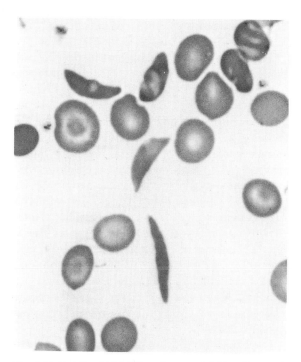

Fig. 5.13 Peripheral blood film of a case of sickle cell anaemia. Sickle cells and target cells are present.

May–Grünwald–Giemsa stain × 940

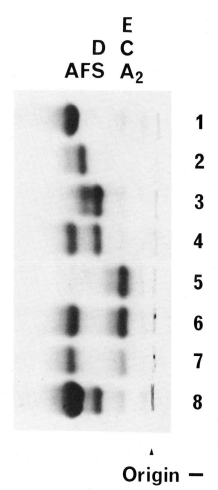

Fig. 5.14 Cellulose acetate electrophoresis (pH 8.5) of haemolysates from the following: (1) normal adult; (2) normal neonate (cord blood); (3) sickle cell anaemia (with 20% HbF); (4) sickle cell trait; (5) homozygous HbC disease; (6) HbC trait; (7) HbE trait; (8) HbD trait. HbE has the same electrophoretic mobility as HbC and HbO Arab. HbD Punjab and Hb Lepore have the same mobility as HbS. HbE can be distinguished from HbC, and HbD Punjab from HbS by electrophoresis in citrate agar at pH 6.0 (Fig. 5.15). HbD Punjab and Hb Lepore do not cause sickling of red cells.

fever.[39] Many older individuals with the sickle cell trait have an impaired ability to concentrate urine. Furthermore, the trait may sometimes cause haematuria. Rarely renal papillary necrosis develops. During pregnancy the incidence of bacteriuria and pyelonephritis is increased in comparison with controls. Other rare associations are central retinal artery occlusion and priapism. An association with rhabdomyolysis and acute renal failure[40] and with sudden death[41] following vigorous exertion at altitude has been suspected. Cases of sickle cell trait have normal haemoglobin levels, MCVs and reticulocyte counts and usually have perfectly normal-looking blood films. However, occasional cases show a few target cells. The diagnosis requires the demonstration of a positive haemoglobin solubility test ('Sickledex test') and is confirmed by haemoglobin electrophoresis which shows both HbA and HbS with more HbA than HbS (Figs 5.14 and 5.15).

Sickle cell anaemia.[42,43] Individuals with this disorder are homozygous for the HbS gene, hav-ing inherited one HbS gene from each parent. Their red cells contain mainly HbS, usually with about 5% but sometimes with up to 20% HbF. There is no HbA (Figs 5.14 and 5.15). The red cells contain sufficient HbS for sickling to take place at the Po_2 found in tissue capillaries *in vivo*. Dehydration, acidosis and fever are thought to facilitate sickling *in vivo*. Initially, the sickling process reverses when the cells enter the arterial

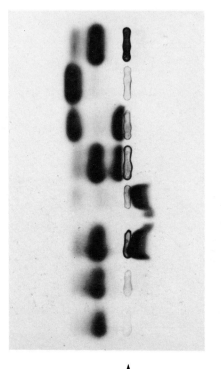

E
D
A₂
F A S C

1

2

3

4

5

6

7

8

▲

—   **Origin**   **+**

Fig. 5.15 Citrate agar electrophoresis (pH 6.0) of haemolysates from the following: (1) normal adult; (2) normal neonate (cord blood); (3) sickle cell anaemia (with 20% HbF); (4) sickle cell trait; (5) homozygous HbC disease; (6) HbC trait; (7) HbE trait; (8) HbD trait. HbE has the same electrophoretic mobility as HbA. HbD Punjab runs very slightly more slowly than HbA.

circulation (with a high P_{O_2}), but eventually irreversibly sickled cells (with irreversibly deformed membranes) are formed. The clinical manifestations of sickle cell anaemia result from the sickling of red cells *in vivo* leading to chronic haemolytic anaemia and recurrent episodes of tissue infarction. The haemolytic anaemia is caused by a decreased deformability of sickled red cells (and of unsickled cells containing polymerized deoxy HbS[44]) which culminates in both extravascular and intravascular haemolysis. The

tissue infarction is caused by obstruction of small or medium-sized vessels by sickled cells.

The severity of the symptoms associated with sickle cell anaemia varies markedly in different patients and some patients may merely have a moderate haemolytic anaemia with few or no infarctive episodes. The factors responsible for this variation are not fully understood; patients with a high percentage of HbF are usually mildly affected. When high HbF levels are present, this may sometimes be due to the inheritance of a gene for the hereditary persistence of HbF (HPFH gene) (p. 143). Neonates have high levels of HbF and relatively little HbS and are therefore asymptomatic. Symptoms usually begin after the first six months of life when the HbF levels have fallen considerably. Coexistence of an α-thalassaemia gene may also reduce the severity of sickle cell anaemia probably by causing a decrease of the MCHC.

The haemoglobin usually varies between 6 and 9 g/dl. However, as HbS has a low oxygen affinity, the degree of tissue hypoxia is less than that suggested by the haemoglobin level. The reticulocyte count is raised (10–20%) and some erythroblasts may be present in the circulation. The MCV may be normal or raised (see p. 115). The blood film shows target cells and varying numbers of poikilocytes. The latter may be banana-shaped with rounded ends or typical sickle cells with pointed ends (Fig 5.13). There is usually a neutrophil leucocytosis. The platelet count is normal or elevated. Many patients eventually display features of hyposplenism (i.e. Howell-Jolly bodies and increased numbers of both target cells and circulating erythroblasts). The red cell life-span is about 10–15 days ($T_{\frac{1}{2}}$Cr, 8–12 d). The bone marrow shows gross erythroid hyperplasia and this may cause skeletal deformities (see p. 117 and Fig 5.4). Bone marrow hyperplasia in vertebrae may be sufficient to reduce mechanical strength and cause partial vertebral collapse. Red haemopoietic marrow is present in marrow cavities that are usually non-haemopoietic (e.g. shafts of the femora). Histological sections may show sickle-shaped red cells and sludging of red cells within marrow sinusoids. Extramedullary haemopoiesis may be present.

Rarely the haemoglobin level may fall rapidly

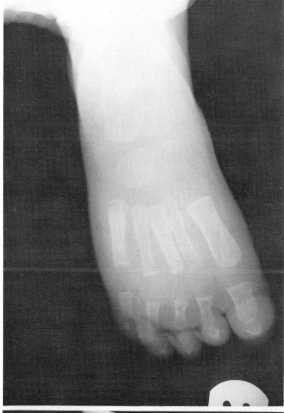

(a)

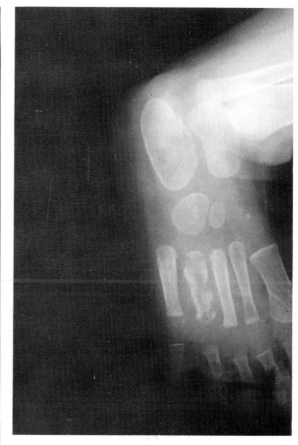

(b)

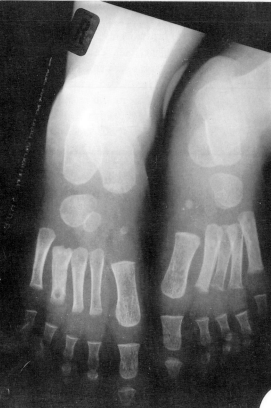

(c)

Fig. 5.16a–c X-ray appearances of the right foot of a 10-month-old infant with sickle cell anaemia who developed the hand-foot syndrome. (**a**) Radiograph after 2 weeks of fever and swelling of hands and feet. No radiological changes are evident. (**b**) X-ray repeated 2 weeks after that shown in (**a**), at a time when the swelling of the hands and feet had subsided. There is necrosis of the right fourth metatarsal. (**c**) Radiograph taken 6 weeks after that shown in (**b**). There is a remarkable degree of regeneration of the right fourth metatarsal. However, the structure is a little sclerotic and the shaft a little thickened when compared with the corresponding bone in the left foot.

Courtesy of Professor T.E. Oppé, Department of Paediatrics, St Mary's Hospital Medical School, London, UK.

due to a secondary folate deficiency (see p. 179) or a transient pure red cell hypoplasia (see p. 190). A high proportion of episodes of red cell aplasia appear to be due to infection by a parvo virus.[45] In young children whose spleens have not yet atrophied a sudden fall of Hb may be due to sequestration of red cells in the spleen.

Different tissues are particularly prone to infarction at different ages. Children between the ages of 6 months and 5 years tend to suffer from infarction of the bones of the hands and feet (hand-foot syndrome) (Fig 5.16). This may be followed by short metacarpals, metatarsals and phalanges due to failure of growth of infarcted bones. The characteristic 'painful crises' usually begin between the ages of 5 and 15 years. They usually consist of attacks of pain, often severe, particularly in the limbs, back, chest and abdomen. The pain probably arises from multiple microinfarcts in joints, bones and bone marrow. The crises are acute in onset and are accompanied by low-grade fever and increased numbers of leucocytes and irreversibly sickled cells in the blood. Infarction of bone marrow may be followed by embolization of necrotic bone marrow to the lungs; this complication has an increased likelihood during pregnancy (possibly attributable to further hyperplasia of the bone marrow during pregnancy) and may cause death (see p. 94). Large infarcts may also occur in many sites. Older children and adults may suffer from segmental avascular necrosis of the heads of the femora or humeri and of the diaphyses of long bones. Vertebral necrosis and collapse may occur. Patients with sickle cell anaemia may also suffer from various lung and cerebral syndromes due to pulmonary and cerebral infarction. These include a pneumonia-like picture, chronic restrictive lung disease, pulmonary hypertension and cor pulmonale,[46] and hemiplegia, convulsions and coma. Infarction of the retina may cause proliferative lesions and repeated vitreous haemorrhages. Venous obstruction in the corpora cavernosa may cause recurrent and severe priapism.

Chronic leg ulcers may develop over the malleoli (Fig 5.17).

Splenomegaly is common under the age of 5 years, but becomes progressively less frequent

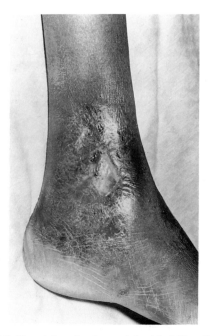

Fig. 5.17 Chronic leg ulcer in an adult with sickle cell anaemia. Note the increased pigmentation of the skin around the ulcer.

thereafter due to increasing fibrosis resulting from recurrent infarction; it occurs in less than 10% of adults. Occasionally, infants and small children with enlarged spleens suffer from the 'splenic sequestration syndrome' in which a marked increase in splenic enlargement and severe anaemia result from the sudden and massive trapping of red cells within the splenic sinusoids. Hypovolaemic shock and death may occur within a few hours. Sequestration in the liver may also occur.

There is an increased susceptibility to infections which appears to be due to a defect of opsonization as well as to hyposplenism secondary to autosplenectomy. Pneumococcal sepsis (meningitis, pneumonia, septicaemia) is an important cause of mortality. Salmonella osteomyelitis is common in some parts of the world, probably being due to proliferation of salmonellae in infarcted tissue.

There is impairment of renal function from early childhood. This impairment can be initially corrected by blood transfusion but becomes irreversible in later life. Haematuria due to papillary necrosis may occur. Renal lesions include not only complications of vascular obstruction (focal scarring, glomerular sclerosis, interstitial fibrosis and papillary necrosis) but also proliferative glomerular lesions. There is mesangial hyperplasia and hypertrophy with electron-dense deposits in the mesangium, focal fusion of foot processes and duplication of the glomerular basement membrane. The nephrotic syndrome may occur. Haemosiderin deposition may be marked in the proximal convoluted tubules. Chronic renal failure is an important cause of death in adults.

Cardiomegaly and flow murmurs are usually present. Subclinical ventricular dysfunction is frequently present, as judged by echocardiography and systolic time intervals.[47] However, death due to congestive cardiac failure is uncommon, often being secondary to complications such as renal hypertension, cor pulmonale or renal failure with pericarditis. At autopsy,[47] the weight of the heart may be increased and both ventricles may be hypertrophied and dilated. The myocardium may appear pale and flabby. Histological findings are usually unimpressive and include vacuolation of myocardial cells, interstitial oedema and, rarely, microfocal fibrosis and haemosiderosis. There may be some degree of haemosiderosis of other organs, even in patients who have been given few or no transfusions.

The chronic haemolysis is associated with an increased incidence of gall stones, the incidence being higher in American than African cases.[48] Various pathological lesions may be seen in the liver.[49] Hepatomegaly is a common finding. Erythrophagocytosis by Kupffer cells may be very prominent. Intrahepatic cholestasis may occur. Patients who survive into the third and fourth decades may develop micronodular or macronodular cirrhosis; cirrhosis is related to iron overload as well as to fibrosis following infarction. Some patients develop liver failure.

Males may be subfertile with a reduction of sperm density and motility and an increase in morphologically abnormal forms.[50]

Pregnancy increases the frequency of sickling crises. In addition, sickle cell anaemia has an adverse effect on the outcome of pregnancy;[51,52,53] stillbirths and neonatal deaths have been reported in 13–22% of pregnancies. Surviving babies may be of low birth weight due to placental insufficiency. Some but not all studies have shown that there is also an increased early fetal loss from abortions.

The prognosis of sickle cell anaemia appears to depend both on environmental factors and on the standard of health care available. A high proportion of patients living in rural Africa die during infancy and childhood so that relatively few patients survive to adult life. This early mortality appears to be much less marked in patients living in the Caribbean and USA where the proportion dying in the first two years of life has been estimated to be 13–14%.[54] The most frequent causes of death in infants and young children are meningitis and other infections (including malaria) and the splenic sequestration syndrome.

Haemoglobin SC disease. Some individuals who are heterozygous for both HbS and HbC are asymptomatic. Others have symptoms similar to those in mildly or moderately affected cases of sickle cell anaemia. About 60% of adult patients have splenomegaly. Ocular complications are more common than in sickle cell anaemia. The incidence of large bone infarcts seems to be the same as in sickle cell anaemia, but fatal bone marrow embolism appears to be much commoner, particularly in pregnancy. Some cases live a normal life-span. The haemoglobin level is usually in the range 10.0–13.5 g/dl and the reticulocyte count varies between about 1.5 and 5.0%. The blood film shows many target cells but few or no irreversibly sickled cells. Most of the haemoglobin consists of HbS and HbC, in roughly equal quantities. The red cell survival is moderately reduced.

Sickle cell β-thalassaemia. This results from the inheritance of an HbS gene from one parent and a β-thalassaemia gene (either β^+ or β^0) from the other. The clinical course varies markedly; some cases are asymptomatic and others have the features of moderately severe sickle cell anaemia. Splenomegaly occurs in over half the adults. Most of the haemoglobin consists of HbS. Patients with the β^+ gene have 15–30% HbA and generally run a more benign course than those with the β^0 gene who have no HbA. Haemoglobin F levels do not differ in the two types being about

5-6% (range, 0.5-20%). The haemoglobin levels and MCVs tend to be higher and the reticulocyte counts lower in those with the β^+ gene (the HbA type) than those with the β^0 gene (the non-HbA type). The abnormalities in the blood film include microcytosis, hypochomia, anisocytosis, poikilocytosis, target cells and sickled cells but the severity of these changes varies markedly from case to case. The reticulocyte count is usually raised and in the range 3-20%. The bone marrow shows erythroid hyperplasia and poor haemoglobinization of the cytoplasm. Electron microscopy reveals intracellular α-chain precipitates in the late polychromatic erythroblasts and marrow reticulocytes, the extent of precipitation being similar to that in heterozygous β-thalassaemia.

Haemoglobin C trait and homozygous haemoglobin C disease

Haemoglobin C ($\alpha_2\beta_2^{6Glu \rightarrow Lys}$) is frequently found in West Africans and is present in 2-3% of American Blacks. The proportion of individuals with HbC is 22% in Northern Ghana, 9% in Southern Ghana and 7% in Nigeria. Individuals with HbC trait (i.e. heterozygotes for the HbC gene) are asymptomatic and have no anaemia. They have 6-40% (mean, 20%) target cells in their blood (Fig. 5.18) and 30-40% HbC (Figs 5.14 and 5.15). Individuals with homozygous HbC disease[55] are usually asymptomatic but may have intermittent episodes of abdominal discomfort or pain, poorly-localized arthralgia without overt arthritis, and mild jaundice. Occasional cases have suffered from haematuria, haemoptysis, epistaxis and bilateral periorbital haemorrhage. Virtually all homozygotes have splenomegaly. They usually have a mild anaemia but may develop severe anaemia during pregnancy. The MCV is low (in the range 55-80 fl) in about 70% of cases. The blood film shows 10-90% (mean, 50%) target cells and some dense poikilocytes (irregularly contracted cells) (Fig. 5.19). Occasional red cells with rhomboidal crystals of HbC are present particularly after splenectomy. The

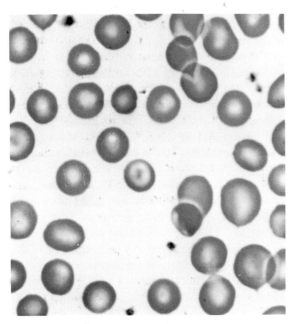

Fig. 5.18 Blood film of an individual with haemoglobin C trait showing an occasional target cell.

May-Grünwald-Giemsa stain   × 940

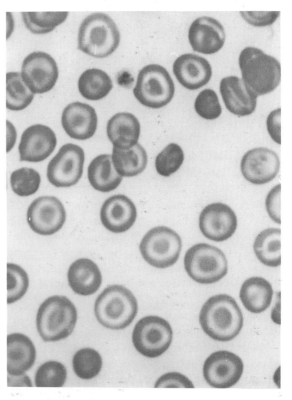

Fig. 5.19 Blood film of a patient with homozygous haemoglobin C disease showing numerous target cells and some dense, irregularly-contracted red cells.

May-Grünwald-Giemsa stain   × 940

reticulocyte count is sometimes raised but is usually less than 6%. Most of the haemoglobin consists of HbC (Figs 5.14 and 5.15). The serum bilirubin is slightly raised (17–34 μmol/l) in some cases. The marrow shows erythroid hyperplasia and some of the polychromatic erythroblasts show indistinct or ragged nuclear outlines. Electron microscopy reveals prominent dyserythropoietic changes. The characteristic finding is the occurrence of substantial numbers of polychromatic erythroblasts in which the nuclei are grossly disorganized, with extensive intranuclear clefts, loss of parts of the nuclear membrane, oozing of nuclear material into the cytoplasm and alterations in both the structure and electron-density of the nuclear chromatin (Fig. 5.20).

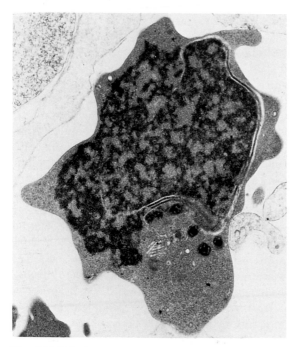

Fig. 5.20 Polychromatic erythroblast from a homozygote for haemoglobin C, showing multiple long intranuclear clefts, loss of part of the nuclear membrane and a peculiar abnormality of the appearance of the nuclear chromatin (compare with normal erythroblast in Fig. 3.8).

Uranyl acetate and lead citrate × 14 825

The anaemia is due to a combination of peripheral haemolysis[56, 57] ($T_\frac{1}{2}$ Cr, 19–24 d) and increased ineffectiveness of erythropoiesis.[58] The peripheral haemolysis is caused by two mechanisms. Firstly, the red cells of homozygotes are less deformable than normal because deoxygenated HbC exists in very small aggregates. Secondly, intracellular crystals of HbC tend to form within erythrocytes (at Hb concentrations greater than 45 g/dl) and these crystal-containing cells are removed by the spleen. The mechanisms underlying the dyserythropoiesis and ineffective erythropoiesis are uncertain.

Haemoglobin E trait and homozygous haemoglobin E disease[59, 60]

HbE ($\alpha_2\beta_2^{26Glu \rightarrow Lys}$) is very common in South-East Asia, its prevalence approaching or exceeding 50% in many areas. The gene for HbE is thought to be present in 30×10^6 people. Individuals who are heterozygous for the HbE gene are asymptomatic. They are usually not anaemic but display the haematological features of mild thalassaemia. All of them have a low MCV (59–78 fl) and about half have a mild erythrocytosis. The blood film shows microcytosis, occasional densely-staining poikilocytes and, sometimes, a few target cells. The level of HbE ($+$HbA$_2$) is 21–33% (Figs 5.14 and 5.15). Homozygotes for the HbE gene are mildly anaemic and may have erythrocytosis. They have a low MCV, many target cells and some dense poikilocytes. There is no HbA produced; virtually all of the haemoglobin is HbE. The microcytosis found in individuals with HbE appears to be caused by inefficient production of mRNA for the β^E chain due to the presence of an alternative splicing site in the primary transcript (i.e. in HnRNA for β^E chains). This leads to imbalance in globin chain synthesis and, in homozygotes, to the intraerythroblastic precipitation of α chains. The extent of this precipitation is similar to that seen in heterozygous β-thalassaemia. The bone marrow of homozygotes shows erythroid hyperplasia.

Haemoglobin E/β-thalassaemia[60]

Patients with this disorder have a variable degree of anaemia (Hb, 2–11 g/dl; mean, 6.4 g/dl) and usually suffer from the clinical and haematological features of thalassaemia intermedia or (less frequently) of thalassaemia major (see p. 140 and Fig. 5.30b). As β^E chains are synthesized inefficiently, the interaction between the HbE gene and a β-thalassaemia gene leads to considerable chain imbalance, precipitation of α chains within early and late polychromatic erythroblasts and a marked increase of ineffective erythropoiesis. The ultrastructure of the bone marrow and the pathophysiology of the anaemia are similar to that in homozygous β-thalassaemia.[61]

Unstable haemoglobins[62]

A number of amino acid substitutions and some deletions (affecting either the α or β chain) result in instability and intraerythrocytic precipitation of haemoglobin molecules. Some substitutions and the deletions generate instability by distorting the tertiary structure of the globin molecule and causing increased dissociation of the tetrameric haemoglobin into its subunits. Other substitutions (i.e. those affecting amino acids in the haem pocket) cause instability by leading to the loss of haem from the affected globin subunits. The precipitated haemoglobin forms inclusions (Heinz bodies) which bind to the red cell membrane probably by disulphide bridges. The spleen removes these inclusions by a 'pitting' action and releases the inclusion-free cells back into the circulation. The process of pitting leads to a reduced MCH and MCHC as well as to membrane damage and the latter causes a shortening of red cell life-span. Examples of some unstable haemoglobins are listed in Table 5.8. The degree of instability (and hence of haemolysis) varies markedly, being mild in Hb Genoa and Hb Freiburg and severe in Hb Bristol and Hb Hammersmith. Hb Zürich causes only drug-induced haemolysis.

Affected individuals are heterozygous for the unstable haemoglobin. The disorder varies considerably in severity. Some patients suffer from anaemia, jaundice, splenomegaly and dipyrroluria (from the catabolism of the haem in the Heinz bodies). Both the anaemia and jaundice are aggravated by infections or the administration of oxidant drugs (see Table 5.6, page 122). Occasionally there may be cyanosis due to a severely decreased oxygen affinity (e.g. Hb Hammersmith) or to methaemoglobinaemia.

The haemoglobin level varies from normal to very low; a minority of unstable haemoglobins have a high oxygen affinity and cause polycythaemia. The blood film indicates a non-spherocytic haemolytic state or anaemia. The red cells show anisocytosis, poikilocytosis and, usually, hypochromia. Following splenectomy, a high proportion of the erythrocytes contain Heinz bodies which can be seen after staining with a supravital dye for 10 min. Heinz bodies are not usually seen in the circulating red cells of non-splenectomized patients, but may be induced *in vitro* by incubating blood for 24–48 h. The diagnosis is made by demonstrating instability of the haemoglobin using the isopropanol precipitation test, or by a (less sensitive) heat-denaturation test. Some, but not all, unstable haemoglobins can be detected by the routine methods of haemoglobin electrophoresis; abnormal bands on haemoglobin electrophoresis may also be caused by the presence of haem-depleted haemoglobin or free α chains.

The marrow shows erythroid hyperplasia. In patients with very unstable haemoglobins, precipitation occurs within erythroblasts as well as erythrocytes. Under the electron microscope, the intraerythroblastic precipitates appear very similar to the α-chain precipitates present in homozygous β-thalassaemia (see Fig. 5.22). The precipitate-containing erythroblasts show a variety of ultrastructural abnormalities indicative of dyserythropoiesis.

Thalassaemia syndromes

There are two main groups of thalassaemia syndromes. These are the α- and β-thalassaemia

Table 5.8 Some unstable haemoglobins which cause haemolytic anaemia

Hb Zürich (β63 His→Arg)

Hb Genova (β28 Leu→Pro)

Hb Freiburg (β5 Val deleted)

Hb Köln (β98 Val→Met)

Hb Philly (β35 Tyr→Phe)

Hb Gun Hill (β91–97 deleted)

Hb Bristol (β11 Val→Asp)

Hb Hammersmith (β42 Phe→Ser)

syndromes in which there is a depression of the rate of synthesis of the α- or β-globin chains respectively. Several different primary biochemical lesions have been shown to be responsible for the depression of globin chain synthesis in both these groups of thalassaemias. In most Asian and Black (Jamaican and American) patients with α thalassaemia, one or more α-chain genes are deleted. However, particularly in some non-Asian, non-Black patients (Cypriot, Sardinian, Turkish, Italian, Saudi Arabian), there may also be dysfunctional α genes with partial deletions or non-deletion defects. By contrast, most patients with β-thalassaemia show no deletion of β-chain genes when investigated by restriction enzyme analysis of DNA. However, the use of newer techniques has revealed that at least some cases show single nucleotide substitutions in the β-chain gene. The genetic change in β-thalassaemia results in biochemical lesions such as absence or reduced production of β-chain mRNA due either to a defect of transcription or to an abnormality in the processing of β-chain HnRNA, production of functionally abnormal β-chain mRNA and, possibly, defective translation of a normal β-chain mRNA (see p. 124 for steps involved in globin chain synthesis). A thalassaemia-like syndrome may also be caused by the production of a structurally abnormal globin chain which is synthesized at a slower than normal rate or of an abnormal haemoglobin which is markedly unstable (see p. 125).

The depression of the synthesis of one of the two types of globin chain in HbA but not of the other leads to an imbalance between α and non-α chain synthesis both in erythroblasts and blood reticulocytes. The demonstration of this imbalance has in the past been used in the diagnosis of thalassaemia. The degree of imbalance can be estimated by incubating blood reticulocytes with ^{3}H-leucine and then measuring the radioactivity in the α and non-α chains after a biochemical separation of these chains. In normal blood reticulocytes, the ratio of the radioactivity in the α chains to that in the β chains ($\alpha : \beta$ ratio) is about 1, indicating that globin chain synthesis is more or less balanced. By contrast, this ratio is greater than 1 in the β-thalassaemia syndromes, indicating the synthesis of an excess of α chains relative

to β chains. In the α-thalassaemia syndromes, the $\alpha : \beta$ ratio is less than 1 due to the synthesis of an excess of β chains. The unbalanced globin chain synthesis leads to an expansion of the intracellular soluble α- or β-chain pool and the precipitation of some of the excess globin chains within erythropoietic cells (Figs 5.21 and 5.22). In the

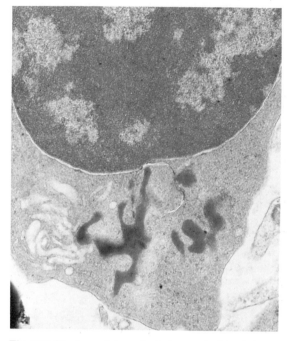

Fig. 5.21 Electron micrograph of a late erythroblast from a patient with HbH disease. The cell contains an electron-dense stellate intracytoplasmic inclusion, probably consisting of precipitated β chains.

Uranyl acetate and lead citrate $\times 21\,875$

case of the α-thalassaemias, some of the excess non-α chains may form soluble tetramers of γ chains in the fetus and neonate and of β chains in the adult. γ_4 is known as Hb Bart's and β_4 is known as HbH. As will be explained later, both the intracellular precipitation of globin chains and the formation of HbH play an important role in the pathogenesis of the anaemia in thalassaemia. Another consequence of the depression of globin chain synthesis which is common to all thalassaemias is a reduction of the amount of haemoglobin produced per developing red cell and consequently a reduced MCV and MCH in circulating red cells. However, if the extent of

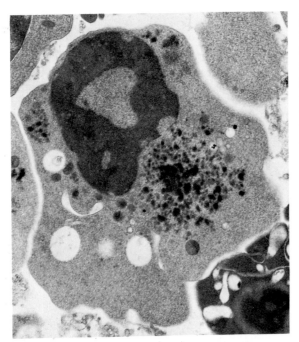

Fig. 5.22 Electron micrograph of a late erythroblast from a homozygote for β-thalassaemia. The cytoplasm contains multiple small rounded masses of electron-dense material some of which have fused together to form larger masses. The masses probably consist of precipitated α chains.

Uranyl acetate and lead citrate $\times 11\,625$

depression of globin chain synthesis in a particular thalassaemia syndrome is very small, the MCV and MCH of most cases may remain within the normal range, even though the average values for a group of patients with that syndrome may be lower than the average values for a group of normal individuals.

Although, for the sake of convenience, all thalassaemia syndromes are considered here under the heading of 'haemolytic anaemias', patients with some forms of thalassaemia have little or no anaemia and show only small reductions in red cell life-span. Peripheral haemolysis is the predominant cause of anaemia in the α-thalassaemia syndrome, HbH disease. By contrast, ineffective erythropoiesis is the main cause of anaemia in the β-thalassaemia syndromes.[63]

α-thalassaemia syndromes[38]

As the α genes are duplicated in most individuals, there are usually four α genes per cell (i.e. two

genes on each chromosome number 16). The normal genotype with respect to α genes could therefore be designated $\alpha\alpha/\alpha\alpha$. Four α-thalassaemia phenotypes can be recognized which result from the deletion of one, two, three or all four of the α genes. These are called α-thalassaemia 2 trait, α-thalassaemia 1 trait, HbH disease and Hb Bart's hydrops fetalis syndrome, respectively. The $\alpha:\beta$ chain synthesis ratios in blood reticulocytes are slightly reduced below the normal limits in some cases of α-thalassaemia 2 trait and are reduced with an average value of 0.7 in α-thalassaemia 1 trait and 0.5 in HbH disease.

The Hb Bart's hydrops fetalis syndrome occurs most commonly in South-East Asia, particularly in Thailand, the Malay peninsula, Indonesia and Southern China. Some cases have also been reported from Mediterranean countries. HbH disease, α-thalassaemia 1 trait and α-thalassaemia 2 trait are seen in all of the above regions as well as in the Middle East and have been reported sporadically in many other countries. Some of the highest figures for the frequency of α-thalassaemia syndromes have been reported from Thailand. In that country the prevalence of the α-thalassaemia 2, α-thalassaemia 1, HbH disease and hydrops fetalis phenotypes are respectively, 8–17, 4–12, 0.2–1.0 and 0.2–0.4%. Recent studies have shown that about 25% of Blacks have the α-thalassaemia 2 phenotype and about 3% the α-thalassaemia 1 phenotype. Nevertheless, HbH disease is extremely rare and the hydrops fetalis syndrome does not occur in Blacks. The different patterns of α-thalassaemia syndromes in South-East Asians and Blacks appear to result from the fact that the α-thalassaemia 1 phenotype could result from two different genotypes, either the deletion of both α genes on the same chromosome ($--/\alpha\alpha$) or the deletion of one of the two α genes on both homologous chromosomes ($-\alpha/-\alpha$). The former seems to account for most cases of α-thalassaemia 1 trait in South-East Asians and the latter in Blacks. The infrequency of HbH disease in Blacks results from the rarity of the genotype $--/\alpha\alpha$ in this population, the usual genotype of HbH disease being $--/-\alpha$.

α-thalassaemia 2 trait (*absence or abnormality of one gene*). This is an asymptomatic condition

which is difficult to diagnose. The diagnosis can frequently be suspected from family studies of established cases of HbH disease but in any given individual it can only be reliably made by direct studies of the number and structure of the α genes. Some cases show mild elevations of Hb Bart's (in the range 0.5–3%) at birth. However, HbH cannot be detected in adults either by electrophoresis or using the property of HbH to form characteristic inclusions after red cells are incubated with redox dyes (e.g. brilliant cresyl blue, new methylene blue) for 1–2 h (see Fig. 5.25). In most cases, the haemoglobin levels and red cell indices are within the normal range; about 15% of cases show slight reductions in the MCV and MCH.

α-thalassaemia 1 trait (absence and/or abnormality of two genes). This condition is also difficult to diagnose with certainty without analysis of α-globin genes. Affected individuals are asymptomatic and have normal or slightly-reduced haemoglobin levels. However, they usually have typical thalassaemic red cell indices, namely a low MCV and MCH and a high red cell count. About 4–8% of Hb Bart's is present at birth and some cases (particularly those from South-East Asia) show redox-dye-induced HbH inclusions within 0.03–0.1% of the red cells. The HbA₂ level is normal.

HbH disease (absence and/or abnormality of three genes). The clinical severity of this disorder varies markedly from an asymptomatic mild chronic haemolytic anaemia to a more severe haemolytic anaemia with bone deformities due to marked erythroid hyperplasia (i.e. a picture resembling β-thalassaemia intermedia; see p. 140). The condition can be diagnosed at birth by the finding of 19–27% Hb Bart's in cord blood but is usually diagnosed during or after the first year. Hepatomegaly and splenomegaly are seen in 70–80% of cases and the latter may occasionally become gross. Severe haemosiderosis does not develop. The haemoglobin is usually in the 8–11 g/dl range but may be as low as 3–4 g/dl. The MCV and MCH are very low. The blood film shows marked microcytosis and hypochromia as well as anisocytosis, poikilocytosis and target cells (Fig. 5.23). The reticulocyte count is usually 4–5%. The anaemia is frequently aggravated by inter-

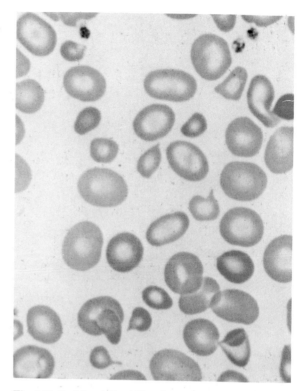

Fig. 5.23 Peripheral blood film of a non-splenectomized patient with HbH disease. The red cells show a marked degree of hypochromia together with anisochromia, anisocytosis and poikilocytosis. There are some misshapen microcytes.

May–Grünwald–Giemsa stain   × 940

current infections or the administration of oxidant drugs and by pregnancy. The diagnosis can be made in older children and adults by the demonstration of 2–40% of HbH in the blood (Fig. 5.24). Some cases also have small amounts of Hb Bart's. On Hb electrophoresis at alkaline pH, both HbH and Hb Bart's move faster than HbA, HbH running slightly ahead of Hb Bart's. The presence of HbH can also be demonstrated by incubating blood with the redox dye, brilliant cresyl blue, for 1–2 h. When stained in this way, cells containing HbH take on a golf-ball-like appearance (Fig. 5.25) due to the formation of many spherical or biconvex masses of denatured HbH which are attached to and which bulge the membrane[64] (Fig. 5.26). In HbH disease 30–85% of erythrocytes form redox-dye-induced inclusions.

The erythroblasts of cases of HbH disease syn-

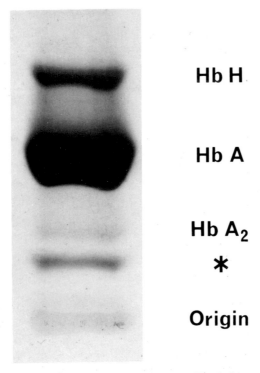

Hb H

Hb A

Hb A₂

∗

Origin

Fig. 5.24 Cellulose acetate electrophoresis (pH 8.5) of a haemolysate from a patient with HbH disease, demonstrating the presence of HbH. ∗ = carbonic anhydrase

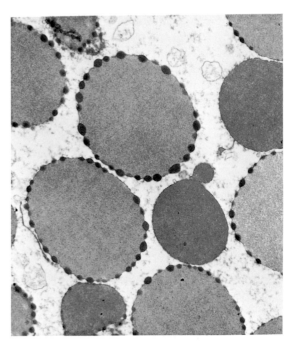

Fig. 5.26 Ultrastructure of red cells from a case of HbH disease after incubation with brilliant cresyl blue for 1 hour. The HbH-containing cells show membrane-bound, redox-dye-induced masses of denatured HbH.

Uranyl acetate and lead citrate × 6650

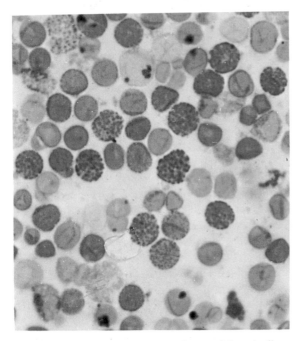

Fig. 5.25 Golf-ball-like appearance of many of the red cells of a case of HbH disease after supravital staining with brilliant cresyl blue.

thesize a considerable excess of β chains relative to α chains. Some of the excess β chains form stellate intraerythroblastic precipitates (Fig. 5.21) and the remainder form soluble tetramers (i.e. HbH). The intraerythroblastic precipitates do not seem to impair cellular function to a major extent.[65] Nevertheless, they are associated with some increase of ineffective erythropoiesis. The major cause of the anaemia, however, seems to be peripheral haemolysis. The latter results from the intracellular precipitation of HbH as red cells age within the circulation. The spleen removes the masses of precipitated HbH (Heinz bodies) without actually destroying the inclusion-containing cells but during this process appears to damage the red cell membrane and thereby considerably shorten red cell life-span. In splenectomized patients, many red cells contain one or more Heinz bodies, usually attached to the cell membrane, and these can be demonstrated by supravital staining with a basic dye (e.g. methyl violet) for 10 min (Fig. 5.27).

HbH disease with Hb Constant Spring (geno-

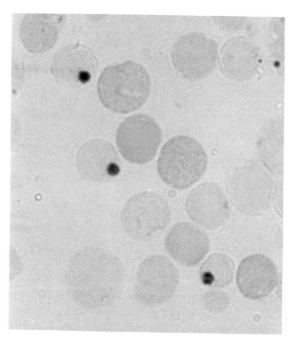

Fig. 5.27 Blood film of a splenectomized patient with HbH disease. The smears were made after supravital staining of venous blood with an equal volume of 0.5% methyl violet in normal saline for 10 minutes. Three of the red cells in the photomicrograph contain a membrane-bound Heinz body which had formed *in vivo*.

×1500

type: --/α^{CS}α). In South-East Asia and southern China, a clinical and haematological picture similar to HbH disease is seen as the result of the inheritance of Hb Constant Spring (see p. 125) together with α-thalassaemia 1 trait.

Hb Bart's hydrops fetalis syndrome (absence and/ or abnormality of four genes). The deletion of all four α genes or a combination of deletions and non-deletion defects affecting all four α genes is incompatible with extra-uterine life. The pregnancy continues for 30-40 weeks (average 34 weeks) and results either in a stillbirth or in the death of the baby within about one hour of birth. Affected babies are pale and oedematous and have ascites, pleural and pericardial effusions, massive hepatomegaly and a variable degree of splenomegaly. Jaundice is not marked. The placenta is very large. There is extramedullary haemopoiesis in the liver, spleen and other sites. The haemoglobin ranges from 4-10 g/dl. The blood film shows marked anisocytosis and poikilocyto-

sis, macrocytosis, hypochromia, reticulocytosis and numerous erythroblasts. About 80-90% of the haemoglobin consists of Hb Bart's (γ_4) and about 10% of the embryonic haemoglobin, Hb Portland ($\zeta_2\gamma_2$). There are also traces of HbH (β_4) but not HbA.

β-thalassaemia syndromes[38]

There are two main types of β-thalassaemia gene which are designated β^+ or β^0 depending on whether the gene is associated with some or no β-chain synthesis respectively. Individuals may be heterozygous or homozygous for the β-thalassaemia gene. The α:non-α-chain synthesis ratios in blood reticulocytes are high, being 1.5-2.5 in heterozygotes for β-thalassaemia and 1.5-30 in homozygotes.

β-thalassaemia occurs in a broad belt stretching from the Mediterranean basin through the Middle East and India to the Far East. The β-thalassaemia genes are particularly common in Italy, Greece, Sardinia, Cyprus and Crete; in some parts of these countries such genes are present in as many as 15-30% of the population. In most parts of India the gene frequency is between 1 and 8% and in Thailand the overall frequency is about 5%. The β^+ gene predominates in Cyprus, both genes occur in Greece, and the β^0 gene predominates in South-East Asia.

Heterozygous β-thalassaemia. Most individuals with this condition are asymptomatic. A few have splenomegaly. The haemoglobin levels are either normal (thalassaemia minima) or slightly reduced (thalassaemia minor) and are usually not lower than 8-9 g/dl. However, there is an exaggerated fall in the haemoglobin level during pregnancy due to a failure to increase red cell production adequately. In addition, there may be a greater frequency of folate deficiency during pregnancy. The MCV and MCH are both reduced in the vast majority of heterozygotes and may sometimes be as low as 55-60 fl and 15-18 pg, respectively. The red cell count is high and could be over 6×10^{12}/l. The reticulocyte count may be slightly raised. The blood film shows microcytosis and anisocytosis and, in some cases, target cells and basophilic stippling. The diagnosis is usually established by the demonstration of raised HbA₂ levels, in the range 3.5–7.0%. About half the cases also have a slightly elevated HbF level (1–5%). The HbF is heterogeneously distributed within the red cell population. When not complicated by co-existing iron deficiency, the serum iron and total iron binding capacity are normal.

There is a moderate degree of erythroid hyperplasia in the bone marrow. Many late polychromatic erythroblasts have very condensed nuclei and ragged cytoplasm, sometimes with basophilic stippling. Electron microscopy reveals precipitated α chains within the most mature of the late polychromatic erythroblasts and within marrow reticulocytes.[66] Red cell survival is not substantially shortened and the anaemia results largely from an increased degree of ineffective erythropoiesis. The latter probably stems from various deleterious effects of free and precipitated α chains on erythroblast function.

Homozygous β-thalassaemia. This condition causes two clinical syndromes known as thalassaemia major and thalassaemia intermedia, which essentially differ only in clinical severity. Thalassaemia major is characterized by the onset of severe anaemia (Hb = 2.5–6.5 g/dl) between the second and twelfth months of life and less frequently during the second year or later. If not treated with blood transfusions, it results in death during infancy or childhood. Thalassaemia

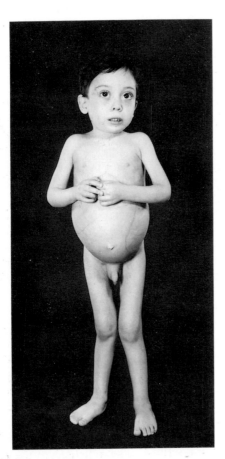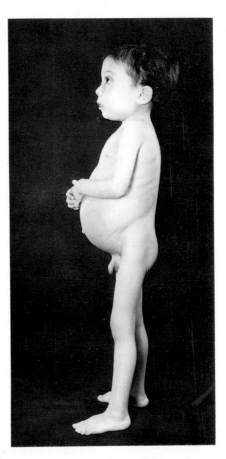

Fig. 5.28 Under-transfused Greek boy with homozygous β-thalassaemia showing a protuberant abdomen due to massive hepatosplenomegaly. He also shows poorly-developed limb muscles and a characteristic facial appearance with prominent malar bones, a depressed nasal bridge and exposure of the upper teeth (due to expansion of the marrow spaces of the maxillary bones).

Courtesy of Dr P.J.N. Cox, Paddington Green Children's Hospital, London, UK.

intermedia is a less severe but symptomatic form of the disease in which a variable degree of anaemia (Hb = 5–10 g/dl) develops, usually after the age of 1–2 years. Few or no blood transfusions are required and the condition is compatible with survival to adult life.

Cases of β-thalassaemia major present (usually during the first year of life) with failure to thrive, feeding problems, pallor, progressive enlargement of the abdomen due to increasing hepatosplenomegaly (Fig. 5.28), mild jaundice, and recurrent attacks of fever. If regular blood transfusions are not administered, affected children subsequently show retarded growth as well as characteristic skeletal deformities due to a massive expansion of erythropoietic tissue (Fig. 5.28). The skeletal deformities include bossing of the frontal and parietal bones, expansion of the maxillary bones leading to severe dental deformities and malocclusion of the teeth, and expansion of the zygomatic bones. The changes in the frontal and zygomatic bones result in a 'Mongoloid' slant of the eyes. Many bones show a thinning of the cortex due to the expansion of the marrow and fractures may follow minor trauma. Massive splenomegaly develops in some cases. Cardiac dilatation is frequent. Occasional clinical manifestations include leg ulcers, various compression syndromes caused by masses of extramedullary haemopoietic tissue, hyperuricaemia, and secondary gout.

Patients who are regularly and adequately transfused do not develop bone deformities because the high haemoglobin level suppresses erythropoietin production and decreases total erythropoietic activity. However, as one unit of blood contains about 250 mg of iron (in haemoglobin), regular transfusion causes the development of progressively increasing degrees of iron overload in tissues. Properly transfused children remain reasonably well until they are 10–12 years old, but then develop various problems due to haemosiderosis. These include endocrine abnormalities such as failure of sexual development or diabetes mellitus, cardiac dysfunction and hepatic cirrhosis. Most patients seem to die of sudden cardiac arrhythmias or congestive cardiac failure during the second or third decade. However, it now appears that some prolongation of

life is achieved if the iron loading is decreased by the regular administration of the iron chelator, desferrioxamine.

Most patients with β-thalassaemia intermedia are relatively well and only require blood transfusion when the anaemia is worsened by infections. Increasing splenomegaly may eventually require splenectomy. Some cases develop severe skeletal deformities (Figs 5.29, 5.30a), masses of extramedullary haemopoietic tissue, leg ulcers and hyperuricaemia. There is haemosiderosis of tissues due to increased iron absorption. Tissue dysfunction due to iron overload may be seen after the third or fourth decades.

Homozygotes for β-thalassaemia have both a low MCV and a low MCH. Their erythrocytes

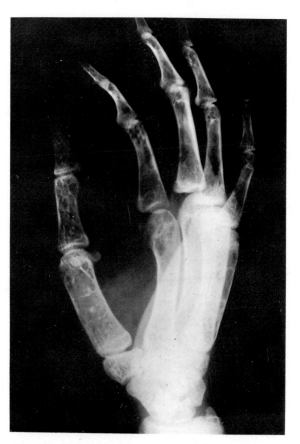

Fig. 5.29 Radiograph of the left hand of a patient with homozygous β-thalassaemia and the clinical syndrome of thalassaemia intermedia. Bone resorption has occurred as a consequence of marked erythroid hyperplasia. The cortices are thinned and residual bone trabeculae are apparent between the rarefied areas.   *Courtesy of Dr S. Abdalla.*

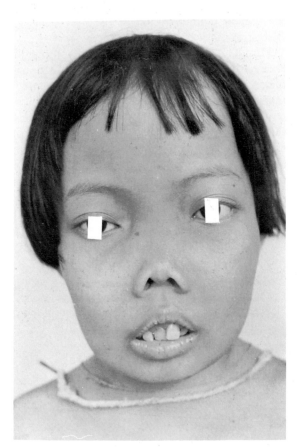
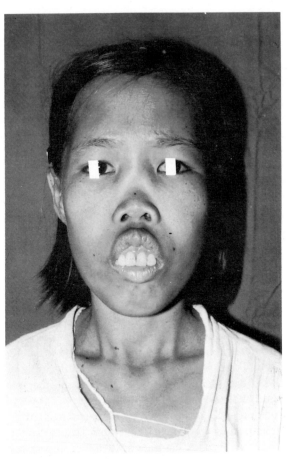

(b)

Fig. 5.30a, b Facial appearances of two untransfused Thai patients with thalassaemia intermedia showing the consequences of erythroid hyperplasia in the facial bones, particularly the maxillae. Both patients show prominent cheek bones, a depressed nasal bridge, widening of the distance between the inner canthi of the eyes and protrusion and exposure of the teeth of the upper jaw. (a) 19-year-old female with homozygous β-thalassaemia. (b) 30-year-old female with HbE/β-thalassaemia.

Courtesy of Professor Prawase Wasi, Department of Medicine, Siriraj Hospital, Bangkok, Thailand.

show microcytosis, marked hypochromia and marked anisopoikilocytosis. Small, irregularly-shaped, red cell fragments are often seen in the blood film and there are numerous thin target cells. Circulating erythroblasts are almost invariably present and increase after splenectomy (Fig. 5.31). Reticulocyte counts are in the range 5–15%. There may be a neutrophil leucocytosis with some myelocytes. However, neutropenia and severe thrombocytopenia may develop in cases with a very large spleen. Untransfused patients with homozygous β^0-thalassaemia have only HbF and HbA$_2$; they have no HbA. Untransfused patients with homozygous β^+-thalas-

saemia have HbF, HbA and HbA$_2$; the percentage of HbF usually exceeds 50%. However, the interpretation of HbF levels early in infancy is complicated by the fact that there is 55–90% HbF in normal cord blood. In normal infants, the HbF level falls to less than 10%, after the age of 4 months.

In both thalassaemia major and intermedia, the bone marrow shows intense erythroid hyperplasia with an absence of fat cells. The late polychromatic erythroblasts have poorly-haemoglobinized ragged cytoplasm and unusually pyknotic nuclei. Marrow smears stained by Perls' method reveal increased quantities of stainable

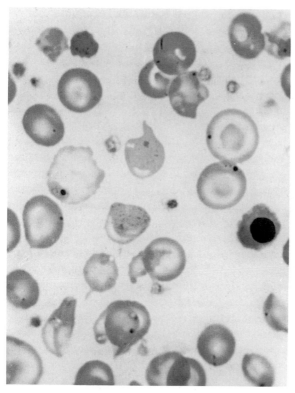

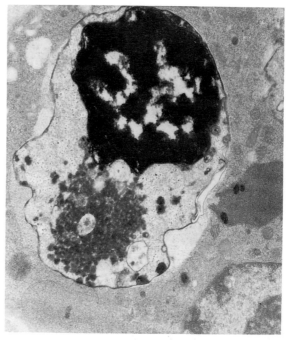

Fig. 5.32 Bone marrow macrophage from a case of homozygous β-thalassaemia. The macrophage contains a phagocytosed late erythroblast within which intracytoplasmic α-chain precipitates can be recognized.

Uranyl acetate and lead citrate   ×11 150

Fig. 5.31 Photomicrograph of a peripheral blood film of a transfusion-dependent, splenectomized patient with homozygous β-thalassaemia. There are transfused normochromic, normocytic cells together with the patient's hypochromic cells which show marked variations in shape and size. One late polychromatic erythroblast and two target cells are also seen. Some of the patient's cells contain Howell–Jolly bodies as a result of the splenectomy.

May–Grünwald–Giemsa stain   ×940

Hereditary persistence of fetal haemoglobin (HPFH)

iron in the bone marrow macrophages and abnormally coarse siderotic granules in the erythroblasts. There are intracellular α-chain precipitates in many of the early and late polychromatic erythroblasts and marrow reticulocytes[67] (Fig. 5.22). The presence of an expanded free α-chain pool or precipitated α chains or both causes a failure of cell proliferation in the early polychromatic erythroblasts (with a pile-up of cells in G_1) and of protein biosynthesis in the late polychromatic erythroblasts.[67] The anaemia is largely caused by a massive degree of ineffective erythropoiesis; phagocytosed erythroblasts can be seen within bone marrow macrophages (Fig. 5.32). The red cell life-span is moderately reduced.

This is a heterogeneous group of inherited conditions in which unusually high levels of HbF persist throughout life; except in one of the forms of HPFH affecting Blacks (mentioned below), there are no obvious haematological changes. HbF may be present in all red cells, though with some variability in the amount per cell (pancellular distribution) or may be present only in a proportion of cells (heterocellular distribution). Pancellular HPFH appears to be a form of δβ-thalassaemia in which the decreased production of HbA and HbA₂ is, for some reason, completely compensated for by increased production of HbF. Heterocellular HPFH, however, does not appear at the moment to be a thalassaemic disorder.

Pancellular HPFH has been described predominantly in Blacks and Greeks. In one form of the Black type of pancellular HPFH, in which a deletion of β and δ genes has been demonstrated, homozygotes and heterozygotes have 100% and 17–36% HbF, respectively, and have microcytic red cells. In another form caused by deletions of parts of the $^A\gamma$ and β genes and the region between them, heterozygotes have 4.5–10.5% HbF and 5.5–27% of Hb Kenya (which has $\gamma\beta$ fusion chains). Heterozygotes for other forms of the Black type of pancellular HPFH, have HbF levels between 15 and 25% and heterozygotes for the Greek type of pancellular HPFH have HbF levels of 10–20%.

There also seems to be more than one type of heterocellular HPFH. Heterozygotes for the Swiss type and the less common British type of HPFH have 1–5% and 4–12% HbF, respectively.

Genes for HPFH may coexist with thalassaemia genes or genes for abnormal haemoglobins such as HbS and cause unexpectedly high HbF levels for individuals with such genes.

ACQUIRED HAEMOLYTIC ANAEMIAS

The acquired haemolytic anaemias can be subdivided into those in which the destruction of red cells is mediated by immunological mechanisms and those in which it is mediated by non-immunological mechanisms.

Immune haemolytic anaemias[16, 68]

In this group of disorders, the haemolysis is usually caused by the presence of antibody or complement components or both on the surface of red cells. It is also theoretically possible that rarely red cells are lysed directly by the cytotoxic effect of specifically sensitized T-lymphocytes in the absence of immunoglobulin or complement on the red cell surface.

Red cells which are coated with small amounts of IgG antibody are selectively removed by the spleen and those coated with large amounts are removed both by the liver and the spleen. This removal of IgG-coated red cells is dependent on their interaction with splenic and hepatic macrophages which have receptors for IgG1 and IgG3 but not for IgM. The ability of the spleen to remove cells coated with small amounts of IgG may be related to the considerable haemoconcentration which occurs in this organ which would result in a greater chance of interaction with macrophages. The coated red cells may be either completely or partially phagocytosed by the macrophages of the spleen and liver. When the phagocytosis is only partial, the unphagocytosed part of the cell may detach from the macrophage and circulate as a spherocyte. Sometimes the unphagocytosed part of the cell may undergo immediate intravascular lysis, presumably as a result of the leak of enzymes from an incomplete phagosome. Circulating spherocytes tend to become sequestered and phagocytosed in the spleen because of their inability to deform adequately in order to enter from the Billroth cords into the splenic sinusoids via the small fenestrations in the sinusoidal walls.

Some IgM antibodies and the Donath-Landsteiner antibody (see p. 148) activate the entire complement sequence (see p. 28) and lead to the binding of C8 and C9 to the red cell membrane. The latter causes the appearance of holes (with a diameter of 10 nm) in the membrane and results

Table 5.9 Immune haemolytic anaemias

Haemolytic transfusion reactions (see p. 31)

Haemolytic disease of the newborn (see p. 34)

Autoimmune haemolytic anaemias
1. *Warm-reactive antibodies*
   Idiopathic
   Secondary (chronic lymphocytic leukaemia, lymphoma, other malignant tumours, systemic lupus erythematosus, thyrotoxicosis, Hashimoto's thyroiditis, myasthenia gravis, ulcerative colitis, rheumatoid arthritis, scleroderma, idiopathic thrombocytopenic purpura, Wiskott-Aldrich syndrome)
2. *Cold-reactive antibodies*
   Cold haemagglutinin disease (CHAD)
   Idiopathic
   Secondary (*Mycoplasma pneumoniae* infection, infectious mononucleosis, lymphomas)
   Paroxysmal cold haemoglobinuria
   Idiopathic
   Secondary (measles, chickenpox, mumps, influenza, other viral infections, congenital and tertiary syphilis)

Drug-related immune haemolytic anaemia

Paroxysmal nocturnal haemoglobinuria

in intravascular haemolysis. Many IgM and some IgG antibodies activate only part of the complement sequence and, therefore, do not cause intravascular lysis. Red cells which have reacted with this type of antibody have activated C3 on their surface and interact with macrophages via C3 receptors present on the surface of these phagocytes; this interaction usually leads to complete phagocytosis.

Some lymphocytes (K cells, p. 18) are capable of lysing antibody-coated red cells *in vitro* but the importance of antibody-dependent cell-mediated cytotoxicity in the causation of the haemolysis seen in the immune haemolytic anaemias remains to be determined.

The immune haemolytic anaemias are listed in Table 5.9. Haemolytic transfusion reactions and haemolytic disease of the newborn are caused by alloantibodies and are discussed on pages 31 and 34 respectively.

Autoimmune haemolytic anaemia (AIHA) with warm-reactive antibodies[68, 69]

This type of anaemia occurs at all ages but is most common over the age of 50 years. Some cases are idiopathic and others are associated with various disorders such as chronic lymphocytic leukaemia, lymphoma, systemic lupus erythematosus and, less frequently, with other tumours, other autoimmune disorders and the Wiskott–Aldrich syndrome (see Table 5.9). Although haemolysis may develop very acutely it is usually insidious in onset. The rate of haemolysis varies considerably so that some cases with relatively mild haemolysis show no anaemia and others with marked haemolysis suffer from a severe anaemia. There may be mild splenomegaly in idiopathic cases and more marked splenomegaly in cases secondary to a lymphoid malignancy. Hepatomegaly and lymphadenopathy may also occur, even in idiopathic cases. The reticulocyte count is raised, sometimes to over 30%, and there may be circulating erythroblasts. Spherocytosis is a characteristic finding (Fig. 5.33). Neutrophil leucocytosis and a leucoerythroblastic blood picture are often present in severely anaemic patients but the neutrophil count may be normal or reduced in others. Blood monocytes occasionally show erythrophagocytosis. The platelet count is usually normal but may be increased or decreased; occasional patients appear to have both AIHA and severe autoimmune thrombocytopenic purpura (Evans' syndrome). The serum bilirubin level is usually in the range 17–51 μmol/l. Haemoglobinuria is rare. The bone marrow usually shows normoblastic erythroid hyperplasia.

The haemolysis is caused by a warm-reactive polyclonal IgG antibody (sub-classes IgG1 and IgG3) which may in some cases be detected in the serum using an indirect antiglobulin test or enzyme-treated cells (see p. 30). In virtually all cases IgG, complement components, or both IgG and complement, can be detected on the surface of red cells using the direct antiglobulin test (DAGT); the approximate frequencies with which these three patterns of reaction are found are 30, 10 and 50%, respectively. Occasionally IgA or IgM may be present on the cell surface. About 2–4% of cases give a negative DAGT, usually because the number of antiglobulin molecules per red cell is too low to be detected by this method. The patterns of reaction with the DAGT are not useful in elucidating the causes of AIHA, except that both IgG and complement are invariably found in AIHA associated with SLE. Studies of antibody eluted from red cells frequently reveal specificity within the Rh system (e.g. anti-e, anti-c or anti-Rh precursor substance). Sometimes the autoantibodies react against a very common red cell antigen such as Wr^b or En^a. Most cases show no increase in the cold agglutinin titre ($< 1:32$ at $4°C$) but some show a moderate increase up to $1:512$. Patients with warm-reactive AIHA commonly have low IgA levels. They also tend to develop alloantibodies following blood transfusion more easily than patients with other disorders.

Some patients with a very acute onset of severe anaemia die rapidly of cardiovascular collapse. However, most cases show some response to high doses of corticosteroids within three weeks. Following this initial response, the reduction of haemolysis can be maintained with low doses of steroids in about 50% of cases. The response to steroid therapy results from a rapid blocking of the phagocytic activity of macrophages, a rapid

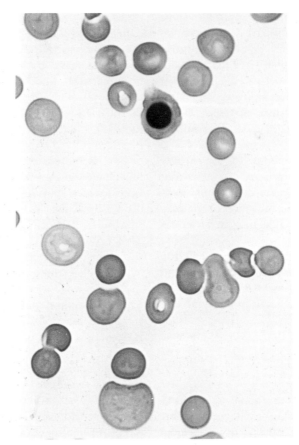

Fig. 5.33 Peripheral blood film from a patient with idiopathic autoimmune haemolytic anaemia showing spherocytes formed by the action of a warm-reactive IgG autoantibody. In addition to spherocytes, the photomicrograph shows a circulating erythroblast and several large polychromatic red cells.

May-Grünwald-Giemsa stain   × 940

reduction of the number of IgG molecules per red cell and a gradual diminution of the rate of production of autoantibody. Splenectomy may be beneficial in about 40% of the cases in which the disease cannot be controlled by steroid therapy. Immunosuppressive therapy (with cytotoxic drugs) may also be of benefit.

Autoimmune haemolytic anaemia with cold-reactive antibodies[68]

The antibody responsible for this type of AIHA rarely reacts at 37°C, normally reacting best at low temperatures (usually below 20°C). Two distinct syndromes are recognized, cold haemagglutinin disease and paroxysmal cold haemoglobinuria.

Cold haemagglutinin disease (CHAD)[70] (see also p. 305). This syndrome is characterized by haemolytic anaemia aggravated by cold weather, a positive direct antiglobulin test due to the presence of complement (C3d and C4d) on the red cell surface and high titres of anti- red-cell antibodies causing maximal agglutination at 0–5°C. Acrocyanosis and splenomegaly may be seen particularly in chronic CHAD. The cold-reactive antibodies combine with red cells and mediate complement fixation in the cooler peripheral circulation but dissociate from the red cells in the warmer central circulation, leaving only complement on the red cell surface. Haemolysis is predominantly intravascular with haemoglobinaemia, haemoglobinuria and haemosiderinuria. The anaemia is usually mild to moderate, the reticu-

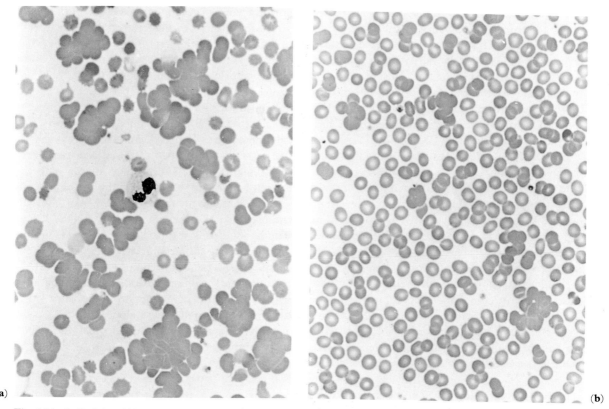

(a)

(b)

Fig. 5.34a, b Peripheral blood smears spread at room temperature showing red cell agglutinates caused by cold-reactive antibodies. (**a**) Idiopathic cold haemagglutinin disease. (**b**) Cold haemagglutinin disease secondary to infectious mononucleosis.

May–Grünwald–Giemsa stain　　×940

locyte count is raised and spherocytes are not usually present. Characteristically, the thinner areas of blood films made at room temperature show large red cell agglutinates (Fig. 5.34). This agglutination may generate falsely-high MCVs together with falsely-low red cell counts on automated blood counting machines and, particularly when blood is stored in a refrigerator, may cause the red cells to form into a single clot-like mass. Blood films may also show white cell agglutinates. CHAD may develop acutely as a rare and self-limiting complication of *Mycoplasma* pneumonia or infectious mononucleosis. The cold agglutinins in these two conditions are polyclonal IgM antibodies, usually with anti-I and anti-i specificity, respectively. A chronic form of CHAD occurs in elderly patients either as an idiopathic disorder or secondary to lymphomas. The cold agglutinin in chronic CHAD consists

of a monoclonal IgM antibody, usually with κ light chains and anti-I specificity. The anti-I titre, which in healthy people is usually less than 1:10–40 at 4°C, may be as high as 1:2000–1:500000. The bone marrow of patients with chronic idiopathic CHAD may show increased numbers of plasmacytoid lymphocytes (see p. 305).

Treatment of chronic idiopathic CHAD consists of maintaining warmth, particularly in the extremities, and avoidance of exposure to cold. Some cases benefit from immunosuppressive agents such as chlorambucil or cyclophosphamide. Occasional cases terminate with malignant lymphoma.

Paroxysmal cold haemoglobinuria (PCH). This is a rare form of AIHA in which episodes of massive intravascular haemolysis are provoked by exposure to cold. These episodes are characterized by marked haemoglobinuria and are some-times accompanied by pains in the back, abdomen and limbs, headache, vomiting, diarrhoea, fever with chills and rigors, urticaria and acrocyanosis. The DAGT shows the presence of complement on the red cells during episodes of haemolysis but not in the intervals between episodes. The autoantibody responsible for the haemolysis is the Donath–Landsteiner antibody. This is an IgG antibody capable of binding complement and it usually has the specificity anti-P. The antibody combines with red cells and the early complement components at the low temperatures (usually below 20°C) encountered in superficial vessels during severe chilling. When the antibody- and complement-coated red cells return to the central circulation (i.e. to 37°C), the antibody dissociates from the red cells. By contrast, the early complement components remain and react with later components, thereby causing lysis. Similarly, haemolysis occurs *in vitro* when the patient's cells and serum are cooled to 0–4°C and then warmed to 37°C. PCH may occur as an idiopathic condition or may develop as a rare complication of various viral and bacterial infections including congenital and tertiary syphilis (see Table 5.9). The haemolysis associated with the non-syphilitic form of the disease is usually transient, rarely paroxysmal and frequently unrelated to cold exposure.[71, 72]

Drug-related immune haemolytic anaemia[73]

Drugs often serve as haptens and, after combination with proteins (e.g. in the plasma or on cell membranes), induce the formation of antibodies against drug-protein complexes. Nevertheless, only a relatively small proportion of individuals receiving certain drugs have been shown to develop an immune haemolytic anaemia. Drug-related immune haemolytic anaemia may be caused by one of three mechanisms. In the first mechanism, small amounts of the drug become firmly fixed to the red cell membrane and drug-specific antibodies provoked by previous exposure to the drug react with red cells coated with the drug. The patient's red cells give a positive DAGT usually with antisera against IgG but not against complement components. This mech-

anism operates in some patients receiving 10×10^6 units or more of penicillin per day and leads to a slowly developing anaemia which is frequently due to extravascular haemolysis. The cephalosporins and some other drugs may also rarely behave in this way. In the second mechanism (known as the 'innocent bystander' mechanism), the drug is not firmly bound to the red cell membrane. Red cell damage is induced by the passive attachment to the red cell membrane of circulating drug-antibody complexes and the subsequent activation of the complement sequence on the membrane. The DAGT reveals the presence of complement on red cells. Drugs which act in this way include stibophen, quinidine, quinine, aminosalicylates, isoniazid, phenacetin, paracetamol (acetaminophen), chlorpropamide and sulphonamides. Affected patients usually give a history of previous exposure to the drug and rapidly develop moderate to severe anaemia, frequently with spherocytosis and haemoglobinuria; renal failure is common. In the third mechanism, which is seen with methyldopa and less frequently with levodopa and mefenamic acid, exposure to the drug for at least 3–4 months appears to cause the production of an autoantibody. Between 15 and 20% of patients taking methyldopa develop a positive DAGT without anaemia and about 1% develop a haemolytic anaemia; the probability of developing an anaemia is related to the daily dosage of the drug. The clinical and haematological picture of affected patients is indistinguishable from that seen in autoimmune haemolytic anaemia due to a warm-reacting antibody and the haemolysis may persist for many months after drug withdrawal. The antibody provoked by the drug sometimes has a specificity within the Rh system (e.g. anti-e, anti-c, etc.). In patients with haemolysis induced by the first two mechanisms but not the third, the antibody in the patient's serum will only react with normal red cells in the presence of the drug.

The anaemia due to drug-related immune haemolysis usually resolves completely within a few weeks of discontinuation of the causative drug. However, in the case of drugs like methyldopa, which cause the production of autoantibodies, the DAGT may remain positive for as long as 7 to >48 months after recovery from the anaemia.

Paroxysmal nocturnal haemoglobinuria (PNH, Marchiafava–Micheli syndrome)[74, 75]

This acquired disorder results from the presence of an abnormal clone of multipotent haemopoietic stem cells which gives rise to mature blood cells (erythrocytes, platelets and leucocytes) whose cell membranes are abnormally susceptible to lysis by the terminal complement complex (C5-C9). BFU-E, CFU-E and CFU-GM (see Chapter 3) also show increased susceptibility to complement-induced lysis.[76] The proportion of abnormal erythrocytes varies from 1-90% and may vary considerably in the same patient at different times.

The disease may affect individuals of any age, shows a peak incidence at 25-35 years and varies considerably in severity. It is characterized by chronic anaemia due to intravascular haemolysis and, in severe cases, a tendency to develop thrombosis in the hepatic veins (causing the Budd–Chiari syndrome) and less commonly in the mesenteric, splenic, portal, cerebral, femoral and iliac veins. Renal dysfunction may occur due to recurrent microthrombi.[77] The haemolysis is usually relatively mild and unaccompanied by haemoglobinuria. About 25% of cases, however, suffer from recurrent episodes of acute haemolysis during sleep, with the passage of red or brown urine (haemoglobinuria) on waking. In severely affected cases the haemoglobinuria may persist throughout the day. The haemoglobinuria may be associated with constitutional symptoms such as fever, headache, drowsiness, lumbar and abdominal pain. It is sometimes precipitated by exercise, menstruation, infection, the administration of iron (particularly parenterally), transfusion or surgery. The PNH defect may develop during the course of Fanconi's anaemia (p. 187), idiopathic marrow hypoplasia or aplasia, or drug-induced aplastic anaemia. Occasionally the PNH defect may precede the development of marrow aplasia or develop after recovery from aplasia. The PNH defect may also be associated with (usually followed by) idiopathic myelofibrosis, Ph[1]-negative chronic myeloid leukaemia,

erythraemic myelosis, acute myeloblastic leukaemia or myelomonocytic leukaemia.

The blood count shows anaemia, which is sometimes severe. The MCV may be raised but may also be decreased due to the development of iron deficiency as a consequence of haemoglobinuria and haemosiderinuria. The reticulocyte count is moderately raised but is usually less than that expected for the degree of anaemia. There may be circulating normoblasts and a neutropenia. A mild thrombocytopenia is common. The serum bilirubin level is elevated and there is chronic haemosiderinuria. During episodes of haemolysis, there is haemoglobinaemia and methaemalbuminaemia. The leucocyte alkaline phosphatase score is often decreased. The bone marrow usually shows normoblastic erythroid hyperplasia, even in many of the cases with pancytopenia. Some cases with pancytopenia have a hypocellular marrow.

Red cells with the PNH defect are best detected by their susceptibility to undergo haemolysis when incubated either in acidified fresh ABO-compatible normal serum or in acidified fresh autologous serum but not when incubated in acidified heat-inactivated serum (acidified serum lysis test or Ham test). The acidification of fresh serum activates the alternative complement pathway and thus causes complement-mediated lysis of the abnormal red cells. PNH erythrocytes also undergo lysis when incubated in sucrose, which reduces the ionic strength and thereby activates the classical and the alternative complement pathways (sucrose lysis test). The red cells of patients with congenital dyserythropoietic anaemia type II (p. 191) differ from those of patients with PNH in that the former are not lysed by acidified fresh autologous serum, are lysed by the acidified fresh serum of only a proportion of normal individuals, and do not give a positive result with the sucrose lysis test.

There is no specific treatment. As the infusion of plasma exacerbates haemolysis, washed red cells must be used when transfusions are indicated. Patients who suffer thrombosis can be safely treated with oral anticoagulants; heparin therapy is also probably safe. Androgens may be beneficial in patients with a hypoplastic marrow. The median survival is about 10 years; important causes of death are pulmonary embolism, cerebral thrombosis and thrombosis of the hepatic veins. There is increased susceptibility to infection, which causes some deaths. A few cases undergo complete clinical remission.

Non-immune acquired haemolytic anaemias

The life-span of the red cell may be decreased through non-immunological processes in a variety of acquired conditions. These processes include: (1) perturbations of erythropoiesis resulting in the production of structurally abnormal red cells; and (2) damage to circulating red cells by mechanical trauma, heat, drugs and other chemicals, infections and venoms and a prolonged passage through an enlarged spleen.

Acquired dyserythropoiesis

In many conditions in which anaemia is associated with acquired dyserythropoiesis, there is a modest reduction of red cell life-span; nevertheless, the anaemia is primarily caused by impaired bone marrow function rather than haemolysis. These conditions include iron deficiency anaemia, megaloblastic anaemia, sideroblastic anaemia, the anaemia of chronic disorder, leukaemia, myelodysplastic states and the chronic myeloproliferative disorders. One syndrome in which acquired dyserythropoiesis results in a marked reduction of red cell life-span is paroxysmal nocturnal haemoglobinuria. This disorder is discussed on p. 149.

Haemolysis caused by mechanical trauma or heat

Red cell fragmentation syndromes. Red cells may undergo fragmentation when subjected to excessive trauma within some part of the cardiovascular system. The resulting intravascular haemolysis and anaemia vary considerably in severity and are characterized by the presence of red cell fragments (schistocytes) in the blood film (Fig. 5.35). Red cell fragmentation may occur in patients with aortic and (less commonly) mitral valve prostheses, patients with severe aortic valve disease who have not been operated on, and in

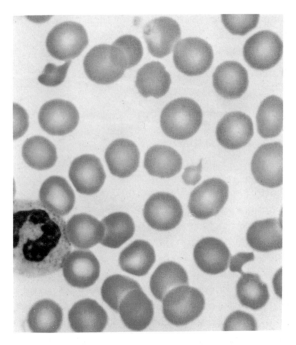

Fig. 5.35 Peripheral blood film from a patient with the red cell fragmentation syndrome caused by a malfunctioning aortic valve prosthesis. Schistocytes are present.
May–Grünwald–Giemsa stain   × 940

patients with teflon patches over ostium primum defects.[78, 79] The development of haemolysis in these conditions is probably largely related to haemodynamic disturbances at the site of the prosthesis (e.g. the regurgitation of blood through or around a valve prosthesis) rather than to the presence of the prosthesis itself. Haemolysis due to red cell fragmentation also occurs in a variety of diseases affecting the small blood vessels; if anaemia results it is designated microangiopathic haemolytic anaemia (MAHA). MAHA is seen in the haemolytic uraemic syndrome (p. 281), in thrombotic thrombocytopenic purpura (p. 280), in association with metastatic malignancy (particularly diffuse intracapillary carcinomatosis in the lungs and elsewhere—e.g. complicating carcinoma arising in the stomach),[80] in disseminated intravascular coagulation (DIC) (particularly chronic tumour-associated DIC), following the administration of fluorouracil plus mitomycin, in severe pre-eclampsia and in eclampsia, in malignant hypertension, and in association with generalized vasculitis and malformations of blood vessels.[81] In at least some of these conditions, the red cell fragmentation may be caused by fine fibrin strands within small vessels. Thrombocytopenia due to consumption of platelets commonly accompanies MAHA.

March haemoglobinuria.[82] This is a rare condition in which haemoglobinuria occurs soon after walking or running over long distances, Bongodrumming or hand-strengthening karate exercises. Anaemia is uncommon and there are no fragmented red cells in the circulation. The haemoglobinuria results from traumatic rupture of red cells in the microcirculation of the soles (in the case of walking and running) or other parts of the body subjected to repeated trauma. The few marathon runners who develop march haemoglobinuria have been observed to differ from the majority, who do not, in having a forceful stamping gait. Recent work has suggested that the red cell membranes of individuals developing march haemoglobinuria are structurally abnormal but this remains to be confirmed.

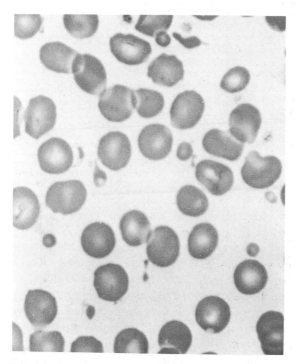

Fig. 5.36 Peripheral blood film of a patient with extensive burns. The red cells have formed microvesicles and fine filamentous structures.

May–Grünwald–Giemsa stain   × 940

Burns. Thermal damage to red cells in vessels close to severe burns results in intravascular haemolysis. The damaged red cells become spherocytic and generate microvesicles[83] (Fig. 5.36).

Haemolysis induced by drugs and other chemicals[84]

Normal red cells contain enzymes (G6PD and enzymes of the glutathione system) concerned with generating reducing substances which protect red cell components against oxidative damage (see p. 121). This reducing power is permanently impaired in some people who are congenitally deficient in one of these enzymes and is relatively poor in the normal newborn. Such individuals are especially susceptible to suffer from haemolysis when exposed to oxidant drugs (Table 5.6). The same drugs may cause oxidative haemolysis in normal adults if given in unusually high doses or in patients with renal failure in whom conventional doses may result in abnormally high drug levels in the blood. Other drugs and chemicals are sufficiently powerful oxidants to cause haemolysis in some or all individuals with normal red cell enzyme levels. Although many drugs which cause haemolysis do so by acting as oxidants, it is possible that some act, at least in part, by non-oxidative mechanisms.

Haemolysis which is unrelated to any red cell enzyme deficiency is seen in most patients receiving drugs such as dapsone, sulphasalazine, phenylhydrazine and acetyl phenylhydrazine. It occurs in very occasional patients taking conventional doses of phenacetin: these patients display a genetically-determined impairment of the oxidation of phenacetin to the pharmacologically active analgesic compound paracetamol (acetaminophen) and, consequently, convert abnormally large amounts of the drug to the oxidant metabolite 2-OH phenetidine.[85] Water-soluble vitamin K analogues may cause haemolysis in premature infants. Naphthalene or betanaphthol found in moth-balls and some nappy (diaper) sterilizers may be absorbed through the skin and thus cause haemolysis in infants. Exposure of normal adults to arsine (which may be generated during smelting, galvanizing, etc.) or nitrobenzene derivatives (which form the basis of some munitions) also causes haemolysis, as does the ingestion of p-nitroaniline (previously present in red and orange crayons) and of sodium or potassium chlorate (found in certain weed-killers). Copper ions are toxic to red cells and the entry of substantial amounts of copper into the blood accounts for the haemolytic episodes which occur during the early stages of Wilson's disease (hepatolenticular degeneration) and after the incorrect use of copper-containing haemodialysis equipment. The contamination of haemodialysis fluid with toxic concentrations of zinc, chloramine, nitrate or formaldehyde (and the use of hypertonic or overheated dialysis fluid) has also caused haemolysis.[86] Certain nitrites used as 'recreational drugs' by homosexuals are oxidants and cause haemolysis.[87] Acute haemolysis has followed contrast angiocardiography with Urografin 370 (a high-iodine-content preparation of diatrizoates).[88]

Intravascular haemolysis has been caused by the entry of water into the circulation in people who have nearly drowned in fresh water and in some patients subjected to transurethral prostatectomy whose bladders were irrigated with distilled water. It has also resulted from the accidental use of hypotonic dialysis fluid.

The degree of haemolysis and the extent of anaemia induced by different drugs and chemicals vary considerably. Extravascular haemolysis predominates with certain substances and intravascular haemolysis with others. The blood film frequently contains red cells with circumscribed 'empty' areas immediately adjacent to the cell membrane (Fig. 5.37). The empty areas probably result from the removal of Heinz bodies (precipitated haemoglobin) in the spleen. Heinz bodies may rarely be seen within a very few red cells after appropriate supravital staining (p. 138), and are only found within large numbers of cells in splenectomized patients or when the oxidative damage is extensive. Spherocytes and schistocytes may also be present, and in cases of severe intravascular haemolysis there may be circulating red cell ghosts. The acute intravascular haemolysis caused by certain chemicals (e.g. arsine or chlorates) may be accompanied by DIC and acute renal failure.

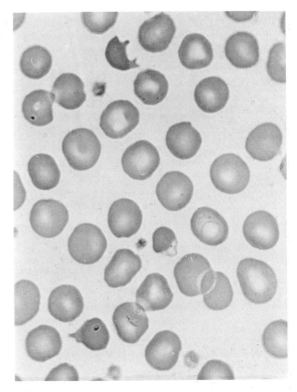

Fig. 5.37 Peripheral blood smear of a patient treated with dapsone for dermatitis herpetiformis. The patient did not suffer from G6PD deficiency. Three of the erythrocytes show evidence of drug-induced damage, being abnormally densely-staining and irregular in shape. One of these red cells shows poorly-staining areas just beneath the cell membrane.
May–Grünwald–Giemsa stain   × 940

Haemolysis caused by infections and venoms

Although the life-span of red cells is slightly reduced in most infections, the anaemia which develops in infected patients is usually largely caused by a depression of erythropoiesis. Nevertheless, in some instances it is primarily caused by severe haemolysis rather than by inhibition of bone marrow function. Examples of infections which cause haemolysis by provoking the formation of autoantibodies have been mentioned elsewhere (pp. 147 and 148). Infections may also induce substantial degrees of haemolysis by non-immunological or as yet undefined mechanisms.

Infections precipitate or aggravate haemolysis in patients with G6PD deficiency or unstable

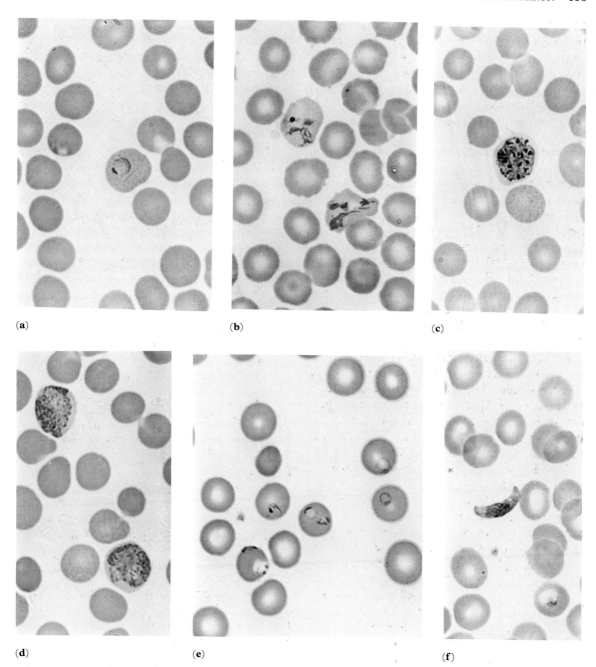

(a)   (b)   (c)

(d)   (e)   (f)

Fig. 5.38a–f Peripheral blood films from two patients, one infected with *Plasmodium vivax* and the other with *Plasmodium falciparum*. (**a**) Ring form (early trophozoite) of *Plasmodium vivax*. The ring is large and the infected red cell is both enlarged and stippled. (**b**) Two amoeboid late trophozoites of *Plasmodium vivax*. The parasitized red cells are enlarged. (**c**) Schizont of *Plasmodium vivax* containing about 16 merozoites. The parasitized red cell is enlarged. (**d**) Two gametocytes of *Plasmodium vivax*. The parasites contain many granules of pigment and the infected red cells are enlarged. (**e**) Ring forms of *Plasmodium falciparum*. The rings are small and delicate. Several erythrocytes are infected and there are two parasites within each of two of the infected cells. In one such erythrocyte one of the parasites has a double chromatin dot and the other is marginated along the red cell membrane. None of the parasitized red cells is enlarged. (**f**) Sickle-shaped gametocyte of *Plasmodium falciparum*. The infected red cell is very pale and not discernible.

May–Grünwald–Giemsa stain   × 940

haemoglobins, presumably by the generation of oxidant substances which act on the abnormal red cells.

Septicaemias (e.g. pneumococcal septicaemia) may cause red cell fragmentation secondary to disseminated intravascular coagulation.

Certain bacterial infections seem to cause haemolysis by a direct effect of the organism or one of its products on the red cell. For example, very occasional patients with septicaemia due to various cocci (particularly *Streptococcus pyogenes*) develop a severe haemolytic anaemia which probably results from the action of haemolysins produced by the infecting organisms. Septicaemia due to *Clostridium perfringens* (*welchii*) frequently causes severe intravascular haemolysis, with marked spherocytosis due to the action of bacterial phospholipases on the red cell membrane. Leptospirosis may also be associated with fulminant haemolysis due to red cell membrane damage.[89] Patients with Oroya fever

regularly suffer from a severe anaemia due to extravascular haemolysis.[90] This infection, which is caused by *Bartonella bacilliformis*, is found in Peru and is transmitted by a sandfly. The organisms can be seen in Romanowsky-stained blood films as red coccobacilli about 1-2 μm long, which are present on or just within the red cell membrane.

The anaemia associated with acute malaria, and particularly with acute *Plasmodium falciparum* malaria, is also mainly caused by haemolysis (see also p. 194). Parasitized red cells (Figs 5.38 and 5.39) rupture during the release of merozoites from mature schizonts. Unparasitized red cells also appear to have a shortened survival, perhaps because of the presence of C3d or IgG on their surface or because of hyperactivity of the mononuclear phagocyte system or both. The morphological appearances of the intraerythrocytic forms of the four species of plasmodia which cause malaria in humans are summarized

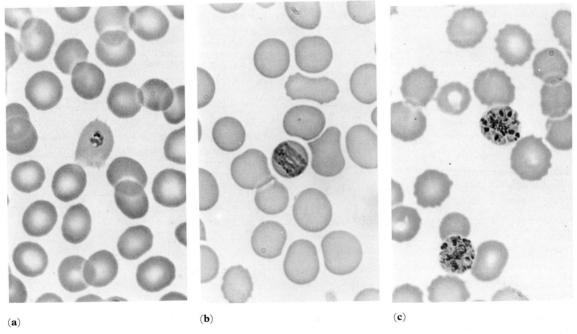

(a) (b) (c)

Fig. 5.39a-c Parasitized red cells from the peripheral blood films of two patients, one infected with *Plasmodium ovale* and the other with *Plasmodium malariae*. (**a**) Ring form (early trophozoite) of *Plasmodium ovale*. The ring is thick and the parasitized red cell is oval with a fimbriated margin. (**b**) Band form of *Plasmodium malariae*. The parasitized red cell is not enlarged. (**c**) Two schizonts of *Plasmodium malariae*. The schizont in the middle of the picture has about seven developing merozoites at its periphery and a collection of small discrete pigment granules at its centre. Each merozoite contains a coarse chromatin dot.

May-Grünwald-Giemsa stain × 940

Table 5.10 Appearances of various species of human malarial parasites within infected red cells in thin blood films (see also Figs 5.38, 5.39)

Characteristic	Plasmodium falciparum	Plasmodium vivax	Plasmodium ovale	Plasmodium malariae
Infected erythrocytes				
Enlarged	−	+	±	−
Oval with a fimbriated margin	−	−	+	−
Stain poorly	−	+	+	−
Many fine red granules around parasite (Schüffner's dots)	−	+	+	−
Few red clefts (Maurer's clefts)	+	−	−	−
Parasites				
Infection of individual erythrocytes by more than one parasite	+	Rare	−	−
Stages seen in venous blood	Usually only ring forms and gametocytes	All stages	All stages	All stages
Proportion of parasitized red cells	Often high	Usually moderate	Usually moderate	Usually small
Early trophozoites	Small delicate rings, some with double chromatin dots, some accolé forms (marginated forms)	Large coarse rings, double chromatin dots rare, accolé forms rare	Large coarse rings	Large coarse rings
Late trophozoites	Rounded and compact, rarely seen in blood	Large and amoeboid	Large and amoeboid, occasional band forms	Rounded and compact forms and band forms
Mature schizont	8–24 merozoites, rarely seen in blood	12–24 (usually 16) merozoites	6–12 (usually 8) merozoites	6–12 merozoites
Gametocytes	Crescent-shaped	Rounded or oval	Rounded or oval	Rounded

in Table 5.10; all four species are transmitted by the bite of an infected anopheline mosquito or, rarely, by the transfusion of blood containing parasites. The syndrome of blackwater fever, in which there is gross haemoglobinuria and acute tubular necrosis, occurred in Europeans who had suffered from recurrent attacks of *Plasmodium falciparum* malaria and had taken quinine irregularly. The relative importance of the role of malaria and of quinine therapy in the pathogenesis of this disorder is uncertain as quinine itself may cause haemolysis either in G6PD-deficient individuals or by an antibody-mediated mechanism. This serious syndrome is now quite rare.

Intrauterine infection with another protozoan, *Toxoplasma gondii*, may result in a clinical picture resembling hydrops fetalis due to severe hae-molytic disease of the newborn. Affected babies are either stillborn or die shortly after birth and have a severe anaemia with erythroblastaemia and hepatosplenomegaly. The mechanisms underlying the haemolysis are obscure.

Babesiosis (piroplasmosis),[91] a protozoan infection affecting cattle, dogs and various wild animals, may, rarely, affect humans. The infection in humans is characterized by fever, severe intravascular haemolysis and hepatosplenomegaly and is particularly prone to affect splenectomized individuals. The causative organisms, *Babesia microti* or *Babesia divergens* (*Babesia bovis*), invade and grow within circulating red cells and superficially resemble the ring form of *Plasmodium falciparum*. Some affected patients have been visitors to the island of Nantucket (off Massachusetts, USA) but cases have been reported from other areas of the world (e.g. Yugoslavia, Ireland, Russia, Scotland, California). The natural reservoir of infection appears to be in field mice, deer mice and other wild animals. The organism is transmitted to humans through the bites of ticks of the family Ixodidae which have become infected by feeding on the blood of infected animals. In the tick, the organism may be transmitted vertically by transovarian passage.

The venoms of certain species of spiders, snakes, bees, wasps and hornets[92, 93] may sometimes cause intravascular haemolysis, presumably by a direct effect of lytic enzymes present in these venoms.

Hypersplenism[94, 95, 96]

Normal red cells show a slight reduction in lifespan when transfused to patients with moderate or massive splenomegaly due to any cause. The anaemia which may be found in such patients is, however, not primarily haemolytic in type; it is caused by a combination of increased pooling of red cells in the spleen and an expanded plasma volume.

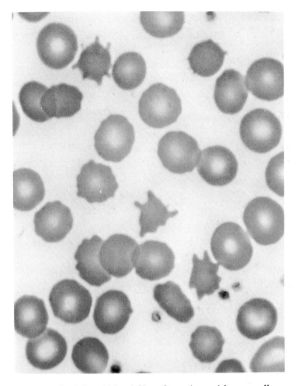

Fig. 5.40 Peripheral blood film of a patient with spur cell anaemia showing acanthocytes. The film also contains some echinocytes.
May–Grünwald–Giemsa stain   × 940

Other causes of haemolysis

Haemolysis in alcoholics. Three syndromes associated with varying degrees of haemolysis have been described in individuals taking excessive quantities of ethanol. Acute alcoholism may be accompanied by a transient haemolytic state associated with an increased number of stomatocytes.[97] Patients with alcohol-induced fatty change in the liver (with little or no cirrhosis) may develop recurrent episodes of haemolysis associated with mild fever, vomiting, upper abdominal pain, hypercholesterolaemia and hypertriglyceridaemia (Zieve's syndrome).[98] Such episodes are related to an excessive intake of alcohol and cease on abstaining from alcohol. During the acute episodes, there is an increase of cholesterol and other lipids in the red cell membrane, and an increase in the osmotic fragility of red cells. A third type of haemolytic syndrome (spur cell anaemia, or acanthocytic haemolytic anaemia) develops in alcoholics with advanced cirrhosis of the liver. This syndrome is characterized by chronic and sometimes severe haemolysis which is associated with the formation of acanthocytes[99, 100, 101] (Fig. 5.40). The latter results from the action of non-dialysable plasma 'factors' on red cells which leads to an increase of cholesterol and of the cholesterol:lecithin ratio in the red cell membrane. Although spur cell anaemia usually occurs in alcoholic cirrhosis, it has also been described in neonatal hepatitis.

The pathogenesis of the haemolysis in the above-mentioned syndromes is uncertain and may be complex. The red cell membrane could be damaged both directly by ethanol or its active metabolite, acetaldehyde, or indirectly via changes in the composition of the plasma secondary to an alcohol-induced impairment of the function of hepatocytes or other cell types.

Vitamin E deficiency.[102, 103] Vitamin E (α-tocopherol) appears to combine with free radicals and thus prevent oxidative damage to the lipids of cell membranes. A deficiency of this vitamin may develop in premature infants fed on diets rich in polyunsaturated fats. It causes a haemolytic anaemia which is associated with acanthocytosis, low serum tocopherol levels, and an abnormal susceptibility of red cells to undergo haemolysis in the presence of H_2O_2 *in vitro*. The condition responds to treatment with tocopherol.

Haemolysis due to hypophosphataemia.[104] Very low serum phosphate concentrations may be complicated by a haemolytic anaemia. The latter appears to be caused by decreased red cell deformability due to a reduction of intracellular ATP levels. This complication may follow starvation, prolonged antacid abuse and total parenteral nutrition with solutions inadequate in phosphate.

IMPAIRED RED CELL FORMATION

The conditions in which the anaemia is largely due to impaired red cell formation are listed in Table 5.11.

Table 5.11 Main groups of anaemias resulting largely from impaired red cell formation

Iron deficiency anaemia

Anaemia of chronic disorders

Anaemia of chronic renal failure

Anaemia of chronic liver disease

Sideroblastic anaemias

Macrocytic anaemias

Endocrine deficiency

Bone marrow infiltration

Aplastic anaemia

Pure red cell hypoplasia

Thalassaemia syndromes

Congenital dyserythropoietic anaemias

Chronic *Plasmodium falciparum* malaria

Protein-energy malnutrition

Anorexia nervosa

IRON DEFICIENCY ANAEMIA[105, 106]

Iron metabolism

Distribution of iron

There are two types of iron-containing compounds in the body: (1) those in which the iron is present within a haem moiety; and (2) those in which no haem is present, the iron being directly associated with the protein. The haemoproteins include haemoglobin and myoglobin which are concerned with the transport and storage, respectively, of oxygen. They also include some enzymes (various cytochromes, catalase and peroxidase) which are involved in electron transport. The iron-containing non-haem proteins consist of transferrin, ferritin, haemosiderin and some enzymes. Transferrin is a specific iron-binding β globulin found in plasma and tissue fluids. It transports iron to and from various cells of the body. Ferritin and haemosiderin represent the two forms in which iron is stored. Ferritin is water-soluble and is therefore usually lost during normal histological processing. By contrast, haemosiderin is insoluble and may be seen as brownish granules in ordinary sections or as bluish-green granules in sections stained by Perls' acid ferrocyanide method. Prolonged treatment of trephine biopsies of bone with certain decalcifying solutions may result in the removal of some or all of the stainable haemosiderin. The iron-containing non-haemoprotein enzymes include xanthine oxidase, aconitase, NADH dehydrogenase and ribonucleotide reductase.

The total amount of iron in the body of an adult varies between 2 and 5 g, being greater in males than in females. About two-thirds of this iron is in the haemoglobin of circulating red cells, there being about 250 mg of iron per 500 ml of whole blood. There are about 0.4 g of iron in myoglobin, 25 mg in cytochromes and catalase and 8 mg in transferrin. Most of the remainder is found stored in the form of ferritin dispersed in the cytosol of hepatocytes and muscle cells and as ferritin and haemosiderin in the macrophages of the liver, spleen and bone marrow. Small amounts of ferritin are also present in all other types of mammalian cells. The amount of storage iron in a healthy adult male is about 0.5–1.5 g.

Less storage iron is present in women and many healthy women have virtually no iron stores.

Absorption

Iron is present in a wide variety of foods; mainly in the form of haemoglobin and myoglobin in the case of animal foods and in the form of non-haem compounds in green vegetables and fruit. About 0.75–1.5 mg (i.e. 5–10%) of the average daily dietary iron intake of 15 mg may be absorbed in individuals with normal iron stores. The amount absorbed depends partly on the composition of the diet; a higher percentage of the iron is absorbed from foods such as liver and meat than from wheat, spinach and corn; some foods enhance or impair the absorption of iron from others. The amount absorbed increases with decreasing iron stores and with increases in total erythropoietic activity. The absorption of iron takes place mainly in the duodenum and in the upper part of the jejunum. Ionized iron and haem are released from food as a result of peptic digestion. Some of the ionized iron, particularly the ferrous iron, remains in solution at the low pH of the gastric juice and part of this is absorbed after conversion to soluble small molecular weight complexes by reaction with substances such as amino acids, sugars and ascorbic acid. The haem is absorbed intact and its iron released within the intestinal cell by the action of the enzyme haem oxygenase. Iron which is taken up by the intestinal epithelial cells but not transferred to the plasma is converted into ferritin and excreted in the faeces as a result of the shedding of the epithelial cells at the end of their 3–4 day life-span. The mechanisms which regulate the quantity of iron transferred into the plasma are still uncertain.

Excretion

In normal males, about 0.9 mg of iron are lost per day. About 0.7 mg of this is lost in the stools; 0.3–0.4 mg is lost per day from slight gastrointestinal haemorrhages and the remainder in the bile and in desquamated epithelial cells. Less than 0.1 mg iron is lost in the urine per day. In menstruating females there is an additional loss of iron, the magnitude of which depends on the quantity of menstrual blood loss. The menstrual loss varies between 2 and 200 ml of blood per period (average 43 ml) and is equivalent to an additional daily loss of 0.03–3.33 mg (average, 0.7 mg) iron per day. The total loss of iron in menstruating women may, therefore, vary between about 0.9 and 4.2 mg (average, 1.6 mg) per day.

Iron balance

In normal adult males, there is a balance between the loss of iron from the body and the absorption of iron from the diet which tends to keep the total body iron content more or less constant. No mechanisms exist for the regulation of iron excretion and the balance is achieved entirely by the regulation of iron absorption. The absorption of 0.75–1.5 mg of iron per day from an average diet nicely balances the daily losses of about 0.9 mg in males. Larger quantities of iron have to be absorbed from the diet to balance the greater iron losses in menstruating women, and when adequate iron is not absorbed a negative iron balance and eventually iron deficiency develop.

Utilization

Although iron is present in all cells, most of the iron in the body is in the erythron. Consequently the kinetics of iron are largely connected with erythropoiesis. There are about 4 mg iron in the plasma and this is bound to transferrin. The plasma iron turnover is about 30 mg per day and about two-thirds of the iron involved in this turnover is derived from the destruction of senescent red cells. Some iron also enters the plasma from intestinal absorption and from ferritin, haemosiderin and metabolic iron pools in various cells. About 85% of the iron leaving the plasma is taken up by erythropoietic cells; the remainder is taken up by other tissues, particularly the liver, muscle and skin.

Causes of iron deficiency

Iron deficiency develops when an individual does not absorb sufficient iron from the diet to (1) balance the losses of iron from the body and (2) meet the need for an increase in total body iron associated with growth. The causes of iron deficiency include inadequate dietary intake, pregnancy and lactation, chronic blood loss, malabsorption and, rarely, chronic haemoglobinuria and haemosiderinuria (Table 5.12). Since about

Table 5.12 Causes of iron deficiency

1. Reduced total body iron at birth: prematurity and low birth weight, early cord clamping

2. Inadequate intake
   Prolonged breast or bottle feeding without iron supplementation, vegetarian diets, poverty

3. Pregnancy and lactation

4. Chronic haemorrhage
   (a) Uterine: menorrhagia (dysfunctional or due to neoplasm), metrorrhagia
   (b) Gastrointestinal: haemorrhoids, salicylate ingestion, peptic ulceration, hiatus hernia, diverticulosis, neoplasm, oesophageal varices, hereditary telangiectasia, Meckel's diverticulum, ulcerative colitis, post-gastrectomy, hookworm infestation, cow's milk sensitivity in infants
   (c) Repeated blood-letting
   (d) Others: lesions (neoplasms, stones, inflammatory disease) of the kidneys, ureter or bladder; recurrent haemoptysis due to vascular anomalies, neoplasms or pulmonary hypertension secondary to heart disease; idiopathic pulmonary haemosiderosis;* Goodpasture's syndrome

5. Malabsorption
   Gluten-induced enteropathy (coeliac disease), post-gastrectomy

6. Chronic haemoglobinuria and haemosiderinuria
   e.g. paroxysmal nocturnal haemoglobinuria, chronic intravascular haemolysis secondary to intracardiac myxomas and valvular prostheses

* In this condition, sequestration of iron within pulmonary macrophages may lead to iron-deficient erythropoiesis without a decrease of total body iron

two-thirds of the body's iron is in the circulating red cells, chronic blood loss can rapidly deplete the iron stores, and cause anaemia. In some Western countries iron deficiency anaemia has been reported in up to 25% of infants, 0–5% of children, 1–3% of male adolescents, 15% of females between the menarche and menopause and 30% of pregnant women. The prevalence of iron deficiency anaemia is considerably higher in poorer countries due both to a much lower dietary intake of iron and to chronic gastrointestinal blood loss from hookworm infestation.

Inadequate dietary intake

A poor diet may cause or contribute to the development of iron deficiency. Since the absorption of iron from vegetable foods is generally less efficient than that from animal foods, iron deficiency tends to develop in individuals living on an inadequate and predominantly vegetarian diet.

The susceptibility of infants, children and adolescents to iron deficiency results from an increased requirement of iron during the growing period. A full-term baby has about 300 mg of iron in the body at birth. Because most of this is acquired from the mother during the last trimester of pregnancy, the iron content of a newborn premature baby is less than that of a full-term baby and is related to the degree of prematurity. A considerable increase in body iron must occur during infancy, childhood and adolescence to enable the adult levels of 2–5 g to be achieved. This requires an average absorption of 0.5 mg iron per day in addition to the amount necessary to replace the inevitable daily losses. Iron deficiency results if the appropriate quantity of iron cannot be absorbed from the diet. As the rate of growth is maximal during the first year of life, iron deficiency anaemia is particularly prone to develop during this period. Milk is a very poor source of iron and anaemia usually develops in babies fed for more than six months on either human or cow's milk alone. Premature infants may become iron-deficient as early as 10–12 weeks after birth if liquid iron supplements are not given. The growth spurt in adolescents of both sexes and the onset of menstruation in females operate to increase the iron requirements and precipitate the development of iron deficiency anaemia in some adolescents.

Pregnancy and lactation

As has been mentioned, the fetus extracts about 300 mg (200–370 mg) of iron from the mother during the pregnancy. In addition, the mother loses 30–170 mg of iron in the placenta and 100–250 mg in the blood lost during delivery.

Although these losses are partly offset by the amenorrhoea during pregnancy, the nett loss of iron from a mother during a pregnancy works out to be about 500 mg. Thus, a single pregnancy and particularly two or more closely spaced pregnancies may deplete the iron stores of a woman and lead to anaemia. About 1 mg iron may be lost per day as a result of lactation.

Chronic blood loss

Menorrhagia is a frequent cause of iron deficiency anaemia in women between the menarche and menopause. A high proportion of women losing more than 80 ml blood per period are anaemic.

In well-nourished adult males and post-menopausal females, iron deficiency is usually due to chronic blood loss from lesions in the gastrointestinal tract and, less frequently, in other sites. Several of these lesions are listed in Table 5.12. Clearly some of them may also be responsible for iron deficiency in children and pre-menopausal women. The commonest causes of gastrointestinal haemorrhage in Europe and North America are haemorrhoids, salicylate ingestion, peptic ulceration, hiatus hernia and colonic diverticulosis. The commonest cause elsewhere in the world is infestation with the hookworms, *Ankylostoma duodenale* and *Necator americanus*. Self-induced haemorrhage may rarely underlay an iron deficiency anaemia of obscure origin.

Other causes

Iron deficiency anaemia may be found in diseases affecting the upper part of the small intestine and this is partly due to malabsorption of dietary iron. In coeliac disease, loss of iron from the increased exfoliation of intestinal epithelial cells may also contribute to the iron deficiency. About 20-30% of patients subjected to partial gastrectomy develop iron deficiency anaemia from 1-12 years after the operation and this appears to be due to malabsorption in some patients and to gastrointestinal blood loss in others. Large quantities of iron may be lost in the urine of patients with chronic haemoglobinuria and haemosiderinuria and this may cause anaemia.

Haematological changes

The sequence of events associated with the progressive depletion of body iron is usually as follows. Initially, the iron stores are gradually used up to maintain the serum iron concentration within the normal range of 13-32 μmol/l (70-180 μg/dl) and to supply an adequate quantity of iron to the erythropoietic cells. During this period the serum ferritin level falls in proportion to the reduction of the iron stores (the normal range for serum ferritin is 12-300 μg/l) and iron absorption is increased (other causes of alterations in the serum ferritin level are given in Table 5.13). When iron deficiency develops in patients

Table 5.13 Causes of alterations in the serum ferritin level

Low serum ferritin

Reduced or absent storage-iron

High serum ferritin

Increased storage-iron (e.g. post-transfusion, idiopathic haemochromatosis)

Infections

Inflammatory disease (e.g. rheumatoid arthritis)

Malignant disease (e.g. acute myeloid leukaemia, acute phase of chronic myeloid leukaemia, acute lymphoblastic leukaemia, multiple myeloma, Hodgkin's disease, non-Hodgkin's lymphoma, carcinoma)

Acute and chronic liver disease

Chronic renal failure

Protein-energy malnutrition

Lysinuric protein intolerance[107]

with chronic inflammation, malignant disease, acute and chronic liver disease and chronic renal failure, the ferritin level falls less. After the iron stores are exhausted, the serum iron level becomes subnormal, the total iron binding capacity (TIBC) rises above the normal range of 50-70 μmol/l (280-400 μg/dl), the transferrin saturation falls (the normal range for the transferrin saturation is 20-50%, mean 35%) and red cell protoporphyrin levels rise. However, despite these biochemical changes, a normal haemoglobin level is maintained for some time. Anaemia eventually develops, usually when the transferrin saturation is below 16%. It is initially normochromic and normocytic in type, with anisocytosis and an increased proportion of microcytic cells. Subsequently it becomes hypochromic and microcytic. However, in some patients a low MCV may be found when the haemoglobin is still within the normal range.

The red cell count is frequently near or within the normal range until the haemoglobin falls below 8–9 g/dl. Both the MCV and MCH may be within the normal range in some patients with mild anaemia and in an occasional patient with moderate anaemia. Even when the MCV is within the normal range, iron therapy causes increases in both the Hb and MCV, suggesting that the initial MCV was subnormal for that particular patient. Patients with severe anaemia invariably have both a low MCV and a low MCH and also a low MCHC. In established iron deficiency anaemia, the blood film shows microcytosis, hypochromia, anisocytosis and poikilocytosis (Figs 5.41 and 5.42); target cells may be present in modest numbers. The severity of these changes is, in general, proportional to the degree of anaemia. The poikilocytes are frequently elliptical

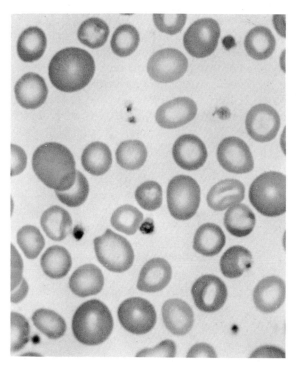

Fig. 5.42 Blood smear from a patient with iron deficiency anaemia treated with ferrous sulphate tablets for three weeks. The red cells are dimorphic with a mixture of iron-deficient hypochromic microcytic cells and recently-formed normochromic normocytic cells.

May–Grünwald–Giemsa stain   × 940

in shape and some elongated pencil-shaped forms may be present. The reticulocyte percentage is usually normal or reduced but may be between 2 and 5%, especially after a haemorrhage. Small numbers of circulating normoblasts may be seen after a haemorrhage or in severely anaemic patients.

The neutrophil and platelet counts are usually normal but may be increased in patients who are bleeding. The platelet count may also be increased in the absence of any evidence of bleeding or malignant disease.[108] Severely anaemic patients may show thrombocytopenia which responds to iron therapy. Hypersegmented neutrophils are sometimes seen in cases of iron deficiency anaemia. However, it is not yet certain whether this change results from the iron deficiency itself or a concomitant masked folate deficiency.

The percentage of erythroblasts in the marrow

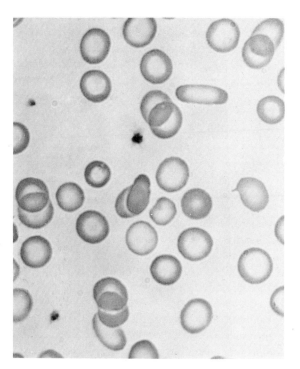

Fig. 5.41 Peripheral blood film from a patient with untreated iron deficiency anaemia. Hypochromic microcytes, elliptocytes and an elongated poikilocyte are present.

May–Grünwald–Giemsa stain   × 940

is usually increased in moderately or severely anaemic patients and the M/E ratios are reduced to 0.5–2.0 : 1. The late polychromatic erythroblasts are smaller than normal and hence erythropoiesis is described as being micronormoblastic. The cytoplasm often stains irregularly and has a ragged border. An abnormally high proportion of the late erythroblasts have pyknotic nuclei. In addition, the late erythroblasts show an increased frequency of dyserythropoietic changes such as basophilic stippling, irregularities in nuclear shape and karyorrhexis. Marrow smears stained by Perls' acid ferrocyanide method show a complete or nearly complete absence of stainable iron in the marrow fragments and a few or no (0–10%) sideroblasts. A proportion of the erythroblasts show slight to strong PAS positivity. Giant metamyelocytes may be found in patients in whom there is no evidence of associated folate or vitamin B_{12} deficiency.

Tissue changes[106, 109]

Changes which are probably related to the reduced activities of various iron-containing enzymes occur in a variety of tissues throughout the body. Such changes usually occur in chronic severe iron deficiency anaemia but may occasionally be seen in non-anaemic patients. The nails become spoon-shaped (koilonychia) and brittle (Fig. 5.43). The tongue may loose its papillae and its epithelium may become thin, smooth and shiny (glossitis). There may be cheilitis, angular stomatitis and both atrophy and abnormal keratinization of the buccal mucosa. The epithelium of the pharynx and oesophagus may also be atrophic. Some authors have attributed the Plummer–Vinson syndrome (Patterson–Kelly syndrome) to epithelial iron deficiency. This syndrome, which consists of glossitis, dysphagia and anaemia, usually affects middle-aged women and may precede the development of post-cricoid carcinoma. It has been suggested that the dysphagia results from recurrent inflammatory episodes in an atrophic pharyngeal mucosa followed by scarring, keratinization and the formation of a post-cricoid diaphragm or web (Fig. 5.44). In Caucasians as well as in Indians, iron deficiency may be associated with superficial gastritis or even gastric atrophy. Children, but not adults, with iron deficiency anaemia show partial atrophy of the duodenal villi and a minor degree of malabsorption. Recent studies have confirmed that tissue iron deficiency leads to various functional changes such as a reduction in exercise

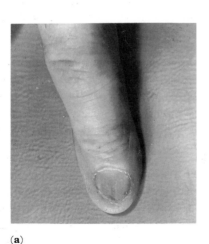

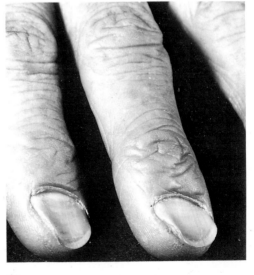

(a)   (b)

Fig. 5.43a, b Concave or spoon-shaped nails (koilonychia) in two patients with iron deficiency anaemia.

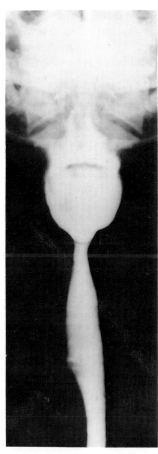

Fig. 5.44 X-ray (barium swallow) showing a post-cricoid web in a patient with the Plummer–Vinson syndrome.

tolerance and work capacity in adults and impairment of mental development in infants.

Pathophysiology of erythropoiesis

The red cells of patients with iron deficiency anaemia have a reduced life-span of about 40–90 days, due to an intracorpuscular defect. The anaemia of iron deficiency results from a failure of the marrow to adequately increase effective erythropoiesis to compensate for this slight or moderate reduction of red cell life-span. The inadequate marrow response is a consequence of a substantial degree of dyserythropoiesis and ineffective erythropoiesis in the non-dividing late polychromatic erythroblasts. The proliferating erythroblasts appear to be more or less normal; they are normally distributed in the different

stages of interphase[11] and show no impairment of the incorporation of various radioactive precursors into DNA and RNA.[110]

ANAEMIA OF CHRONIC DISORDERS[111, 112]

A mild to moderate anaemia develops during the course of a variety of chronic disorders such as chronic infections (e.g. tuberculosis), rheumatoid arthritis and other collagen vascular diseases and various malignant diseases (carcinoma, lymphoma, leukaemia and multiple myeloma). In general, the severity of this anaemia is a function of the severity or extent of the chronic disorder as judged by systemic manifestations such as fever, weight loss and the extent of elevation of the erythrocyte sedimentation rate. The anaemia is usually normochromic and normocytic in type but may be hypochromic and microcytic with MCVs which are sometimes as low as 60 fl. Other characteristics of the anaemia of chronic disorder are a decreased serum iron concentration, a reduction of the total iron binding capacity of the serum, a decreased transferrin saturation, a reduction in the percentage of sideroblasts in the marrow (normal range, 20–90%), a normal or increased quantity of iron in bone marrow macrophages, a normal or raised serum ferritin level, a raised serum copper level and caeruloplasmin concentration, and an increase in free erythrocyte protoporphyrin (normal range, 140–790 μg/l of red cells). The absolute reticulocyte count is either normal or at most twice normal. Serum erythropoietin levels may be inappropriately low for the haemoglobin concentration. Thyroxine levels may be reduced. When uncomplicated by iron or folate deficiency, the anaemia does not respond to any of the usual haematinics. However, if iron is given parenterally rather than orally some response may be seen. The blood picture only returns to normal with successful treatment of the underlying disorder. Not infrequently, the anaemia of chronic disorders is complicated by various factors such as chronic blood loss, infiltration of the bone marrow by malignant cells, drug-induced impairment of bone marrow function and secondary folate deficiency. When iron deficiency develops in a patient with the anaemia of chronic disorders, the total iron binding capacity may not be elevated, and although the serum ferritin level falls it may not fall below the lower limit of normal.

The anaemia of chronic disorders appears to be largely due to an impairment of erythropoiesis. The red cell life-span is either normal or shows a modest reduction due to an extracorpuscular defect. The explanation for the impairment of erythropoiesis is still uncertain. There seems to be a block in the release into the plasma of the iron derived from the degradation of senescent red cells. Such a block could impair the supply of iron to erythroblasts and account for the low serum iron level, the reduction in the proportion of sideroblasts and the formation of hypochromic microcytes. However, the anaemia of chronic disorders does not respond to oral iron therapy and it therefore seems likely that other disturbances of erythropoiesis exist. Theoretical possibilities include impaired regulation of erythropoiesis (there is often a failure of serum erythropoietin levels to increase in proportion to the degree of anaemia) and increased ineffective erythropoiesis. Recent studies have shown that patients with anaemia due to rheumatoid arthritis have a factor in their serum which directly or indirectly suppresses the proliferation of an early erythroid progenitor cell (BFU-E) *in vitro*.[113] Inhibition of erythroid colony formation by autologous bone marrow macrophages has also been reported.[114]

ANAEMIA OF CHRONIC RENAL FAILURE[115]

Anaemia regularly accompanies chronic renal failure irrespective of the nature of the renal pathology. Its severity correlates roughly with the degree of impairment of renal function as judged by the glomerular filtration rate, the serum creatinine level or the blood urea level. Mild anaemia may be detected when the glomerular filtration rate falls below 30% of the normal value, the plasma creatinine rises above 180–350 μmol/1 (2–4 mg/dl) and the blood urea increases above about 8 mmol/1 (50 mg/dl). As the blood urea rises from 8 to 40 mmol/l, the haemoglobin falls by about 2 g/dl for every 8 mmol increase in blood urea. In general, for a given degree of renal failure, patients with polycystic disease of the kidneys are less anaemic and those with an underlying microangiopathy are more anaemic than other patients. The red cells are usually normochromic and normocytic but are occasionally mildly macrocytic. The blood film may contain keratocytes and echinocytes and some schistocytes (Fig. 5.45). (Patients with a

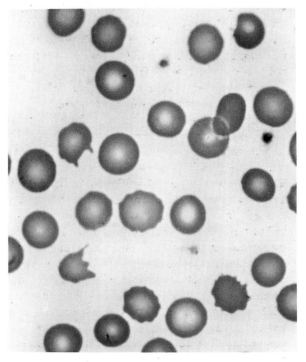

Fig. 5.45 Photomicrograph of a blood film from a patient with chronic renal failure showing two keratocytes (usually termed burr cells in the British literature) and two echinocytes.
May-Grünwald-Giemsa stain   × 940

microangiopathy show a much more striking degree of red cell fragmentation than others, see pp. 150 and 281) The reticulocyte percentage may be normal or increased to 4–10%. The neutrophil and platelet counts are normal or slightly increased and there may be hypersegmentation of the neutrophils which is unrelated to folate deficiency. The bone marrow usually shows normal or increased cellularity. Erythropoiesis is normoblastic and there may be some erythroid hyperplasia. Characteristically the degree of hyperplasia is mild despite a moderate or severe degree of anaemia. Erythroid hypoplasia may also be found, particularly when renal failure develops relatively rapidly.

The main disturbance of bone marrow function in chronic renal failure is an impaired response of the marrow to anaemia. This is caused by two mechanisms: (1) a suboptimal production of erythropoietin by the diseased kidneys; and (2) the presence in the plasma of low molecular weight inhibitors of BFU-E and CFU-E (these are removed, to a large extent, by haemodialysis). These inhibitors may consist of polyamines such as spermine. There is usually a mild to moderate reduction of red cell life-span which is mainly caused by an unidentified non-dialysable 'uraemic toxin' in the plasma. Patients on chronic ambulatory peritoneal dialysis have higher haemoglobin levels when compared with patients on haemodialysis, suggesting that the 'uraemic toxin', responsible for shortening the red cell life-span, may consist of 'middle molecules' (low molecular weight substances are more effectively cleared by haemodialysis whereas the larger 'middle molecules' are more effectively cleared by peritoneal dialysis).[116] Patients with infected or inflamed kidneys may also display the disturbances in iron metabolism which occur in the anaemia of chronic disorders (p. 163). The anaemia of chronic renal failure is largely due to a reduced red cell mass, but the haemoglobin concentration may be further lowered by an increase of the plasma volume which commonly occurs.

ANAEMIA OF CHRONIC LIVER DISEASE[117, 118]

Anaemia develops in a high proportion of patients with chronic liver disease. It is generally of mild to moderate severity, with haemoglobin levels above 9 g/dl. The red cells are often normochromic and normocytic but may be macrocytic with MCVs in the range 100–115 fl. The macrocytosis is usually unrelated to vitamin B_{12} or folate deficiency[119] and is caused either by some folate-independent effect of chronic alcoholism on the bone marrow (p. 182) or, less commonly, by some ill-understood effect of hepatic failure on erythropoietic cells. The macrocytosis is occasionally caused by a dietary folate deficiency. Some patients have a hypochromic microcytic anaemia as a result of iron deficiency secondary to bleeding from oesophageal varices or haemorrhoids. Patients with most types of chronic liver failure have target cells in their blood; however, such cells are more numerous in patients with obstructive jaundice uncomplicated by hepatocellular failure. The target cells result from an increase of surface area secondary to the accumulation of both cholesterol and lecithin in the red cell membrane. The accumulation of lipids occurs from the plasma. Other features of the blood count in chronic liver disease include a normal or increased reticulocyte percentage and, in some cases, a mild thrombocytopenia or pancytopenia due to hypersplenism.

The bone marrow is usually normocellular or moderately hypercellular, with normoblastic or macronormoblastic erythropoiesis. There is often a mild degree of erythroid hyperplasia. Some patients show micronormoblastic erythropoiesis due to iron deficiency and others show frankly megaloblastic haemopoiesis due to folate deficiency.

The normocytic and macrocytic types of anaemia are caused by a combination of a mild to moderate reduction of red cell life-span and an inadequate response of the marrow to the anaemia. The biochemical processes underlying both these disturbances are unknown. The reduction of red cell life-span is not related to the formation of target cells (which have a more or less normal survival) and is probably only partly explained by hypersplenism secondary to congestive splenomegaly.

An unusual degree of haemolysis occurs in Zieve's syndrome and spur cell anaemia, both of which are associated with alcohol-induced liver damage. These syndromes are described on page 156.

SIDEROBLASTIC ANAEMIA[120, 121, 122]

The sideroblastic anaemias are characterized by the presence of a perinuclear ring of abnormally

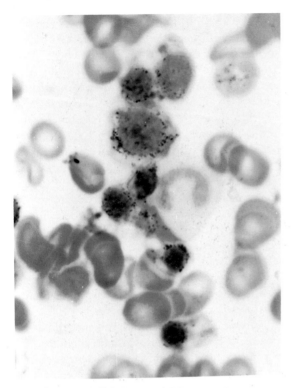

Fig. 5.46 Marrow smear from a patient with primary acquired sideroblastic anaemia showing several ringed sideroblasts.

Perls' acid ferrocyanide stain   × 940

coarse siderotic granules in a substantial proportion of the erythropoietic cells examined after staining by Perls' acid ferrocyanide method (Fig. 5.46). Electron microscope studies have revealed that the majority of the siderotic granules consist of iron-laden mitochondria. The iron-containing material is found between the mitochondrial cristae (Fig. 5.47). The affected mitochondria sometimes display degenerative changes such as the loss of some or all of the cristae and the presence of abnormally electron-lucent areas in the mitochondrial matrix.

Studies of haem synthesis have shown different defects in various patients, the two most commonly observed being reduced activity of the enzymes aminolaevulinic acid (ALA) synthetase and ferrochelatase. However, as the enzymes concerned with haem synthesis are located in the mitochondria, it is not yet certain whether the impairment of haem synthesis is a cause or a consequence of the iron-laden mitochondria.[11]

The sideroblastic anaemias occur as inherited or acquired conditions. The inherited conditions include hereditary sideroblastic anaemia, in which the sideroblastic erythropoiesis and its complications are the only pathological changes, and two syndromes, thiamine-responsive anaemia and the Wolfram-Tyrer syndrome, in which the haematological abnormalities are associated with other congenital abnormalities. Only some cases of thiamine-responsive anaemia and of the Wolfram-Tyrer syndrome appear to be associated with sideroblastic erythropoiesis. Hereditary sideroblastic anaemia is much rarer than the acquired sideroblastic anaemias and may be first diagnosed any time between the ages of 1 and 30 years, usually in adolescence. In most affected families the disease appears to have been transmitted as an X-linked recessive condition and in these families the anaemia is usually confined to males; female carriers usually show only minor changes in the blood and marrow. However, some anaemic females have been reported in whom the inheritance appears to be autosomal. The acquired sideroblastic anaemias can be subdivided into (a) primary (idiopathic) acquired sideroblastic anaemia (see also p. 240) and (b) secondary sideroblastic anaemia. The former accounts for about one-third of the cases of sideroblastic anaemia and usually affects the elderly. The average age at diagnosis is about 70 years (range, 37–86 years). In the secondary sideroblastic anaemias, the sideroblastic erythropoiesis is present as a usually rare manifestation or complication of a variety of diseases and of drug therapy. The many conditions reported to have been associated with sideroblastic erythropoiesis are listed in Table 5.14; the commonest is undoubtedly alcoholism.

Some cases of hereditary and primary acquired sideroblastic anaemia show a considerable haematological response to pyridoxine administered orally. Patients with sideroblastic erythropoiesis may also develop a secondary folate deficiency and such patients may show some response to folate therapy.

Mild or moderate splenomegaly may occur in hereditary sideroblastic anaemia and mild splenomegaly in the primary acquired type.

The blood picture in hereditary sideroblastic

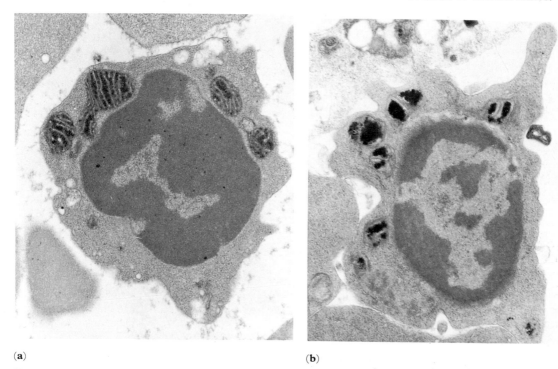

(a)   (b)

Fig. 5.47a, b Electron micrographs of ringed sideroblasts from a case of hereditary sideroblastic anaemia (**a**) and a case of primary acquired sideroblastic anaemia (**b**). Note the presence of very electron-dense iron-containing material between the cristae of the mitochondria.

Uranyl acetate and lead citrate   (**a**) × 20 000; (**b**) × 17 775

anaemia is essentially that of a hypochromic, microcytic anaemia. Some cases have a variable number (up to 50%) of normochromic normocytic red cells. The anaemia may be severe and

Table 5.14 Causes of secondary sideroblastic anaemia

1. Drugs and toxins
   Alcoholism; lead poisoning; therapy with isoniazid, cycloserine, pyrazinamide, chloramphenicol, phenacetin, azathioprine

2. Myeloproliferative disorders*
   Myelofibrosis, polycythaemia vera, thrombocythaemia, chronic myelomonocytic leukaemia, refractory anaemia with excess blasts, acute leukaemia, erythraemic myelosis

3. Miscellaneous
   Malabsorption syndromes, partial gastrectomy, nutritional megaloblastic anaemia, carcinoma, lymphoma, chronic lymphocytic leukaemia, myeloma*, rheumatoid arthritis, polyarteritis nodosa, porphyria cutanea tarda, erythropoietic porphyria, hypothyroidism, hyperthyroidism, chronic haemolytic anaemia, infectious mononucleosis, pernicious anaemia, hypothermia

---

* Although usually classified with secondary sideroblastic anaemias, in these conditions the sideroblastic erythropoiesis is a manifestation of a stem cell abnormality

require treatment with blood transfusion. Both the MCV and MCH are often low, and may be as low as 58 fl and 18 pg respectively. Apart from the microcytosis, there is anisocytosis and poikilocytosis and there may be some target cells. In primary acquired sideroblastic anaemia, the haemoglobin is usually between about 6 and 10 g/dl and the MCV is frequently raised. The blood film is characteristically dimorphic with a major population of well-haemoglobinized, normocytic or macrocytic cells and a second population of hypochromic microcytes which are often misshapen (Fig. 5.48). The percentage of microcytes varies widely from less than 1 to 30. The well-haemoglobinized cell population may also show poikilocytosis and there may be a few target cells. In both the hereditary and primary acquired types, a very few cells displaying basophilic stippling or Pappenheimer bodies and a very occasional circulating erythroblast may be present; the numbers of such cells increase considerably following splenectomy. The red cells

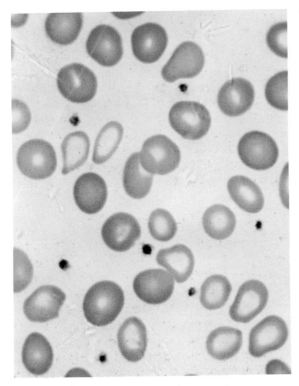

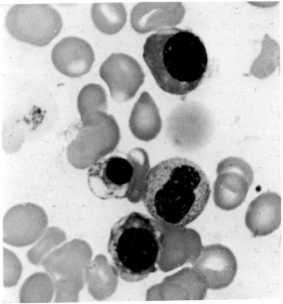

Fig. 5.49 Marrow smear from a patient with primary acquired sideroblastic anaemia showing a late polychromatic erythroblast with feebly-staining ('vacuolated') areas in the cytoplasm, a few coarse basophilic cytoplasmic granules and a pyknotic nucleus.

May–Grünwald–Giemsa stain   × 940

Fig. 5.48 Peripheral blood smear from an untransfused patient with primary acquired sideroblastic anaemia showing both normochromic and markedly hypochromic red cells.

May–Grünwald–Giemsa stain   × 940

of cases of secondary sideroblastic anaemia resemble those of the primary acquired type in being dimorphic with a small population of hypochromic microcytes. Sideroblastic erythropoiesis is associated with a normal or slightly raised (up to 5%) reticulocyte count.

The leucocyte and platelet counts are usually normal but may be slightly reduced both in hereditary and primary acquired sideroblastic anaemia; very occasionally, thrombocytosis may be seen in the primary acquired type.

In many cases of sideroblastic anaemia, the marrow shows erythroid hyperplasia with some increase in the proportion of basophilic erythropoietic cells. These changes are usually both more frequent and more marked in primary acquired sideroblastic anaemia than in the hereditary or secondary types. Erythropoiesis is usually micronormoblastic with poor haemoglobinization of the cytoplasm in the inherited type and either macronormoblastic or megaloblastic in the pri-

mary acquired type. The megaloblastic change is sometimes partly or wholly caused by a secondary folate deficiency but is more often unrelated to folate status. A characteristic finding in all types of sideroblastic anaemia is the presence of some polychromatic erythroblasts with areas of feebly-staining ('transparent' or 'vacuolated') cytoplasm (Fig. 5.49). Such cells may also contain several coarse basophilic granules and pyknotic nuclei which are often irregularly-shaped. Some of these polychromatic erythroblasts have very scanty cytoplasm with indistinct or ragged edges.

The cardinal feature required for the diagnosis of sideroblastic erythropoiesis is the demonstration of many ringed sideroblasts in the marrow. It should be noted that ringed sideroblasts may be present, albeit with a very low frequency, in normal marrow and that the proportion of such cells is slightly increased in many disorders of haemopoiesis. Thus, the diagnosis of sideroblastic erythropoiesis requires the presence of substantial numbers of ringed sideroblasts. Ringed sideroblasts are seen at all stages of erythroblast maturation in primary acquired sideroblastic anaemia and many cases of alcohol-induced sideroblastic anaemia. By contrast they are more or less confined to the late polychromatic erythroblast compartment in hereditary sideroblastic anaemia and most other types of secondary sideroblastic anaemia.

In primary acquired sideroblastic anaemia, the accumulation of large quantities of iron within the mitochondria is associated with and possibly causes: (1) an impairment of proliferation in the early polychromatic erythroblast compartment[123] and (2) a gross suppression of protein biosynthesis in some early and late polychromatic erythroblasts.[124] The anaemia in this disorder is largely the consequence of a high death rate amongst both the early and late polychromatic erythroblasts (i.e. due to a gross degree of ineffective erythropoiesis). By contrast, there is usually a lesser degree of ineffective erythropoiesis in the hereditary sideroblastic anaemias, presumably because in this disorder, marked iron loading of the mitochondria and consequent cell death is more or less confined to the non-dividing late polychromatic erythroblasts.[125] Impaired haemoglobin synthesis and the production of poorly-haemoglobinized microcytes also play a significant role in the pathogenesis of the anaemia in the hereditary disorder.

Some patients with hereditary sideroblastic anaemia die in infancy or childhood; others have a normal life-span. Primary acquired sideroblastic anaemia usually runs a relatively benign course with a median survival of 10 years; these patients often die of conditions related to old age (e.g. pneumonia, cardiac infarction) rather than to the anaemia. In approximately 10% of patients with primary acquired sideroblastic anaemia, the disease evolves into an acute myeloblastic leukaemia.[126] The neutrophils of such patients may show hypogranular cytoplasm, Auer rods, the acquired Pelger-Huët anomaly or a low neutrophil alkaline phosphatase (NAP) score for a considerable period prior to the development of overt leukaemia. The hereditary and primary acquired sideroblastic anaemias may be complicated by haemosiderosis with hepatic, myocardial and pancreatic damage.

MACROCYTIC ANAEMIA[127]

The macrocytic anaemias can be usefully subdivided into two groups: those which are associated with megaloblastic haemopoiesis and those which are associated with normoblastic haemopoiesis (see p. 47). In the former group, the megaloblastic change may be caused by vitamin B_{12} or folate deficiency, disturbances of vitamin B_{12} or folate metabolism, or mechanisms independent of vitamin B_{12} or folate.

Megaloblastic haemopoiesis[11, 128]

The term megaloblast was first used by Paul Ehrlich in 1880 to describe a morphologically abnormal type of erythroblast seen in the bone marrow of cases of untreated pernicious anaemia. Subsequent experience has shown that megaloblasts occur in many other conditions (see Tables 5.15 and 5.16). The two major features of megaloblastic erythropoiesis are that: (1) the erythroblasts are larger than normal at all stages of maturation; and (2) there appears to be a retardation of the normal process of progressive condensation of nuclear chromatin with increasing cell maturation. The latter leads to a dissociation between cytoplasmic and nuclear maturity, early and late polychromatic erythroblasts with well-haemoglobinized (i.e. polychromatic) cytoplasm having nuclei with considerably smaller quantities of condensed chromatin than their normal counterparts (Fig. 5.50). Other features of megaloblastic erythropoiesis include an increased frequency of dyserythropoietic changes (see Table 4.3 on p. 77) in the early and late polychromatic erythroblasts, an increase in the number of basophilic erythropoietic cells relative to more mature erythroblasts and erythroid hyperplasia. The magnitude of all of the morphological changes seen in megaloblastic erythropoiesis increases with increasing severity of the anaemia.

There is a considerably greater degree of ineffective erythropoiesis in megaloblastic marrows than in normoblastic marrows, the extent of ineffectiveness being greatest in the most severely anaemic patients. The ineffectiveness of megaloblastic erythropoiesis results from an abnormality of the red cell precursors which leads to

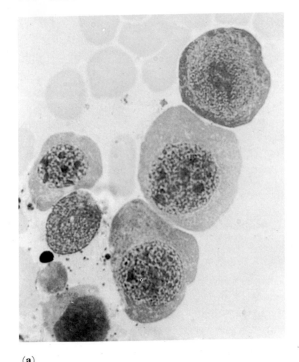

(a)

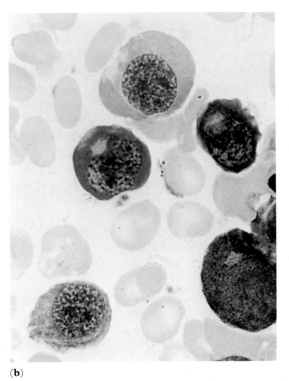

(b)

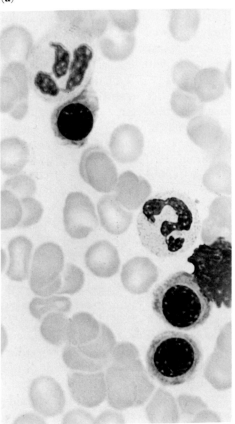

(c)

Fig. 5.50a–c Differences between megaloblastic and normoblastic erythropoiesis as seen in bone marrow smears. (a), (b) Several early polychromatic megaloblasts (and one basophilic megaloblast) from a patient with severe pernicious anaemia. (c) Three early polychromatic normoblasts from a healthy adult.

May–Grünwald–Giemsa stain   × 940

the phagocytosis by bone marrow macrophages of a substantial proportion of the early and late polychromatic megaloblasts. Some vitamin B_{12}-deficient or folate-deficient early polychromatic megaloblasts seem to become arrested at all stages of the cell cycle.

Many patients with megaloblastic erythropoiesis also show morphological abnormalities ('megaloblastic changes') in the granulocytopoietic cells. The two most characteristic changes are the presence of giant metamyelocytes in the marrow (Fig. 5.51) and of hypersegmented neutrophil granulocytes (see Fig. 5.52 and p. 210) in the blood. The giant metamyelocytes may have diameters of 17–30 µm or more and usually have long horseshoe-shaped nuclei, sometimes with one or more bud-like protuberances. In addition,

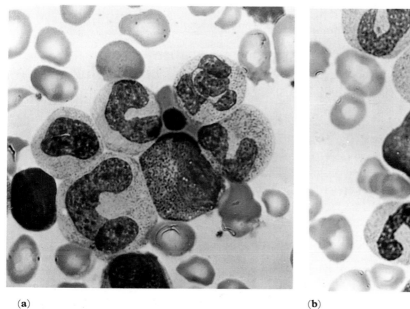

(a)

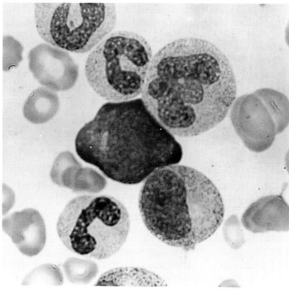

(b)

Fig. 5.51a, b Two photomicrographs of a marrow smear from a patient with pernicious anaemia, each of which contains a giant metamyelocyte adjacent to normal-sized metamyelocytes and band forms. The giant metamyelocyte in (**b**) has an E-shaped nucleus.

May–Grünwald–Giemsa stain   × 940

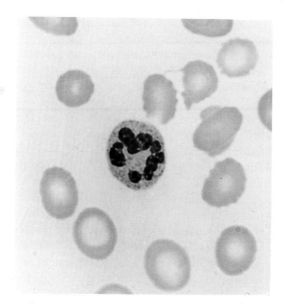

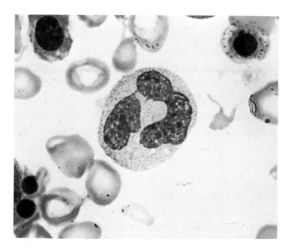

Fig. 5.52 Hypersegmented neutrophil from the blood smear of a patient with pernicious anaemia.

May–Grünwald–Giemsa stain   × 940

Fig. 5.53 Macropolycyte from the bone marrow smear of a patient with pernicious anaemia. The nuclear and cytoplasmic areas of this cell are similar to those of the giant metamyelocytes in Fig. 5.51.

May–Grünwald–Giemsa stain   × 940

some giant metamyelocytes contain cytoplasmic vacuoles, nuclear perforations or poorly-staining chromatin. The giant metamyelocytes seem to result from an abnormal type of development in promyelocytes and myelocytes which have been arrested or retarded during their progress through the cell cycle;[129] they have DNA contents in the entire range between the diploid (2c) and tetraploid (4c) values. Most of these cells appear to be phagocytosed by bone marrow macrophages but a few undergo nuclear segmentation and develop into giant polymorphonuclear leucocytes known as macropolycytes (Fig. 5.53). Such macropolycytes have hyperdiploid DNA contents. By contrast, hypersegmented neutrophils have diploid DNA contents and appear to be derived from normal-looking metamyelocytes with diploid DNA contents.

Megakaryocytes are usually present in normal or increased numbers and may occasionally display markedly hypersegmented nuclei.

Vitamin B_{12}-dependent and folate-dependent causes of megaloblastic anaemia

The vitamin B_{12}-dependent and folate-dependent causes of macrocytosis with megaloblastic erythropoiesis are given in Table 5.15.

Vitamin B_{12}

This vitamin is composed of two parts aligned at right angles to each other: (1) a corrin nucleus (containing four pyrrole rings); and (2) the ribonucleoside of 5,6-dimethylbenzimidazole. A cobalt atom is situated at the centre of the corrin nucleus and is coordinately bonded to the four pyrrole rings and to one of the nitrogen atoms of the ribonucleoside as well as to one of a variety of organic groups such as methyl, deoxyadenosyl, cyano or hydroxo. The two naturally occurring coenzyme forms of the vitamin have the methyl or deoxyadenosyl group and are referred to as methylcobalamin and deoxyadenosylcobalamin, respectively. In nature, vitamin B_{12} is synthesized exclusively by microorganisms. The vitamin is present only in foods of animal origin (including dairy products). Vegetables and fruits are devoid

Table 5.15 Vitamin B_{12}-dependent and folate-dependent causes of macrocytosis with megaloblastic erythropoiesis

1. Vitamin B_{12} deficiency
   (a) Veganism
   (b) Gastric lesions: pernicious anaemia, total or partial gastrectomy, congenital intrinsic factor deficiency, congenitally abnormal intrinsic factor
   (c) Intestinal lesions: stagnant loop syndrome, ileal resection, Crohn's disease, chronic tropical sprue, fish tapeworm, selective malabsorption with proteinuria (Imerslund-Gräsbeck syndrome)
   (d) Congenital transcobalamin II deficiency

2. Folate deficiency
   (a) Inadequate dietary intake
   (b) Malabsorption: coeliac disease, jejunal resection, tropical sprue
   (c) Increased requirement: pregnancy, haemolytic anaemia, malignant disease, ? chronic inflammatory disease
   (d) Complex mechanism: anticonvulsant therapy, ethanol abuse

3. Disturbances of vitamin B_{12} or folate metabolism
   (a) Inactivation of vitamin B_{12} by N_2O
   (b) Methylmalonic aciduria-homocystinuria
   (c) Therapy with dihydrofolate reductase inhibitors (methotrexate, pyrimethamine, trimethoprim and triamterene)
   (d) Congenital disorders of folate metabolism

of vitamin B_{12} except by virtue of contamination by bacteria. A normal diet contains about 5–30 μg vitamin B_{12} per day and 1–3 μg of this are absorbed. The vitamin is released from foods by the action of proteolytic enzymes and attaches to intrinsic factor, a glycoprotein secreted by the parietal cells of the fundus and body of the stomach. The vitamin B_{12}-intrinsic-factor complex, which is resistant to digestion, passes down to the terminal ileum where absorption takes place. Absorption is preceded by attachment of the complex to specific receptor sites on the brush border of the mucosal cells. There is a mucosal delay of a few hours before the absorbed vitamin B_{12} enters the portal blood. Most of the newly-absorbed vitamin B_{12} in portal blood is attached to transcobalamin II (TC II) and most of the vitamin B_{12} in systemic blood to transcobalamin I (TC I). Apparently hepatocytes take up some of the vitamin B_{12} from TC II and either store it or release it into the plasma, bound to TC I.

Most of the body's vitamin B_{12} is found in the

liver, the hepatic stores being 2–5 mg. The absorption of 1–3 μg vitamin B_{12} per day balances an inevitable daily loss of the same magnitude, largely via the urine and faeces. There is an enterohepatic circulation of vitamin B_{12}: about 3–6 μg is excreted daily into the intestinal tract, mainly in the bile, of which all but about 1 μg is reabsorbed in the terminal ileum. If intrinsic factor is absent or ileal absorption is defective there is failure to conserve vitamin B_{12} secreted in the bile.

There is still uncertainty as to the biochemical mechanisms by which vitamin B_{12} deficiency leads to its main clinical consequences of anaemia, peripheral neuropathy and subacute combined degeneration of the spinal cord.[127, 130] There are only two reactions known to require vitamin B_{12} in man. The first is the isomerization of methylmalonyl coenzyme A to succinyl coenzyme A, which is dependent on deoxyadenosylcobalamin; the second is the methylation of homocysteine to methionine, which requires the methyl donor 5-methyltetrahydrofolate (methyl-THF) and the coenzyme methylcobalamin. During the latter reaction the methyl-THF is converted to THF. The impairment of the homocysteine–methionine methyl transferase reaction in bone marrow cells results in defective methylation of deoxyuridylate to thymidylate due to a decreased availability of 5,10-methylenetetrahydrofolate (5,10-methylene-THF) and it is generally considered, though not proven (see p. 179), that defective thymidylate synthesis leads to defective DNA synthesis and, consequently, to the development of megaloblastic haemopoiesis and anaemia. However, there is still controversy as to the mechanism by which an impairment of the transferase reaction results in decreased levels of 5,10-methylene-THF. Some workers consider that this impairment causes trapping of intracellular folates in the form of 5-methyl-THF which cannot be converted to 5,10-methylene-THF. Others have suggested that the important consequence of the impairment of the transferase reaction is the failure of methionine synthesis which in turn results in a paucity of formate and inadequate formylation of tetrahydrofolate, formyltetrahydrofolate being the precursor of 5,10-methylene-THF-polyglutamate. There is considerable doubt about the biochemical mechanisms underlying the neurological damage induced by vitamin B_{12} deficiency. Recent work suggests that the neurological damage may result from a failure to methylate basic proteins in myelin sheaths. This appears to be secondary to a failure of the synthesis of S-adenosylmethionine from methionine as a consequence of the decreased methylcobalamin-dependent conversion of homocysteine to methionine.

The clinicopathological features of subacute combined degeneration of the cord and the peripheral neuropathy caused by vitamin B_{12} deficiency are described in the section on pernicious anaemia (p. 174). These neurological abnormalities have also developed in patients with vitamin B_{12} deficiency due to veganism (p. 173), partial or total gastrectomy (p. 177), congenital intrinsic factor deficiency (p. 177), abnormal small intestinal bacterial flora (p. 177), ileal resection (p. 177) and the Imerslund–Gräsbeck syndrome (p. 178). A severe peripheral neuropathy has been reported in inadequately-treated patients with congenital transcobalamin II deficiency (p. 178).

Causes of vitamin B_{12} deficiency

Veganism.[131, 132] As vitamin B_{12} is only found in foods of animal origin (p. **zzz**), strict vegetarians who do not take appreciable amounts of milk or eggs (vegans) must have a very low dietary intake of this vitamin. The largest group of vegans are the Hindus. Although more than 50% of vegans have low serum vitamin B_{12} levels, most vegans have normal haematological values (including MCVs) and appear to be in good health. Apparently an intact enterohepatic circulation of vitamin B_{12} (see p. 173) together with the very small quantities of vitamin B_{12} absorbed from the diet ensure adequate supplies of the vitamin to marrow and other cells despite the reduced vitamin B_{12} stores. However, some vegans with a low serum B_{12} level develop a megaloblastic anaemia which responds to either oral or parenteral vitamin B_{12} therapy and a few suffer from vitamin B_{12} neuropathy (see page 176). Breast-fed infants of vegan mothers may develop vitamin B_{12} deficiency during the first year of life.

Pernicious anaemia.[127] This is a disorder in which impaired vitamin B_{12} absorption and vitamin B_{12} deficiency result from a severe depression of intrinsic factor secretion secondary to gastric atrophy. The vitamin B_{12} deficiency may lead to anaemia, neurological damage or both. The disease is most common in people of Northern European extraction and is thought to be relatively uncommon in Africans and Asians. However, cases have been reported in most races. Pernicious anaemia is uncommon before the age of 30 but the incidence then increases with advancing age, most patients being between 50 and 70 years old. The overall prevalence in the United Kingdom is about 1 per 1000 of the population, but approaches 1% after the age of 60 years. The male:female ratio is about 1:1.5. A family history of pernicious anaemia is present in about 20% of patients with pernicious anaemia and about 8% of the relatives of patients with this disease have impaired vitamin B_{12} absorption and a low serum vitamin B_{12} level. Autoimmune diseases (thyroid diseases, hypoparathyroidism and hypofunction of the adrenal glands) are commoner in patients with pernicious anaemia and their relatives than in the general population, and patients show a slightly higher than normal incidence of the blood group A. Male patients have an increased incidence of gastric carcinoma.

Symptoms are of slow onset and may include weakness, lassitude, dyspnoea, a sore tongue and gastrointestinal disturbances (anorexia, constipation, diarrhoea, dyspepsia). Some patients have neurological symptoms such as paraesthesiae, difficulty in walking, impotence and impairment of bladder and rectal control. There may be slight jaundice, a low-grade pyrexia and slight enlargement of the spleen. Neurological signs include sensory loss (particularly loss of position and vibration sense), ataxia, positive Romberg sign, impairment of memory and, less commonly, the features of a spastic paraplegia.

Patients diagnosed early have a high MCV (macrocytosis) and high MCH associated with a haemoglobin level within the normal range. Others have both macrocytosis and a mild to severe anaemia. There is a reduction of the red cell count which is more marked than that of the

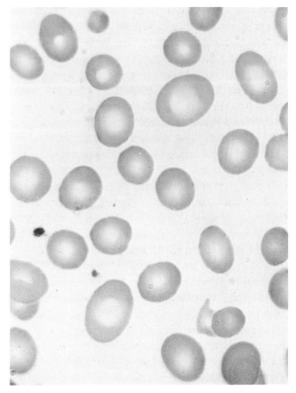

Fig. 5.54 Peripheral blood film of a patient with pernicious anaemia. Oval macrocytes and another poikilocyte are seen. May-Grünwald-Giemsa stain   × 940

haemoglobin level. Usually some of the macrocytes are oval in shape (Fig. 5.54).

With increasing anaemia the red cells also show an increasing degree of anisocytosis and poikilocytosis. The poikilocytes include tear-drop-shaped and irregularly-shaped cells as well as small red cell fragments. There is a rough inverse correlation between the degree of anaemia and the MCV; unusually mild degrees of macrocytosis for the extent of anaemia are found when there are many small red cell fragments (usually in patients with Hb less than 7 g/dl) and in patients with coexistent iron deficiency, chronic disorder (see p. 163, or thalassaemia syndrome. The circulating neutrophil granulocytes of most cases show a tendency towards hypersegmentation of their nuclei, more than 3% of the neutrophils containing five or more nuclear segments. There may be mild neutropenia or thrombocytopenia, particularly in severely anaemic patients.

The bone marrow is hypercellular and in severely anaemic patients there may be an almost complete replacement of fat cells by haemopoietic cells. Haemopoiesis is megaloblastic in type (see p. 169). The M/E ratio is usually reduced but may be increased. The quantity of stainable iron in the marrow fragments is usually normal or increased. There are abnormal sideroblasts but few, if any, ringed sideroblasts (see p. 87).

The serum bilirubin level may be slightly elevated and the serum lactate dehydrogenase is frequently increased. The serum iron is high but falls within 48 h of a single injection of vitamin B_{12}. The serum vitamin B_{12} level is almost invariably below the normal range. However, a low serum vitamin B_{12} level should be considered as presumptive rather than definitive evidence of vitamin B_{12} deficiency as low levels are also seen in about one-third of patients with folate deficiency. Furthermore, low vitamin B_{12} levels may be found in pregnant women or in the elderly, without any haematological, neurological or biochemical disturbances attributable to a deficiency of this vitamin. Red cell folate levels are low in 60% of patients with pernicious anaemia and normal in the remainder. The serum folate level is low in 10% of cases and high in 20%. Parietal cell antibodies are found in the serum in about 85% of patients and IgG intrinsic factor antibodies in 55%. The gastric juice contains an IgA antibody against intrinsic factor in about 60% of cases; there is no correlation between the presence of this IgA antibody and of the IgG antibody.

There is a histamine-fast or pentagastrin-fast achlorhydria. The pH of gastric juice is usually alkaline, but may vary between 6 and 8; after the injection of pentagastrin, the pH usually becomes more alkaline and in any case does not fall by more than 0.5 units. The intrinsic factor content of pentagastrin-stimulated gastric juice is very low, being in the range 0–250 U per hour (normal, >2000 U per hour). Vitamin B_{12} absorption tests, such as the Schilling test, show impaired absorption of an orally-administered physiological dose of ^{57}Co- or ^{58}Co-labelled vitamin B_{12}; this impaired absorption is improved by the simultaneous oral administration of intrinsic factor.

The diagnosis of pernicious anaemia requires the demonstration of a gross impairment of intrinsic factor secretion. This is usually achieved indirectly by performing a Schilling test, with and without intrinsic factor. The vast majority of patients have megaloblastic haemopoiesis and a low serum vitamin B_{12} level, but this combination of abnormalities may occur in other conditions. Furthermore, very occasional patients with a vitamin B_{12} neuropathy may show no morphological abnormalities in either the blood or the bone marrow. The diagnosis of pernicious anaemia cannot be maintained in the absence of a histamine-fast or pentagastrin-fast achlorhydria but this type of severe achlorhydria is not uncommon in elderly subjects with adequate intrinsic factor secretion. Parietal cell antibodies are not specific for pernicious anaemia, being found in a small percentage of healthy individuals (2% of those less than 30 years of age and 16% of those greater than 60 years) and in a higher proportion of individuals with various disorders such as myxoedema, Graves' disease, iron deficiency anaemia and gastritis without pernicious anaemia. By contrast, intrinsic factor antibodies are virtually confined to pernicious anaemia.

At necropsy, untreated cases of advanced pernicious anaemia show pallor and fatty change in most organs. In the heart, the fatty change causes a 'tabby-cat striation' of the myocardium. The liver and spleen are slightly enlarged and contain heavy deposits of haemosiderin as well as foci of extramedullary haemopoiesis. There is replacement of the yellow fatty marrow of long bones by hyperplastic haemopoietic marrow which is deep red in colour. The expansion of the marrow causes a thinning of the bone cortex and loss of trabeculae. There is severe atrophy of the mucosa and muscle coat of the upper two-thirds of the stomach. Histological examination of the mucosa reveals only a few scattered glands and these are lined by mucus-secreting cells (Fig. 5.55). There is a lack of oxyntic and peptic cells with a variable degree of infiltration by lymphocytes and plasma cells. The epithelium of the tongue, oesophagus and intestine is also thinned. Cytological and histological studies show that the epithelial cells lining the buccal cavity, tongue, stomach, jejunum, bronchial tree, urinary tract, vagina, and cervix

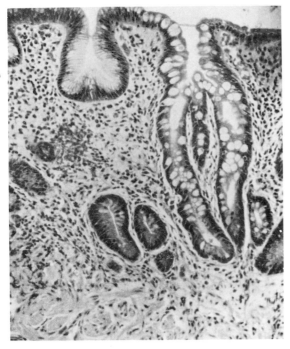

Fig. 5.55 Biopsy of the gastric mucosa in pernicious anaemia showing a paucity of gastric glands. The few glandular elements seen contain mucous-secreting cells. The mucosal layer contains increased numbers of lymphocytes and plasma cells.

Haematoxylin–eosin

From reference 127, courtesy of Dr I. Chanarin, MRC Clinical Research Centre, Northwick Park Hospital, Harrow, Middlesex, UK.

uteri display 'megaloblastic changes'—particularly an increase in cell and nuclear size.

In some patients, the features of subacute combined degeneration of the spinal cord may be seen (Fig. 5.56).[133] There is patchy degeneration of the dorsal columns and pyramidal and spinocerebellar tracts causing a greyish discoloration of the white matter. Usually, the foci of degeneration initially affect (and are most extensive in) the lower cervical and upper thoracic segments of the cord and gradually spread upwards into the upper cervical segments and downwards into the lumbar segments. The dorsal columns and spinocerebellar tracts are most affected in the upper part of the spinal cord and the pyramidal tracts in the lower part. Microscopically, there is marked swelling of the myelin sheaths (giving the affected areas a vacuolated appearance) followed by degeneration of the axons; the degenerating myelin sheaths and axons are removed by phagocytic cells which become laden with lipid. Extensive damage is eventually followed by substantial gliosis. Similar degenerative changes may be present in the posterior nerve roots. Foci of demyelination may also occur in the white matter of the cerebral hemispheres and the medulla oblongata. In long-standing cases, there is secondary degeneration of the long tracts in areas of the spinal cord not directly involved by the disease.

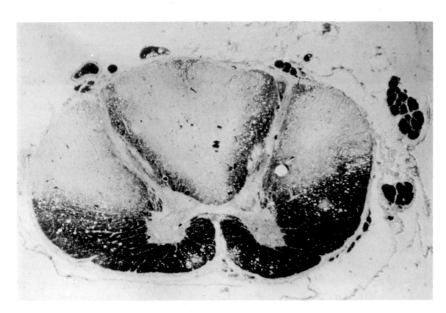

Fig. 5.56 The cervical spinal cord in advanced subacute combined degeneration. The posterior and lateral columns show pale areas, indicating demyelination.
Weigert–Pal method for myelin

Courtesy of Dr R.O. Barnard, Department of Neuropathology, Maida Vale Hospital, London, UK.

The cerebrospinal fluid shows an increase of protein (usually less than 100 mg/dl) in about half the patients with subacute combined degeneration of the cord.

There may be evidence of a peripheral neuropathy with loss of nerve fibres and the muscles may show denervation atrophy.[127, 133] Bilateral optic atrophy has been reported occasionally.

Total or partial gastrectomy.[134, 135] Total gastrectomy results in the removal of the intrinsic-factor-secreting cells and therefore inevitably leads to a megaloblastic anaemia due to vitamin B_{12} deficiency. This anaemia appears 2-10 years after the operation; the long delay represents the time taken for normal vitamin B_{12} stores to run out after the abrupt cessation of vitamin B_{12} absorption.

Anaemia due to iron deficiency develops in about half the cases subjected to partial gastrectomy, and anaemia or neuropathy due to vitamin B_{12} deficiency in about 5% of the cases. The iron deficiency anaemia usually appears during, and the vitamin B_{12} deficiency anaemia after the first five post-operative years. In most cases, the vitamin B_{12} deficiency appears to result from a combination of the loss of intrinsic-factor-secreting mucosa at operation and the subsequent atrophy of the remainder of the gastric mucosa. The probability of developing vitamin B_{12} deficiency is a function of the amount of stomach resected. In a few cases, the vitamin B_{12} deficiency is the consequence of the development of an abnormal intestinal bacterial flora.

Congenital intrinsic factor deficiency.[136] Patients with this rare syndrome present with megaloblastic anaemia, usually during the first three years of life. The syndrome is characterized by the virtual absence of intrinsic factor but the presence of hydrochloric acid and pepsin in gastric juice, a normal-looking gastric mucosa, the absence of parietal cell and intrinsic factor antibodies and an autosomal recessive inheritance. Heterozygotes are clinically normal.

Congenitally abnormal intrinsic factor.[137] A single case has been described in which a severe megaloblastic anaemia was due to homozygosity for the production of a mutant intrinsic factor molecule. This abnormal intrinsic factor bound vitamin B_{12} but failed to promote vitamin B_{12} absorption.

Abnormal intestinal bacterial flora.[138] Vitamin B_{12} deficiency may develop in conditions in which there is small-intestinal stasis. Such conditions include multiple jejunal diverticula, small-intestinal strictures, intestinal involvement in systemic sclerosis, and stagnant intestinal loops resulting either from gastrointestinal surgery or from fistulae complicating regional ileitis or tuberculosis. The intestinal stasis results in the presence of an increased number of bacteria (e.g. enterobacteria, bacteroides, streptococci, lactobacilli and Gram-positive anaerobes) within the proximal part of the small gut. These bacteria convert vitamin B_{12} from ingested food into inactive cobamides and thus decrease the availability of vitamin B_{12} for absorption at the terminal ileum.[139] Patients with vitamin B_{12} deficiency due to the presence of an abnormal intestinal bacterial flora show a decreased absorption of an oral dose of vitamin B_{12} which is not improved when the vitamin is given with intrinsic factor. However, they show a substantial improvement in absorption soon after a course of a broad-spectrum antibiotic such as tetracycline.

Ileal resection,[140] *Crohn's disease and chronic tropical sprue.* As mentioned, vitamin B_{12} is absorbed in the terminal ileum (p. 172). A deficiency of this vitamin due to impairment of its absorption may, therefore, develop in diseases affecting the lower part of the ileum (e.g. Crohn's disease, chronic tropical sprue) or after resections of the terminal ileum.

Megaloblastic anaemia is present in 60-90% of patients with tropical sprue. About 90% of patients with this disease malabsorb vitamin B_{12} and many also malabsorb folate. The absorption of vitamin B_{12} frequently returns to normal after a course of broad-spectrum antibiotics and in the early stages of the disease may improve following therapy with folic acid.

Infestation with the fish tapeworm (Diphyllobothrium latum).[141, 142] Infestation with this tapeworm is seen in people living around the freshwater lakes of Finland, the Baltic States and the Soviet Union. Infestation occurs by eating raw or partly cooked fish containing a larval form. The adult tapeworm may grow to a length of 10 m and is found attached by its head to the mucosa of the ileum. A few per cent of infested humans develop megaloblastic haemopoiesis or neurological abnormalities due to vitamin B_{12} deficiency. The tapeworm causes these effects by extracting vitamin B_{12} from food. Although most fish tapeworms are attached to the distal half of the small intestine, the worms of anaemic individuals seem to be attached much higher up. This observation has led to the suggestion that parasites with a high attachment may extract more vitamin B_{12} than others. Vitamin B_{12} deficiency due to infestation with the fish tapeworm is becoming less common because of pollution of the lakes and a consequent reduction in the population of potentially-infective fish. Whereas in the past about 20% of Finns harboured the fish tapeworm this figure had come down to about 2% in 1977.[143]

Selective malabsorption of vitamin B_{12} with proteinuria (Imerslund-Gräsbeck syndrome).[144] Patients with this rare congenital disorder present with megaloblastic anaemia during the first 2–15 years of life. The anaemia results from a failure of the terminal ileum to absorb vitamin B_{12} from the vitamin-B_{12}–intrinsic-factor complex. The defect of absorption only affects vitamin B_{12}, the absorption of other substances being entirely normal. The gastric juice contains normal quantities of intrinsic factor and the histology of the stomach and terminal ileum is normal. Over 90% of cases have proteinuria (0.02–0.1 g protein/dl urine) but there are usually no other defects of renal function. The disease is inherited as an autosomal recessive characteristic.

Congenital transcobalamin II deficiency.[145] A few children have been reported in whom a megaloblastic anaemia resulted from the complete absence of transcobalamin II (TC II). This transcobalamin is concerned with the active transport of vitamin B_{12} into all cell types and away from the epithelial cells of the terminal ileum (following absorption from the vitamin-B_{12}–intrinsic-factor complex). Most patients present with severe megaloblastic anaemia, leucopenia and thrombocytopenia early in infancy. One patient also had marked hypogammaglobulinaemia. Since most of the vitamin B_{12} in serum is bound to transcobalamin I, the serum vitamin B_{12} level is normal. By contrast, the unsaturated vitamin B_{12}-binding capacity of the serum, which is normally largely dependent on the presence of apotranscobalamin II, is greatly reduced (normal range, 1000 ± 200 pg/ml). There is also a failure to absorb dietary vitamin B_{12} which is not corrected by the administration of intrinsic factor. The anaemia responds to the injection of 1000 μg vitamin B_{12} once or twice a week. These massive doses probably work, despite the absence of the specific transport protein, by causing free vitamin B_{12} to enter cells by passive diffusion. Megaloblastic haemopoiesis caused by a congenitally abnormal TCII molecule has been described.[146]

Malabsorption of vitamin B_{12}, usually without megaloblastic anaemia

Malabsorption of vitamin B_{12} has been demonstrated in patients receiving aminosalicylates, neomycin, colchicine, slow-release potassium chloride, metformin, phenformin, cimetidine, cholestyramine and large doses of vitamin C. Vitamin B_{12} malabsorption has also been described in the Zollinger–Ellison syndrome, severe pancreatic disease and giardiasis. In all of these situations, the malabsorption has usually not been sufficiently severe or has not been allowed to continue for a sufficiently long period to cause the development of megaloblastic anaemia. However, rarely megaloblastic anaemia has developed in severe pancreatic disease and following prolonged treatment with aminosalicylates or metformin.

Folates

The folates are a family of compounds derived from the biologically inactive parent compound pteroyl monoglutamic acid (folic acid). Most intracellular folates are pteroyl polyglutamates with a total of 3–7 (usually 4, 5 or 6) glutamic acid residues linked together by γ-carboxy peptide bonds. By contrast most of the extracellular folates are monoglutamates. Naturally occurring intracellular and extracellular folates are also in the reduced di- or tetrahydrofolate form and, in addition, contain a single carbon unit in various states of reduction (e.g. methyl, formyl, methylene).

Folates are present in all types of animal and vegetable foods; particularly high concentrations are found in yeast, spinach, Brussels sprouts and liver. The folate content of an average diet is about 680 μg/day, and is greatly influenced by the method of preparation of food. Folates are rapidly destroyed by heat and 30–90% may be lost during cooking. About 80% of a 200 μg dose of ^{3}H-pteroylglutamic acid is absorbed; less folate is absorbed from dietary polyglutamates than monoglutamates. The amount of folate absorbed by an adult is 100–200 μg per day. Prior to absorption, dietary pteroyl polyglutamates are first hydrolysed into monoglutamates, probably in the lumen of the gut, by the enzyme folate conjugase. The enterocyte converts the folate monoglutamates into 5-methyltetrahydrofolate before transfer to portal blood. The jejunum and upper part of the ileum absorb folate more actively than the remainder of the small intestine.

The total folate content of the human body is about 6–10 mg; most of this is found in the liver. The daily absorption of 100–200 μg folate is balanced by an equal loss of folate in sweat, desquamated cells (e.g. skin cells) and urine. Because of the relatively large daily requirement, folate stores may become depleted and folate deficiency develop within 3–4 months of taking a folate-depleted diet.

Folate coenzymes are involved in the transfer of single carbon units in a number of reactions. 5,10-methylenetetrahydrofolate is required for the methylation of deoxyuridylate to thymidylate. 10-formyltetrahydrofolate and 5,10-methenyltetrahydrofolate are involved in the supply of carbons 2 and 8 of the purine ring, respectively. 5-methyltetrahydrofolate participates in methionine synthesis (see p. 173). Other folate-dependent reactions in humans include the conversion of serine to glycine and the degradation of histidine through formiminoglutamic acid to glutamic acid.

Folate deficiency causes megaloblastic haemopoiesis but does not lead to neurological damage. Some workers have attributed the haematological changes to impaired DNA synthesis secondary to defective methylation of deoxyuridylate to thymidylate. However, the situation appears to be more complex than this as studies of DNA synthesis have suggested that most folate- (or vitamin B_{12}-) deficient human marrow cells elongate daughter DNA strands at a normal rate and incorporate nucleic acid precursors (other than deoxyuridine) into DNA at normal or even enhanced rates.

Causes of folate deficiency

Inadequate dietary intake. Megaloblastic anaemia due to a dietary folate deficiency tends to occur in the poor, the neglected elderly, the mentally disturbed, chronic alcoholics, and infants fed almost exclusively on goat's milk (which contains little folate). 'Goat's milk anaemia' has been reported in various countries including Germany, Italy, New Zealand and the USA.

Malabsorption. Diseases such as Crohn's disease and tropical sprue, which affect the upper part of the small intestine, often cause anaemia due to malabsorption of folate.

Increased requirement. An increased requirement of folate due to increased nucleic acid turnover may lead to folate deficiency, particularly in those taking suboptimal quantities of folate in their diet. An increased requirement occurs in pregnancy because of the needs of the growing fetus, in chronic haemolytic anaemias because of increased erythropoietic cell proliferation and in premature infants because of the rapid growth during the first 2–3 months. There also appears to be an increased folate requirement in chronic myelofibrosis and various malignant diseases presumably due to increased proliferation of fibroblasts and neoplastic cells respectively.

Before the use of folate supplements during pregnancy, megaloblastic haemopoiesis was found in the latter part of pregnancy in about 25% of women in the UK and in over 50% of women in South India. However, the incidence of megaloblastic anaemia was much lower, being about 0.5–5.0% in the UK. Megaloblastic anaemia is particularly common in twin pregnancies and is most likely to present after the thirty-sixth week of gestation, around the time of delivery or early in the postpartum period.

Patients with active chronic inflammation such as those with tuberculosis or severe rheumatoid arthritis tend to become folate-deficient, probably because of a combination of: (1) inadequate intake (as the result of a poor appetite); (2) increased urinary loss; and (3) an increased requirement to support the increased formation of chronic inflammatory cells.

Anticonvulsant therapy and ethanol abuse. Most patients with macrocytosis associated with anticonvulsant therapy[147] or chronic alcoholism[148] do not suffer from folate deficiency[119] (see p. 181). In those who do, the deficiency seems to be mainly caused by an inadequate diet. However, malabsorption of folate has been described both in treated epileptics and chronic alcoholics, and probably contributes to the development of folate deficiency, as may other unidentified deleterious effects of the intake of anticonvulsants or ethanol.

Disturbances of vitamin B_{12} or folate metabolism

Inactivation of vitamin B_{12} by nitrous oxide.[149] The continuous exposure of patients to a mixture of 50% N_2O and 50% O_2 for 5–6 days or more (once used in the management of severe tetanus) may cause bone marrow aplasia with severe megaloblastic changes in the residual haemopoietic cells.[150] Continuous exposure for 5–24 h (e.g. during the post-operative ventilation of patients who have undergone cardiac bypass surgery) often induces mildly megaloblastic erythropoiesis.[151] It is also possible that the intermittent use of nitrous oxide over long periods (e.g. Entonox—a mixture of equal parts of N_2O and O_2—inhaled for 15–20 min two or three times a day to facilitate physiotherapy) may induce megaloblastic changes.[152] Furthermore, neuropathy resembling that seen in vitamin B_{12} deficiency has been described in dentists repeatedly exposed to

N_2O for prolonged periods.[153] These effects seem to result from the oxidation of methyl cobalamin by N_2O and its consequent inactivation.

Methylmalonic aciduria-homocystinuria.[154, 155] This rare congenital disorder results from an impairment of the conversion of vitamin B_{12} to the two coenzymes methylcobalamin and adenosylcobalamin. The deficiency of these coenzymes results in both homocystinuria and methylmalonic aciduria (see p. 173). The primary defect may lie in a failure to reduce vitamin B_{12} from the cob(III)alamin to the cob(I)alamin form. Clinical features include failure to thrive, mental retardation and, in some cases, megaloblastic haemopoiesis. Impaired methylation of deoxyuridylate in marrow cells has been demonstrated both in patients with megaloblastic and in those with normoblastic erythropoiesis. Nevertheless, it is of interest that despite impairment of both of the only vitamin B_{12}-dependent reactions known in man, haematological abnormalities are not a major feature of the disorder.

Therapy with dihydrofolate reductase inhibitors.[119, 156] The enzyme dihydrofolate reductase, which is present in most mammalian cells, catalyses the reduction of dihydrofolate to tetrahydrofolate. The dihydrofolate which is reduced in this way is derived both from the diet and from the 5,10-methylenetetrahydrofolate-dependent methylation of deoxyuridylate to thymidylate. In the latter reaction the folate coenzyme is oxidized to dihydrofolate. The administration of dihydrofolate reductase inhibitors (such as methotrexate, pyrimethamine and triamterene) appears to cause megaloblastic haemopoiesis by impairing the regeneration of 5,10-methylenetetrahydrofolate from dihydrofolate and thus reducing the rate of methylation of deoxyuridylate. Trimethoprim, which is present in co-trimoxazole (Septrin), is a weak inhibitor of mammalian dihydrofolate reductase: when used in conventional dosage it causes megaloblastic haemopoiesis only in patients with a pre-existing impairment of the methylation of deoxyuridylate due, for example, to a mild degree of vitamin B_{12} or folate deficiency.

Congenital disorders of folate metabolism.[127] Rare cases of megaloblastic haemopoiesis with high serum folate levels have been attributed to decreased levels of dihydrofolate reductase, methyltetrahydrofolate-homocysteine methyltransferase or other (unidentified) enzymes involved in folate metabolism. Mental retardation has developed in some cases.

Vitamin B$_{12}$-independent and folate-independent causes of megaloblastic erythropoiesis (Table 5.16)

Abnormalities of nucleic acid synthesis

Drug-induced impairment of DNA synthesis.[119, 156] A number of drugs interfering with DNA synthesis cause macrocytosis with megaloblastic erythropoiesis. These include mercaptopurine, thioguanine and azathioprine (which interfere with purine synthesis), fluorouracil (which inhibits thymidylate synthetase), cytarabine (which inhibits DNA polymerase), and hydroxyurea (which inhibits ribonucleotide reductase). Other drugs which cause megaloblastic changes by vitamin B$_{12}$-independent or folate-independent mechanisms include cyclophosphamide, procarbazine and acyclovir. Arsenic poisoning also causes megaloblastic changes.

Orotic aciduria.[157] This is a rare inherited disorder of pyrimidine synthesis characterized by severe megaloblastic anaemia, failure to thrive, the excretion of large quantities (0.5–1.5 g/d) of orotic acid in the urine and impaired cellular (but not humoral) immunity. The disorder is caused by a greatly reduced activity of two enzymes, orotidylic pyrophosphorylase and orotidylic decarboxylase, which are involved in the conversion of orotic acid to uridine monophosphate, a precursor of the pyrimidine bases of DNA. Affected patients appear to be homozygotes for an autosomal recessive gene and present between the ages of 3 months and 7 years. The serum vitamin B$_{12}$ and red cell folate levels are normal and there is no response to vitamin B$_{12}$ or folate therapy. Both the anaemia and the failure of growth and development respond well to the daily administration of 1–1.5 g uridine.

Lesch–Nyhan syndrome.[158] This syndrome is characterized by mental retardation, choreoathetosis, self-mutilation (especially biting of the lips and fingers), gout, and a sex-linked recessive inheritance. It is caused by a deficiency of the enzyme hypoxanthine phosphoribosyltransferase, which is involved in purine synthesis. Some cases have shown megaloblastic erythropoiesis.

Children with the Lesch–Nyhan syndrome may also have an increased susceptibility to infection due to defective function of B-lymphocytes. Evidence of B-cell dysfunction includes a reduced number of B-cells, decreased IgG levels, reduced isoagglutinin titres and an impaired response to pokeweed mitogen.

Uncertain aetiology

Anticonvulsant therapy.[119] Some patients who develop megaloblastic erythropoiesis as a consequence of treatment with phenytoin (either on its own or in combination with other anticonvulsant drugs) do not suffer from a folate deficiency or an impairment of the methylation of deoxyuridylate due to any other cause. In these cases, the megaloblastic changes appear to be the result of a folate-independent drug-induced impairment of DNA synthesis and erythroblast proliferation (see also p. 182).

Chronic alcoholism.[119] About 10% of chronic alcoholics display mildly megaloblastic erythro-

---

Table 5.16 Vitamin B$_{12}$-*independent* and folate-*independent* causes of macrocytosis with megaloblastic erythropoiesis

1. Abnormalities of nucleic acid synthesis
   (a) Therapy with antipurines (e.g. mercaptopurine, thioguanine, azathioprine), antipyrimidines (e.g. fluorouracil, azauridine, cytarabine), hydroxyurea, cyclophosphamide, procarbazine, acyclovir. Arsenic poisoning.
   (b) Orotic aciduria, Lesch-Nyhan syndrome

2. Uncertain aetiology
   (a) Anticonvulsant therapy,* chronic alcoholism*
   (b) Myelodysplastic syndromes, erythroleukaemia
   (c) Congenital dyserythropoietic anaemia, types I and III (p. 191)
   (d) Thiamine-responsive anaemia

* See also Table 5.17

poiesis in the absence of evidence of folate deficiency. The megaloblastic changes presumably
result from a direct effect of ethanol (or its metabolites) on erythropoietic cells (see below).

*Myelodysplastic syndromes and erythroleukae-
mia.*[119] The megaloblastic erythropoiesis seen in
these disorders is not primarily caused by vitamin B_{12} or folate deficiency but may occasionally
be complicated by folate deficiency as a result of
an increased requirement for folate (see p. 179).

Thiamine-responsive anaemia.[159] This rare congenital disorder is characterized by sensorineural
deafness, diabetes mellitus, and megaloblastic anaemia which is refractory to vitamin B_{12}, folate
or pyridoxine therapy. Some cases also have sideroblastic erythropoiesis. The anaemia, but not
the deafness, responds to the oral administration
of large doses (20–100 mg/day) of thiamine.
Patients do not show any of the clinical features
of the syndrome (beriberi) produced by a dietary
deficiency of thiamine and appear not to be deficient in this vitamin. They seem to suffer from
a thiamine-responsive disturbance affecting the
erythropoietic cells.

Macrocytosis with normoblastic erythropoiesis[119]

The conditions in which at least a proportion of
the patients with macrocytosis have normoblastic
erythropoiesis are listed in Table 5.17. Chronic
alcoholism is a very common cause of macrocytosis (usually without anaemia) in countries like the
UK and USA. Alcohol-induced macrocytosis is
associated with normoblastic erythropoiesis in
about 70% of the cases and in these the macrocytosis is independent of folate deficiency or an
impairment of the 5,10-methylenetetrahydro-
folate-dependent methylation of deoxyuridylate.
Similarly, phenytoin-induced macrocytosis is occasionally associated with normoblastic erythropoiesis, usually with no evidence of impairment
of the methylation of deoxyuridylate. The mechanism underlying the macrocytosis in both these
conditions is uncertain but may be an impairment

Table 5.17 Causes of macrocytosis with normoblastic
erythropoiesis

Physiological
  Neonates (see Table 1.4)
  Old age* (see Table 1.4)

Smoking

Chronic alcoholism†

Chronic liver disease†

Haemolytic anaemia†

Hypothyroidism (see p. 183)

Therapy with anticonvulsant drugs†

Normal pregnancy†

Chronic pulmonary disease

Primary acquired sideroblastic anaemia† (see p. 165)

Hypoplastic and aplastic anaemia (see p. 187)

* There is a slight but progressive increase in the MCV with
increasing age
† Some cases show megaloblastic erythropoiesis

of cell proliferation by a direct effect of alcohol
or the drug or their metabolites on erythroblasts.
The macrocytosis seen in non-folate-deficient
patients with haemolytic anaemia results from
various erythropoietin-induced alterations in the
kinetics of erythropoiesis; the reticulocytes produced by patients with stimulated erythropoiesis
are considerably larger than normal reticulocytes
and mature into rounded macrocytes. About
25% of cases of hypothyroidism (without associated pernicious anaemia) have macrocytic red
cells and in these the macrocytosis seems to be a
manifestation of a deficiency of thyroid hormones. Even those patients with hypothyroidism
whose MCVs are within the normal range show
some fall in the MCV when they become euthy-
roid.[160] In women who are not iron- or folate-
deficient there is a slight but progressive increase
in the MCV throughout pregnancy and occasionally the MCV may rise above the normal range
for adults.[161] Another cause of macrocytosis with
normoblastic erythropoiesis is chronic pulmonary disease.[162] Here, the macrocytosis is sometimes associated with true polycythaemia secondary to a reduced Po_2 in arterial blood and has
been attributed to a swelling of red cells.

ENDOCRINE DEFICIENCY[163]

The secretions of various endocrine glands play a role in maintaining normal erythropoiesis. Thyroxine, androgens and growth hormone stimulate erythropoiesis partly by an effect on the kidneys which results in an increased production of erythropoietin. Thyroxine also stimulates erythropoiesis by modulating β-adrenergic receptor activity in CFU-E (p. 45) and androgens directly stimulate the proliferation of multipotent haemopoietic stem cells and CFU-E. Corticosteroids enhance erythropoiesis both by a stimulation of erythropoietin production and by a direct effect on the bone marrow. There is some evidence that oestrogens may inhibit erythropoiesis; the sex difference in the haemoglobin levels of adults appears to be largely due to the higher androgen levels in males.

Patients with hypofunction of the thyroid, testes, adrenal glands or anterior lobe of the pituitary gland may suffer from a mild to moderate anaemia which responds only to treatment with the deficient hormone or hormones. Both in hypofunction of the adrenal glands and in hypopituitarism, the anaemia is sometimes partly obscured by a contraction of the plasma volume. The anaemia of endocrine deficiency syndromes results primarily from decreased red cell production. It is usually normochromic and normocytic in type, but in the case of hypothyroidism may be macrocytic. Patients with hypothyroidism may also have acanthocytes in their blood films (Fig. 5.57).

BONE MARROW INFILTRATION (MYELOPHTHISIC ANAEMIA)

Anaemia may develop as a result of the infiltration of the marrow by malignant cells (secondary carcinoma, myeloma, leukaemia and lymphoma), fibrous tissue (myelofibrosis), lipid-laden macrophages (Gaucher's disease, Niemann–Pick disease and Hand–Schüller–Christian disease) or bone (marble bone disease of Albers–Schönberg). The anaemia is usually normochromic and normocytic in type. The blood film shows anisocytosis and, often, a marked degree of poikilocytosis. The percentage of circulating reticulocytes is slightly or moderately increased and the blood may contain erythroblasts, frequently in large numbers. The neutrophil count is usually normal or moderately increased but is sometimes decreased. The blood film may show several neutrophil metamyelocytes, a few myelocytes and an occasional myeloblast. The presence of both erythroblasts and immature neutrophils in the blood, sometimes in large numbers, is a characteristic (but not unique) finding in the myelophthisic anaemias; the resulting blood picture is described as being leucoerythroblastic.[164] A leucoerythroblastic blood picture may also be seen in severe acute blood loss, severe haemolytic states, acute pneumonia, cyanotic congenital heart disease, polycythaemia rubra vera, severe megaloblastic anaemia (before and after treatment) and accompanying bone marrow necrosis.

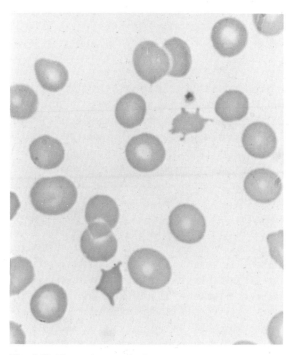

Fig. 5.57 Photomicrograph of a blood film of a 70-year-old man with severe hypothyroidism (Hb 9.1 g/dl; MCV 95 fl). Two acanthocytes are seen.

May–Grünwald–Giemsa stain   × 940

Primary idiopathic myelofibrosis (myelosclerosis, agnogenic myeloid metaplasia)[165,166]

This disorder usually affects the middle-aged and elderly. It is characterized by leucoerythroblastic anaemia, progressive fibrosis of the bone marrow, moderate to gross splenomegaly and extramedullary haemopoiesis. Between 10 and 60% of patients give a definite or suggestive history of polycythaemia rubra vera or essential thrombocythaemia and occasional patients of Ph[1]-positive chronic granulocytic leukaemia. The liver may be enlarged. There is radiological evidence of osteosclerosis, particularly in the axial skeleton and the upper ends of the humeri and femora in about 50% of cases.

Occasional patients may have a true polycythaemia at diagnosis but most are anaemic and the severity of the anaemia increases with time. The anaemia is caused by a combination of a reduced rate of effective erythropoiesis, an expanded plasma volume due to splenomegaly, an increased pooling of red cells within the large spleen and some reduction in red cell life-span. The circulating red cells show marked anisocytosis and poikilocytosis, often with frequent tear-drop-shaped poikilocytes (Fig. 5.58). The number of poikilocytes decreases after splenectomy, suggesting that the spleen plays a role in the production of such cells.[167] The total white cell and platelet counts vary; they may be normal, raised or reduced. There may be abnormally large platelets (Fig. 5.58) and increased numbers of circulating megakaryocytes. Several patients have become folate-deficient due to an increased requirement for folate (p. 179) and such patients may show macrocytosis and megaloblastic erythropoiesis. Serum uric acid and serum vitamin B_{12} levels may be raised, as in polycythaemia rubra vera (p. 196); serum lactate dehydrogenase and bilirubin levels may be increased, reflecting ineffective erythropoiesis, and serum lysozyme may be elevated, indicating increased (often ineffective) granulocytopoiesis. About half the patients show a polyclonal increase of serum immunoglobulins.[168] Other abnormalities found in some patients include positive tests for rheumatoid factor, antinuclear or anti-smooth muscle

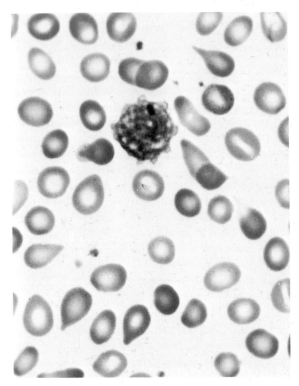

Fig. 5.58 Photomicrograph of a blood film from a patient with primary idiopathic myelofibrosis, showing tear-drop-shaped poikilocytes and a giant platelet.
May–Grünwald–Giemsa stain   × 940

antibodies, a positive direct antiglobulin test, anti-I autoantibody, decreased levels of immunoglobulins or a monoclonal immunoglobulin.[168]

Some patients present with hypercellularity of all haemopoietic cell lines and minimal fibrosis of the marrow (hypercellular panmyelosis phase)[169] and show progressively increasing fibrosis thereafter (Fig. 5.59). Others present with established fibrosis (Fig. 5.60). In the hypercellular phase, large clusters of erythroblasts and many large megakaryocytes are present, reticulin fibres are slightly increased and bone marrow aspiration may be possible. With established fibrosis, bone marrow aspiration is difficult and frequently yields only a little blood ('blood tap') or no aspirate ('dry tap'). Trephine biopsy shows a reduction of haemopoietic tissue and the presence of many fibroblasts and greatly increased quantities of reticulin (Fig. 5.61) and collagen. The reticulin fibres are abnormally coarse and tend to run

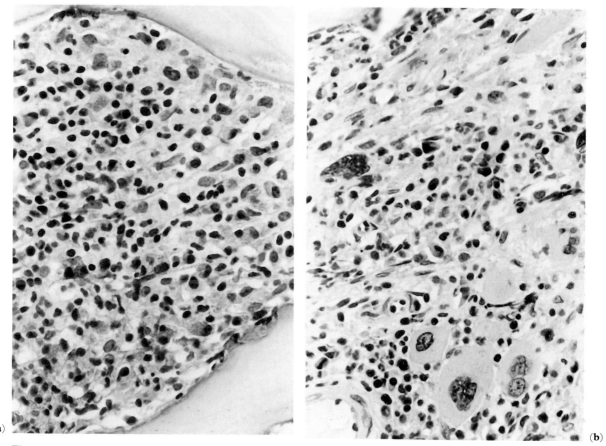

(a)

(b)

Fig. 5.59a, b Trephine biopsies of bone marrow from two patients with primary idiopathic myelofibrosis at an intermediate stage of the disease. Both biopsies show hyperplasia of haemopoietic elements, some increase of fibroblasts and a moderate degree of fibrosis. (**b**) also shows several megakaryocytes.   Haematoxylin–eosin   × 350

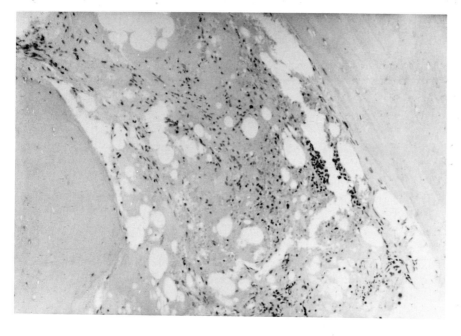

Fig. 5.60 Trephine biopsy of bone marrow from a patient with idiopathic myelofibrosis at the end-stage of the disease. The marrow cells are markedly reduced in number and replaced by fibroblasts and collagen. The bony trabeculae are sclerotic.

Haematoxylin–eosin

×   350

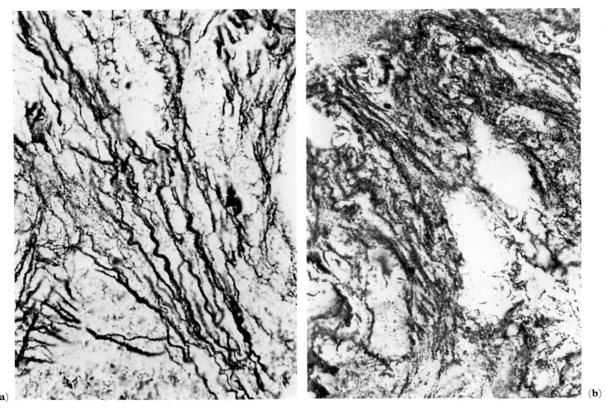

(a) (b)

Fig. 5.61a, b Trephine biopsies of marrow from the posterior superior iliac spines of two patients with primary idiopathic myelofibrosis. There is a moderate increase in the quantity of reticulin fibres in (**a**) and a marked increase in (**b**) when compared with the biopsy of normal marrow shown in Figure 3.2 (p. 43).

Silver impregnation of reticulin   × 375

in parallel bundles. All types of haemopoietic cells may be present in the fibrotic marrow but megakaryocytes are particularly prominent. There may also be patches of hyperplastic hae-mopoietic marrow between the fibrosed areas. In some patients there is a considerable increase in the thickness of bone trabeculae (osteosclerosis). Osteolytic lesions and pathological fractures occur uncommonly. The proliferating fibroblasts do not appear to be derived from the multipotent haemopoietic stem cells. It is now thought that the fibroblastic reaction is induced by mitogenic factors secreted by the increased number of (pos-sibly functionally-abnormal) megakaryocytes and that a similar explanation might underly the les-ser degrees of myelofibrosis which may occur in polycythaemia rubra vera, essential thrombo-cythaemia and chronic granulocytic leukaemia.

Patients show a slow clinical and haematolog-ical deterioration with increasing splenomegaly. Average survival from the time of diagnosis is about 5-7 years but some patients survive much longer. From 10-20% of patients eventually de-velop acute myeloblastic or acute megakaryoblas-tic leukaemia. Other causes of death include in-fection, congestive cardiac failure, bleeding and thrombosis.

At post mortem, the spleen is very large and may show recent or old infarcts. Extramedullary haemopoiesis is seen in the spleen and liver and may also be seen in many other sites including lymph nodes, kidneys, adrenals, peritoneum, gut, pleura, lungs, fatty tissue, skin, breasts, ovaries and thymus; proliferating myeloid cells may form tumour masses. Extramedullary haemopoiesis in the liver may result in cramming of sinusoids with haemopoietic cells;[170] it may be accompanied by periportal fibrosis. Portal hypertension and ascites are not uncommon.[170] Osteosclerosis may be evident.

Secondary myelofibrosis (see also page 92)

Myelofibrosis may occur as a reaction to irradiation of the marrow or to the presence of carcinoma cells (Fig. 4.14), malignant lymphoma cells (especially those of Hodgkin's disease) or tubercle bacilli in the marrow. It may also be seen in a wide variety of other conditions which are listed in Table 4.9 on page 93. The carcinomas that most frequently cause myelofibrosis and myelosclerosis are those of the breast and prostate. Acute myelofibrosis develops in patients with acute megakaryoblastic leukaemia, probably as the result of the action of a mitogenic factor secreted by megakaryoblasts (see p. 235).

APLASTIC ANAEMIA[171, 172]

The term aplastic anaemia is applied to a disorder of haemopoiesis in which anaemia and thrombocytopenia and, usually, leucopenia result from a marked reduction in the number of haemopoietic cells in the marrow. The precise biochemical and cytokinetic disturbances which underly the congenital or acquired aplastic anaemias are still unknown. However, it seems

Table 5.18 Classification of aplastic anaemia

Congenital

Fanconi syndrome

Dyskeratosis congenita

Others (e.g. hypoplastic anaemia with pancreatic insufficiency)

Acquired

Idiopathic

Secondary
  Drugs and chemicals
  Irradiation
  Viral hepatitis (usually, non-A non-B)
  Pregnancy
  Thymoma
  Graft-versus-host disease
  Infectious mononucleosis
  Dengue fever
  Influenza

likely that these disorders result from damage to the multipotent haemopoietic stem cells or to cell types in the bone marrow which provide the appropriate microenvironment for the normal functioning of the stem cells. The damage may result in a decreased number, rate of self-renewal or rate of differentiation of the multipotent stem cells. A classification of aplastic anaemia is given in Table 5.18.

Congenital pancytopenia (familial hypoplastic anaemia, Fanconi syndrome)[173]

This inherited disorder is characterized by pancytopenia which usually develops between the ages of 5 and 10 years. Males are affected twice as frequently as females and more than one member of the family may be affected. The pancytopenia is usually but not invariably associated with various congenital abnormalities. The most common of these are patchy skin pigmentation, microcephaly, short stature, strabismus, genital hypoplasia, skeletal defects (particularly of the thumbs and radii) and renal abnormalities. Less common abnormalities include mental retardation, congenital heart disease, microphthalmia and deafness. Family members may show congenital abnormalities without pancytopenia. The anaemia is normocytic or macrocytic and the absolute reticulocyte count is usually reduced. Target cells may be present due to splenic atrophy. HbF levels are raised. The bone marrow may initially show hyperplasia of haemopoietic cells but eventually becomes hypoplastic or aplastic. Cytogenetic studies of cultured bone marrow cells, lymphocytes and skin fibroblasts show breaks in chromatids, chromatid exchanges between non-homologous chromosomes and an excess of endoreduplicated metaphases. Patients with congenital pancytopenia suffer from a substantially increased prevalence of acute myelomonocytic and monocytic leukaemia and of solid tumours such as carcinomas of the anus, vulva, gums, oesophagus or breast. Hepatomas also occur but may be related to androgen therapy. In addition, occasional patients may develop paroxysmal nocturnal haemoglobinuria. The pancytopenia frequently responds slowly to a combination of androgens and prednisolone but continuous treatment is required to maintain the improvement.

Dyskeratosis congenita[174]

Patients with this rare syndrome resemble those with the Fanconi syndrome in suffering from a delayed onset of marrow failure, abnormal skin pigmentation, stunted growth and an increased tendency to develop carcinoma. Features not found in the Fanconi syndrome include telangiectatic erythema, nail dystrophy, hyperhidrosis, lacrimal duct atresia and leucoplakia of mucous membranes. Renal and skeletal abnormalities do not occur, nor do chromosomal changes. Affected patients are almost exclusively male.

Other constitutional aplastic anaemias

A number of other syndromes in which constitutional aplastic anaemia is a feature have been described in single families or several families (e.g. hypoplastic anaemia with pancreatic insufficiency).[175]

Acquired aplastic anaemia

Acquired hypoplastic or aplastic anaemia is much more common than congenital pancytopenia, affecting about 10 per million of the population. The acquired disorder may follow exposure to some drugs, certain chemicals used in industry or the home, ionizing radiation or the hepatitis virus (usually, non-A non-B) (secondary aplastic anaemia). However, in about 30% of cases, no known causative agent can be discovered (idiopathic aplastic anaemia). Recent *in vitro* work has indicated that the blood and marrow of some patients with acquired aplastic anaemia contain T-cells which cause a pathological suppression of the growth of colonies from autologous and allogeneic CFU-C and CFU-E: this has raised the possibility that an abnormality of T-lymphocytes may play an important role in the causation of the aplasia.[176] This possibility has received some support from the clinical observation that both antithymocyte globulin[177] and immunosuppressive chemotherapy are effective in improving haemopoiesis in some patients with aplastic anaemia.

Some drugs, such as those used in the treatment of malignant disease, regularly cause marrow hypoplasia above certain dosages. However, even with these drugs, different individuals show different degrees of marrow suppression at the same dosage. Other drugs only cause marrow hypoplasia very occasionally (idiosyncratic reaction). Possible mechanisms underlying idiosyncracy to a drug include differences in the rates of metabolism or excretion of the drug, differences in biochemical pathways within haemopoietic stem cells and their progeny, and the development of an immunological response against these cells. A list of drugs which have been clearly shown to occasionally cause aplastic anaemia is given in Table 5.19. Many of the substances

Table 5.19 Some drugs which may cause aplastic anaemia in occasional patients[33]

Anti-inflammatory drugs
  Phenylbutazone, oxyphenbutazone, indomethacin, sodium aurothiomalate

Antibacterial drugs
  Chloramphenicol, trimethoprim-sulphamethoxazole, other sulphonamides, streptomycin, tetracycline, isoniazid, penicillin

Anti-epileptic drugs
  Phenytoin, methoin (mephenytoin), troxidone (trimethadione), paramethadione, phenacemide, methsuximide

Antimalarial drugs
  Mepacrine (quinacrine), chloroquine, pyrimethamine

Antidiabetic drugs
  Chlorpropamide, tolbutamide

Miscellaneous
  Organic arsenicals, chlorpromazine, chlorothiazide, meprobamate, hydralazine, aspirin, allopurinol, potassium perchlorate

listed usually cause only a selective neutropenia (e.g. phenylbutazone and chlorpromazine) or thrombocytopenia (e.g. thiazide diuretics, gold and arsenic compounds) and less frequently cause pancytopenia. Furthermore, neutropenia or thrombocytopenia may precede the development of marrow aplasia. The six drugs which most commonly cause aplastic anaemia are phenylbutazone, oxyphenbutazone, chloramphenicol, indomethacin, sodium aurothiomalate and trimethoprim-sulphamethoxazole. Certain chemicals other than drugs may also cause aplastic anaemia; these include benzene (present in many solvents), trinitrotoluene, insecticides (chlorophenothane [DDT], parathion, chlordane, pentachlorophenol), carbon tetrachloride, various glues and thiocyanate. Aplastic anaemia has been reported in patients with ankylosing spondylitis treated with irradiation, in atomic bomb survivors and in people involved in radiation accidents. Severe aplastic anaemia may also develop following a mild attack of viral hepatitis, usually within 10 weeks.

In acquired aplastic anaemia, the blood count shows a normocytic or macrocytic anaemia. There is slight to moderate anisocytosis and poikilocytosis. The reticulocyte count is usually low but may fluctuate and sometimes be as high as 5%. Most patients show neutropenia and monocytopenia at some stage of the disorder and some also show lymphopenia. The platelet count is invariably low ($<100 \times 10^9$/l). The degree of reduction of the various formed elements of the blood is often reflected in the degree of hypoplasia of the different haemopoietic cell lines in the marrow. In marrow smears from patients with severe aplastic anaemia, marrow fragments usually show a marked reduction of haemopoietic cells and a corresponding increase of fat cells (Fig. 3.28c); the cell trails leading from the fragments show very few cells, most of which consist of lymphocytes, plasma cells and macrophages. The aplasia of haemopoietic cells does not usually affect all areas of the marrow uniformly and even in severely affected patients occasional marrow aspirates may yield normocellular or hypercellular marrow fragments. A proper assessment of cellularity may require several marrow aspirations or a trephine biopsy. The normocellular and hypercellular areas may show erythroid or myeloid activity or both, a high frequency of erythroblasts with dyserythropoietic changes, and a paucity of granulocytopoietic cells beyond the myelocyte stage. The plasma and urinary erythropoietin levels are markedly increased.

The prognosis is very variable; 10–15% of patients die within three months of diagnosis and 50% within 15 months. Some patients survive more than 10 years. Bad prognostic features include a platelet count below 20×10^9/l and a neutrophil count below 0.2×10^9/l. Patients usually die of haemorrhage or infections. Available lines of treatment, after withdrawal of any causative drug or chemical, include stimulation of haemopoiesis using androgens with or without corticosteroids (some workers have reported shorter survival with corticosteroids), and bone marrow transplantation. Response to antithymocyte globulin may occur.[177] In the case of toxicity due to arsenic or gold compounds, treatment with dimercaprol (BAL) may sometimes result in rapid recovery.[178] Very occasional cases of aplastic anaemia subsequently develop leukaemia and about 15% develop paroxysmal nocturnal haemoglobinuria (PNH) or show laboratory evidence of a PNH-like red cell defect (see p. 149).

At necropsy, signs of haemorrhage, infections and anaemia may be found. All of the red haemopoietic marrow is replaced by yellow marrow; however, it may be noted that aplastic marrow occasionally appears red due to marked engorgement of the marrow sinusoids.

PURE RED CELL APLASIA[179]

In some patients an anaemia develops due to a selective hypoplasia or aplasia of erythropoietic cells. The other cell lines in the marrow are unaffected and both the leucocyte and platelet counts in the blood are normal. The bone marrow usually shows a marked deficiency of erythropoietic cells at all stages of maturation or a total absence of erythroblasts. Occasionally there are increased numbers of pronormoblasts and basophilic normoblasts (sometimes with giant forms) and an absence of more mature cells. The blood reticulocyte count is low. Pure red cell aplasia occurs both as a congenital defect (constitutional erythroid hypoplasia) and as an acquired defect.

Constitutional erythroid hypoplasia (congenital erythroblastopenia, Diamond-Blackfan syndrome, erythrogenesis imperfecta)[180, 181]

This syndrome is characterized by the onset at birth or during the first three months of life of anaemia due to selective hypoplasia of the red cell precursors. Most familial cases appear to show an autosomal recessive inheritance. The anaemia, which is normocytic or macrocytic in type, becomes progressively worse and is eventually severe. About 25% of patients have minor congenital abnormalities; these include skeletal anomalies affecting the lateral aspects of the limbs (e.g. triphalangeal thumbs) and webbing of the neck. There are usually no renal abnormalities. The marrow shows few or no erythroblasts but is normal in other respects. The plasma and urinary erythropoietin concentrations are increased but the CFU-E (see p. 45) and proerythroblasts appear to be relatively erythropoietin-unresponsive.[182, 183] About 80% of the patients respond to treatment with corticosteroids, erythroblasts reappearing in the bone marrow. Occasional steroid-responsive and non-responsive patients remit spontaneously, sometimes at puberty.

Acquired pure red cell aplasia

A pure red cell aplasia may develop acutely in various chronic haemolytic anaemias (e.g. hereditary spherocytosis and sickle cell anaemia). The abrupt cessation of erythropoiesis in patients with a markedly shortened red cell life-span leads to a rapid and life-threatening fall in the haemoglobin level. Recovery occurs spontaneously within 1–2 weeks. The erythroid aplasia is usually precipitated by unidentified (presumably viral) infections of the upper respiratory and gastrointestinal tracts. Recent studies have shown that the development of red cell aplasia in sickle cell anaemia is correlated with a parvovirus infection. Transient pure red cell aplasia may also follow a minor febrile illness in individuals with a normal red cell life-span. Such individuals would not be expected to drop their haemoglobin to any appreciable extent after a transient arrest of erythropoiesis and are only recognized, usually accidentally, by an absence of reticulocytes. Rarely, pure red cell aplasia may complicate the course of primary atypical pneumonia, infectious mononucleosis or mumps.

Pure red cell aplasia has followed exposure to benzene and treatment with drugs such as phenytoin, chloramphenicol, azathioprine and sulphonamides.

A chronic form of pure red cell aplasia also occurs. No associated disorder can be found in some cases of chronic acquired pure red cell aplasia. However about 30–50% of cases are associated with the presence of a thymic tumour and a small number of cases with chronic lymphocytic leukaemia, Hodgkin's disease or carcinoma of bronchus, breast or stomach. Other cases have been induced by renal insufficiency and protein-energy malnutrition (see p. 194). Chronic pure red cell aplasia has also been associated with various autoimmune disorders such as myasthenia gravis, systemic lupus erythematosus, rheumatoid arthritis and autoimmune haemolytic anaemia. The association of pure red cell aplasia with thymoma and autoimmune disorders and the response of some cases to corticosteroids or immunosuppressive therapy have suggested the possibility that immunological mechanisms may underly the aplasia in at least some patients. This view is supported by studies in a very few cases which have shown the presence of antibodies directed against erythroblasts, morphologically unrecognized erythroid progenitor cells or erythropoietin. Furthermore, the possibility that alterations in T-lymphocyte subpopulations may underly the aplasia in some patients has been raised by the observation that patients with pure red cell aplasia associated with chronic lymphocytic leukaemia show a reduced number of circulating $T\mu$ (helper) cells, an increased number of $T\gamma$ (suppressor) cells and an impaired capacity of T-cells to stimulate autologous or allogeneic BFU-E.[184]

Apparently-idiopathic pure red cell aplasia may precede the diagnosis of carcinoma by several months or the development of frank leukaemia by several years.

THALASSAEMIA SYNDROMES

The anaemia in homozygous β-thalassaemia is largely caused by a failure to increase adequately the rate of effective erythropoiesis, due to a gross increase of ineffective erythropoiesis (p. 143). There is some increase of ineffective erythropoiesis in the α-thalassaemia syndrome, HbH disease, but the anaemia in this syndrome is primarily caused by increased peripheral haemolysis (p. 138).

CONGENITAL DYSERYTHROPOIETIC ANAEMIAS

These are a group of congenital anaemias of unknown aetiology in which the erythropoietic cells show striking morphological abnormalities indicative of dyserythropoiesis. The anaemia results mainly from a considerable ineffectiveness of erythropoiesis. Most cases can be allocated to one of three types, chiefly on the basis of the types of morphological abnormality that predominate in the bone marrow.[185] The chronic ineffective erythropoiesis may lead to the formation of pigment stones in the gall bladder and, more importantly, to tissue damage (e.g. endocrine abnormalities and cirrhosis of the liver) due to haemosiderosis.

Congenital dyserythropoietic anaemia, type I[186, 187]

This rare disorder is usually diagnosed during the first two decades of life. Affected patients show a mild to moderate macrocytic anaemia (average Hb 10.0 g/dl, range 6.0–12.6 g/dl), mild jaundice, a normal or only slightly raised reticulocyte count and intense erythroid hyperplasia in the marrow. Erythropoiesis is megaloblastic in type. Some of the more mature basophilic erythroblasts and many of the early and late polychromatic erythroblasts show dyserythropoietic features. The most prominent morphological abnormalities are frequent internuclear chromatin bridges connecting pairs of partially separated polychromatic erythroblasts and some increase in the percentage of binucleate polychromatic erythroblasts. The latter often contain nuclei of different size and show partial fusion of the two nuclear masses; the two nuclei within the same cell may display different staining characteristics. The most striking ultrastructural abnormality is the presence of nuclei with a 'Swiss-cheese' appearance in a high proportion of the mono-

nucleate early and late polychromatic erythroblasts; these nuclei have multiple rounded electron-lucent areas within abnormally electron-dense heterochromatin. Nuclei having the 'Swiss-cheese' appearance may also contain nuclear-membrane-lined cytoplasmic intrusions, sometimes with cytoplasmic organelles. An abnormally low percentage of mononucleate early polychromatic erythroblasts synthesize DNA; the non-DNA-synthesizing cells have DNA contents between the 2 c and 8 c values (1 c = the haploid DNA content, i.e. the DNA content of a spermatozoon) and appear to be derived from the maturation of cells which have become arrested during their progress through the cell cycle. There is a marked increase in ineffective erythropoiesis as the result of a high rate of intramedullary destruction of the morphologically abnormal cells. Most of the patients have moderate splenomegaly. Some cases show other congenital abnormalities such as abnormal pigmentation of the skin, syndactyly and aberrations of the bones of the hand. The disorder appears to be inherited as an autosomal recessive character.

Congenital dyserythropoietic anaemia, type II (hereditary erythroblastic multinuclearity with positive acidified serum lysis test, HEMPAS)[185, 188]

This is the commonest type of congenital dyserythropoietic anaemia, and appears to be inherited as an autosomal recessive character. Most of the cases have been reported from North-West Europe, Italy and North Africa. Patients with this disorder present usually during childhood with mild to moderate normochromic, normocytic anaemia (some are not anaemic), mild intermittent jaundice, a normal or only slightly raised reticulocyte count, characteristic morphological abnormalities of the erythroblasts and characteristic serological reactions of the red cells. Most patients have hepatosplenomegaly and a few show mental retardation. Red cells show moderate anisocytosis and poikilocytosis and basophilic stippling. The bone marrow shows normoblastic erythroid hyperplasia. A few of the basophilic erythropoietic cells and early polychromatic erythroblasts and 10–35% of the late erythroblasts

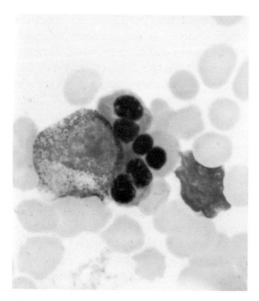

Fig. 5.62 Bone marrow smear of a patient with congenital dyserythropoietic anaemia, type II, showing three binucleate late polychromatic erythroblasts.

May–Grünwald–Giemsa stain   × 940

are binucleate; the nuclei are usually of equal size (Fig. 5.62). In addition, a small proportion of the erythroblasts are trinucleate or multinucleate. Many of the mononucleate and binucleate late erythroblasts have orthochromatic cytoplasm and highly-condensed, structureless nuclei. The anaemia results from ineffectiveness of erythropoiesis, there being a high rate of phagocytosis of mononucleate and binucleate late erythroblasts by bone marrow macrophages.[189] Electron microscope studies reveal a characteristic double membrane (probably endoplasmic reticulum) aligned parallel to and at a distance of 40–60 nm from the cell membrane in a high proportion of the late erythroblasts[190, 191] (Fig. 5.63). The red cells give a positive acidified serum lysis test with about 30% of fresh normal sera but not with the patient's own serum. The reactive sera contain an IgM antibody which combines specifically with an antigen on HEMPAS red cells. This antibody can be removed by absorption with red cells of cases of HEMPAS but not of patients with paroxysmal nocturnal haemoglobinuria.

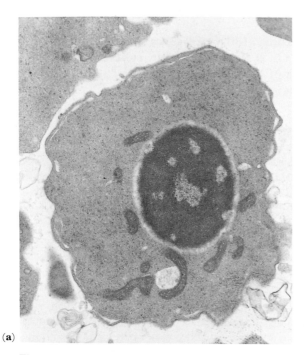

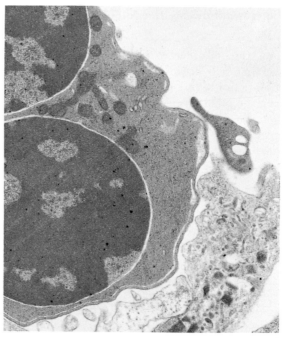

(a)   (b)

Fig. 5.63a, b Electron micrographs of a mononucleate (a) and binucleate (b) late polychromatic erythroblast from a case of congenital dyserythropoietic anaemia, type II. The characteristic double membrane can be seen running parallel to the cell membrane of both erythroblasts.

Uranyl acetate and lead citrate   (a) × 14 525; (b) × 17 725

Congenital dyserythropoietic anaemia, type III[192, 193, 194]

This is the rarest type of congenital dyserythropoietic anaemia. More than one case has occurred in some families. The disorder is characterized by a mild to moderate macrocytic anaemia, normal granulocyte and platelet counts, marked erythroid hyperplasia, megaloblastic erythropoiesis in the absence of vitamin B_{12} or folate deficiency and the presence in the marrow of some large uninucleate erythroblasts with big lobulated nuclei and many giant multinucleate erythroblasts. Some patients have splenomegaly. The acidified serum lysis test is negative. The blood film shows giant erythrocytes, poikilocytosis, fragmented red cells and basophilic stippling. The reticulocyte count is normal or slightly raised. The morphological abnormalities in the marrow may be seen in basophilic erythropoietic cells but are most marked in the early and late polychromatic erythroblast stages. Over 35% of the erythroblasts may be binucleate or multinucleate (Fig. 5.64) and the latter may contain up to 12 nuclear masses and may have total DNA contents up to 40 c (see p. 191). Sometimes the two nuclei of a binucleate cell or two or more of the nuclei within a multinucleate cell are joined together either by a narrow strand of chromatin or over a wide area of contact. The nuclear masses within multinucleate erythroblasts are rounded in outline and equal in size and staining characteristics in some cells but irregular in shape, unequal in size or different in their staining characteristics in others. The giant mononucleate erythroblasts have DNA contents up to 20 c. Other abnormalities affecting erythroblasts include coarse basophilic stippling of the cytoplasm and karyorrhexis of interphase nuclei. Electron microscope studies show a variety of abnormalities including differences in the ultrastructural appearances of different nuclei within the same multinucleate cell (Fig. 5.65). The anaemia results largely from

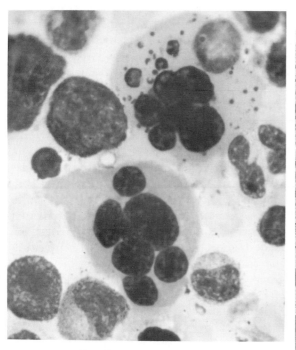

Fig. 5.64 Bone marrow smear of a patient with congenital dyserythropoietic anaemia, type III, showing two giant multinucleate erythroblasts. The upper multinucleate cell contains many Howell-Jolly bodies and one of its nuclear masses stains less intensely than the others.

May–Grünwald–Giemsa stain   × 940

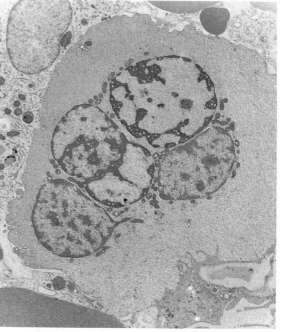

Fig. 5.65 Electron micrograph of a giant multinucleate erythroblast from a case of congenital dyserythropoietic anaemia, type III. Note the different ultrastructural appearances of the different nuclei within the same cell.

Uranyl acetate and lead citrate   × 3 500

ineffective erythropoiesis; both mononucleate and multinucleate cells may be seen within bone marrow macrophages. The disorder runs a relatively benign course; most cases are diagnosed in older children or young adults.

PLASMODIUM FALCIPARUM MALARIA[195]

Some young children with *P. falciparum* malaria have a high proportion of parasitized red cells (usually >8%), an increased absolute reticulocyte count and a mild to moderate anaemia (usually Hb > 8 g/dl) mainly due to increased peripheral haemolysis. Others have a lower proportion of parasitized red cells (<4%) and a severe anaemia (usually Hb < 6 g/dl) predominantly due to a gross increase of ineffective erythropoiesis. The absolute reticulocyte counts of the severely anaemic patients are normal or slightly increased, the degree of increase being inappropriate to the degree of anaemia. Their marrow aspirates show marked erythroid hyperplasia and a high proportion of erythroblasts display dyserythropoietic changes. Some patients have occasional ringed sideroblasts or a few giant metamyelocytes. Iron stores are usually present. The serum vitamin B_{12} and red cell folate levels are normal as is the methylation of deoxyuridylate by marrow cells. The mechanisms responsible for the dyserythropoiesis and ineffective erythropoiesis in *P. falciparum* malaria are unknown; there is no parasitization of erythroblasts.

PROTEIN-ENERGY MALNUTRITION (KWASHIORKOR, MARASMIC KWASHIORKOR AND MARASMUS)

Anaemia is a common finding in children with protein-energy malnutrition (PEM). The Hb is usually only slightly or moderately reduced. The MCV is usually normal but may be elevated. The results of plasma volume and red cell mass measurements suggest that in the early stages of PEM the red cell mass decreases in proportion to the body weight and that the plasma volume is unaltered. In severe PEM, the reduction in red cell mass is greater and there is often a very marked reduction in the plasma volume so that the actual reduction in the red cell mass may be much greater than that suggested by the haemoglobin level.[196, 197] There is a slight reduction of red cell life-span in kwashiorkor and marasmic kwashiorkor ($T_{\frac{1}{2}}$ Cr^{51} values of 11.4–24.0 d; mean 17.12 d) but not in marasmus[198, 199, 200] and this reduction appears to be due both to a corpuscular and an extracorpuscular defect.

The bone marrow often shows erythroid hypoplasia or normocellular erythropoiesis, but sometimes shows erythroid hyperplasia or, rarely, even pure red cell aplasia. Erythropoiesis is usually essentially normoblastic but there are often some giant metamyelocytes. In some patients the erythroblasts display marked dyserythropoietic changes. A few cases show frankly megaloblastic erythropoiesis. Iron stores are present in normal or increased quantities. The number and size of siderotic granules within erythroblasts may be increased and there may be occasional ringed sideroblasts. Serum vitamin B_{12} levels are normal or raised and red cell folate levels are usually within the normal range. Serum erythropoietin levels are normal or increased. Ferrokinetic studies have shown that in severe PEM there is a decrease in both total and effective erythropoietic activity as reflected by the plasma iron turnover and red cell iron utilization, respectively, but that in less severe protein deficiency states there may be an increase in both total and effective erythropoiesis.[200, 201] Except in an occasional patient, the changes in plasma iron turnover (i.e. total erythropoietic activity) are modest, the observed values being between 80 and 120% of the average value in the control group. The above data suggest that the anaemia of severe PEM results primarily from erythroid hypoplasia and that the anaemia in milder cases of PEM results from a failure of the bone marrow to adequately increase red cell production to compensate for a modest reduction in red cell life-span.

The biochemical mechanisms underlying the various haematological disturbances in PEM are still not clear. However, it is likely that the protein deficiency *per se* is primarily responsible for the anaemia. It is theoretically possible that the protein deficiency causes decreased levels of various enzymes within haemopoietic cells and thereby impairs the proliferation and differentiation of these cells. For example, it has recently been shown that the marrow cells of some cases of PEM (with normoblastic or mildly megaloblastic erythropoiesis but normal red cell folate levels) give an abnormal result with the deoxyuridine suppression test, suggesting an impairment of the methylation of deoxyuridylate.[202, 203] Children with PEM may, however, suffer from various problems other than a dietary deficiency of protein. These include: (1) a dietary deficiency of calories, vitamins and minerals; (2) a variety of infectious diseases (e.g. measles, hookworm infestation); and (3) malabsorption.[204] The available data suggest that these factors do not play a major role in the pathogenesis of the anaemia of PEM. The levels of serum ascorbic acid, serum vitamin E, serum iron and plasma copper are low in some untreated patients with kwashiorkor,[205] but there is little evidence that an impaired supply of any of these substances to the erythron contributes significantly to the anaemia. Although the anaemia in children with PEM from some countries (e.g. Nigeria) has been shown to be independent of folate deficiency, it is possible that the importance of folate deficiency in the pathogenesis of the anaemia may vary from country to country.

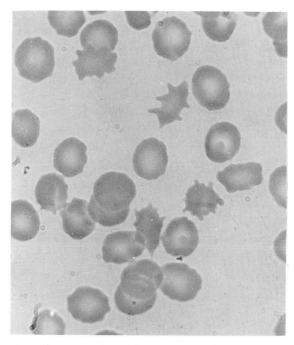

Fig. 5.66 Peripheral blood film of a patient with anorexia nervosa showing acanthocytes.
May–Grünwald–Giemsa stain   × 940

ANOREXIA NERVOSA

Patients with severe anorexia nervosa frequently have a mild anaemia which may be associated with lymphopenia, neutropenia and thrombocytopenia. Their blood films show anisocytosis and poikilocytosis and contain acanthocytes (Fig. 5.66) and, sometimes, a few spherocytes. The reticulocyte count may be reduced despite a slight shortening of red cell life-span. The plasma volume is increased. The bone marrow is hypocellular and often shows gelatinous transformation (see p. 101 and Figs 4.20 and 4.21). The anaemia appears to result from a combination of an increased plasma volume and some suppression of erythropoiesis. The mechanisms by which a severe deficiency of carbohydrates and calories (with a relative sufficiency of protein and fat) causes an impairment of haemopoiesis are unknown.

POLYCYTHAEMIA

The term polycythaemia is now applied when the venous haematocrit or the haemoglobin level are above the normal range. (In some patients with the potential to develop polycythaemia, the haematocrit and haemoglobin may be within the normal range because erythropoiesis is limited by complicating iron or folate deficiency and polycythaemia is only manifest following correction of the deficiency state.) The repeated finding of a venous haematocrit greater than 0.50–0.52 in males and 0.47 in females in samples taken without venous occlusion should be viewed with suspicion and explored further by the measurement of the red cell mass and plasma volume. The values for the red cell mass are usually expressed as ml red cells per kg body weight. However, because fat is relatively avascular and the mass of fat in the body varies considerably from one person to another, the red cell mass is more usefully expressed as ml red cells per kg lean body mass (the lean body mass can be derived from measurements of total body water, e.g. the antipyrine space). In practice, it is adequate to express the total red cell mass in ml obtained in a given patient as a percentage above or below the red cell mass predicted for the height and weight of that patient, using the blood volume formulae of Nadler et al. which take account of the amount of fatty tissue in the body. True (or absolute) polycythaemia may be considered to exist when the measured red cell mass exceeds the patient's own mean predicted normal value by more than 25% in males and 30% in females.[206] Patients

Table 5.20 Classification of patients with elevated venous haematocrit values

True polycythaemia

1. Polycythaemia rubra vera (primary proliferative polycythaemia, Vaquez-Osler disease)

2. Secondary polycythaemia
   (a) *Generalized tissue hypoxia*
       High altitude
       Cyanotic heart disease
       Chronic hypoxic pulmonary disease
       Alveolar hypoventilation due to gross obesity
       Heavy smoking
       Haemoglobins with high oxygen affinity
   (b) *Inappropriate erythropoietin production or renal hypoxia*
       Kidney disease (e.g. carcinoma, cysts, hydronephrosis)
       Renal transplantation[215]
       Hepatocellular carcinoma
       Cerebellar haemangioblastoma
       Massive uterine fibromyomata

3. Idiopathic erythrocytosis

Apparent polycythaemia (relative polycythaemia)

1. Fluid loss, diminished fluid intake

2. Stress polycythaemia (spurious polycythaemia, Gaisböck's syndrome)

with an elevated venous haematocrit whose red cell mass is not increased to this extent are considered to have apparent (or relative) polycythaemia. The disorders associated with true and apparent polycythaemia are listed in Table 5.20.

TRUE POLYCYTHAEMIA [207, 208]

Polycythaemia rubra vera (PRV, primary proliferative polycythaemia, Vaquez–Osler disease)

This is a chronic progressive disease of unknown aetiology in which hyperplastic marrow produces an excess of red cells and, frequently, also of granulocytes and platelets. It is considered to be one of the chronic myeloproliferative disorders (see p. 283). The marrow contains a mutant clone of multipotent haemopoietic stem cells which generates some abnormal erythroid progenitor cells (BFU-E and CFU-E): these, unlike their normal counterparts, form bursts and colonies in the absence of added erythropoietin. In PRV, individual primitive BFU-E may produce only erythropoietin-dependent progeny or a mixture of erythropoietin-dependent and independent progeny.[209] The increased production of red cells results in an increase in the circulating red cell mass and venous haematocrit which, in turn, leads to an increase in whole blood viscosity and a decrease in blood flow through the limbs and brain. For example, cerebral blood flow is low in PRV and doubles as the venous haematocrit is reduced from 0.60 to 0.45.[210] The increase in red cell mass is also frequently associated with an increase of the peripheral vascular bed (i.e. an engorgement of tissues). These haemodynamic changes affect many organs and account for the diversity of symptoms encountered in the disease.

Most cases occur between 40 and 70 years of age and there is a slight preponderance of males. The onset of the disease is insidious. The usual presenting symptoms include headaches, fullness in the head, dizziness, tinnitus, dyspnoea, fatigue, visual disturbance, pruritus, Raynaud's phenomenon, claudication and peripheral gangrene (Fig. 5.67). Some patients present acutely with a thrombotic or haemorrhagic episode. Occasional manifestations include epigastric discomfort, paraesthesiae, bone pain, and depression and other psychiatric disturbances. About 10% of patients suffer from gout as a result of increased urate production secondary to the increased turnover of blood cells and their precursors.

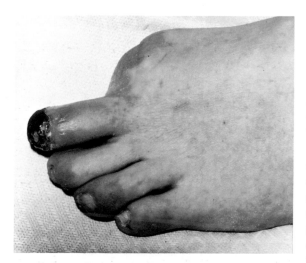

Fig. 5.67 The foot of a patient with polycythaemia rubra vera showing gangrene of the second toe. The big toe had become gangrenous and had been amputated earlier.

Peripheral arterial occlusion, deep vein thrombosis, superficial thrombophlebitis, cerebral thrombosis or haemorrhage and coronary thrombosis are common and account for the high morbidity and mortality of the untreated disease. There may also be mesenteric, splenic, portal or hepatic vein thrombosis. The risk of occlusive vascular episodes (arterial and venous) increases with increasing venous haematocrit. Untreated patients also show an increased frequency of thrombotic episodes post-operatively. The episodes of vascular occlusion appear to result from a combination of increased whole blood viscosity, reduced blood flow and the prevalence of arterial degeneration and hypertension in the affected age group. The risk of vascular occlusion is also related to the platelet count, being higher in patients with thrombocytosis.

Some patients suffer from ecchymoses, epistaxes, or excessive haemorrhage during and after surgery. The haemorrhagic tendency is not fully understood but has been attributed to acquired defects of platelet function.

Examination may reveal a characteristic dusky-red colouration both of the exposed areas of the skin and of mucous membranes. Congestion of conjunctival vessels and marked distension of retinal veins may be present. The spleen is enlarged in 70% of cases and the liver in 40%.

Venous blood[211] is dark and thick and difficult to spread satisfactorily on glass slides. Haemoglobin levels are usually between 18 and 24 g/dl but may be higher. The PCV is frequently over 0.55. Red cell counts are commonly between 6 and $10 \times 10^{12}/l$. These findings are associated with an absolute increase in the red cell mass. The plasma volume may be decreased, normal or increased. The red cells are usually normochromic and normocytic but may be hypochromic and microcytic. The microcytosis is caused by: (1) an absolute iron deficiency due either to repeated venesection or to spontaneous recurrent gastrointestinal blood loss; or (2) a state of relative iron deficiency in which the total body iron is within the normal range but inadequate to cope with the large increase in red cell count. The reticulocyte count is usually $100-250 \times 10^9/l$. An occasional erythroblast may be seen in the blood film. In 75% of the cases the total white cell count is increased, usually being between 12 and $30 \times 10^9/l$. There is a neutrophil leucocytosis with an occasional neutrophil metamyelocyte and myelocyte. The neutrophil leucocyte alkaline phosphatase score is often considerably raised but may be normal. The basophil count may be elevated. The platelet count is raised in two-thirds of the patients; it is usually in the range $400-1000 \times 10^9/l$ and is sometimes as high as $2000 \times 10^9/l$. Some large bizarre platelets are present and the platelets show functional abnormalities. The serum vitamin B_{12} level and the unsaturated vitamin B_{12}-binding capacity may be elevated. The serum lysozyme and serum histamine levels may also be increased. Plasma and urinary erythropoietin levels are decreased. Although early studies indicated that the arterial oxygen saturation is usually normal (saturation >92%), subsequent studies have revealed mild degrees of unsaturation in a substantial proportion of cases, probably due to ventilation perfusion imbalance.[212]

Marrow smears and trephine biopsies[213] show a hyperplasia of the erythropoietic, granulocytopoietic and megakaryocytic elements (Fig. 5.68); the degree of hyperplasia in each cell line usually reflects the degree of increase in the concentration of the corresponding cell type in the peripheral blood. Usually, erythroid hyperplasia is

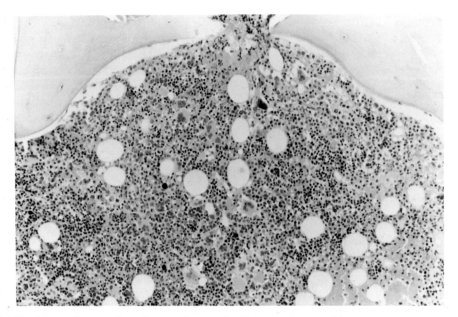

Fig. 5.68 Trephine biopsy of marrow from the posterior superior iliac crest of a man with polycythaemia rubra vera. The section shows increased cellularity and the presence of several megakaryocytes.

Haematoxylin-eosin   × 94

prominent with an M/E ratio of 1 or less and there are increased numbers of large megakaryocytes. A very occasional mononucleate and binucleate micromegakaryocyte may be present (see p. 274). Often lymphocytes, plasma cells and mast cells are also increased. Iron stores are reduced or absent. In 85% of the patients, sections of trephine biopsies show an increase in the area occupied by haemopoietic marrow with a corresponding diminution of the area occupied by fat cells; frequently, haemopoietic cells fill 90% or more of the intertrabecular space. In most cases, the sections also show some increase in reticulin fibres in the marrow parenchyma. The vascularity of the marrow is increased and the sinusoids are hyperaemic. There may be chromosome abnormalities in marrow cells (e.g. aneuploidy or the presence of an extra C group chromosome), even in those patients who have not received ^{32}P or cytotoxic drugs.

A firm diagnosis of polycythaemia rubra vera can usually be made when an increase in the red cell mass is associated with either splenomegaly or at least two of the following abnormalities: neutrophil leucocytosis, thrombocytosis, high neutrophil alkaline phosphatase score and elevated serum vitamin B_{12} level.

The main aim of treatment is to minimize the risk of occlusive vascular episodes by maintaining the PCV at less than 0.45. The median survival of untreated patients is about 18 months from diagnosis. This figure increases to 3–7 years in cases treated by venesection alone and to 8–16 years in those treated either with ^{32}P or alkylating agents. Patients with a high platelet count whose PCV is controlled by venesection alone may continue to suffer from thrombotic or haemorrhagic complications, presumably because venesection does not suppress the platelet count and may actually increase it further. Increasing fibrosis of the marrow and a clinicopathological picture indistinguishable from that of idiopathic myelofibrosis develops in about 30% of patients. Acute leukaemia develops in a proportion of the others. The incidence of acute leukaemia is higher in those treated with ^{32}P or alkylating agents than in those treated by venesection alone but the possibility exists that at least some of this difference results from the longer survival of those treated by the first two methods.

At necropsy all organs show marked vascular engorgement and there are widespread haemorrhages. In untreated patients, dark red haemopoietic marrow is found to have extended far down the shafts of limb bones. Areas of extramedullary haemopoiesis may be seen in the spleen and the liver, both of which are enlarged. The spleen is firm, weighs between 200 and 1200 g and often contains scars from old infarcts. The lymphoid follicles of the spleen are atrophied. The splenic pulp is hypertrophied and its sinusoids are engorged with red cells.

Secondary polycythaemia[214]

In the secondary polycythaemias there is an absolute increase in the red cell mass as a consequence of some identifiable primary disorder. The conditions associated with secondary polycythaemia are listed in Table 5.20. In all these conditions, the polycythaemia probably results from the action of increased concentrations of erythropoietin on normal, erythropoietin-responsive erythroid progenitor cells. The high levels of erythropoietin are usually produced as a physiological response to decreased oxygenation of renal tissue. In the majority of cases, the tissue hypoxia results from a lowering of the oxygen saturation of arterial blood due to inadequate oxygenation in the pulmonary capillaries or the shunting of venous blood from the right side of the heart to the left. Tissue hypoxia may also result from the inheritance of structurally abnormal haemoglobins (see Table 5.21) which have a high oxygen affinity and do not release adequate amounts of oxygen to the tissues.[38, 216] The poly-

Table 5.21 Some haemoglobinopathies associated with increased oxygen affinity and hereditary polycythaemia

Hb Chesapeake (α92 Arg→Leu)

Hb Little Rock (β143 His→Gln)

Hb Ranier (β145 Tyr→Cys)

Hb Capetown (α92 Arg→Gln)

Hb Yakima (β99 Asp→His)

Hb Kempsey (β99 Asp→Asn)

Hb Hiroshima (β21 His→Asp)

cythaemia which develops in some heavy smokers appears to be caused partly by an interaction between carboxyhaemoglobin and unaltered haemoglobin, which results in a shift of the oxygen dissociation curve to the left (i.e. increased oxygen affinity), and partly by a decreased plasma volume.[217] High levels of erythropoietin are present, in the absence of generalized tissue hypoxia, in patients with various tumours and cysts.[218] Extracts of some cerebellar haemangioblastomas, hepatomas, renal cysts and hydronephrotic kidneys have been shown to contain erythropoietin and it is thought that these tumours and abnormal kidneys produce erythropoietin inappropriately. Other tumours may stimulate erythropoietin production as a result of renal hypoxia induced by pressure on renal tissue or the renal blood supply. The erythrocytosis encountered in secondary polycythaemia is rarely associated with increases in the numbers of white cells or platelets or with splenomegaly. The marrow usually shows a selective red cell hyperplasia.

Idiopathic erythrocytosis[219]

In this condition the patient has a high PCV and an increased red cell mass. The diagnosis is based on the absence of splenomegaly or other haematological features considered to be necessary for the diagnosis of polycythaemia rubra vera and the lack of evidence of any of the known causes of secondary polycythaemia. On prolonged follow-up, some patients initially diagnosed as having idiopathic erythrocytosis eventually develop polycythaemia rubra vera. However, others do not make this transition. The aetiology of the polycythaemia in the latter group remains unknown. Patients with idiopathic erythrocytosis may suffer from episodes of vascular occlusion but the frequency of such episodes is lower than that in polycythaemia rubra vera.

APPARENT POLYCYTHAEMIA

This term is applied when a high PCV is associated with a high normal, normal or reduced red cell mass. Apparent polycythaemia may develop acutely as a result of a decrease in the plasma volume secondary to persistent vomiting, severe diarrhoea, profuse sweating, burns, and inadequate post-operative intravenous fluid therapy. Chronic forms of apparent polycythaemia also exist. Some of these cases have been reported under various names such as Gaisböck's syndrome, stress polycythaemia, pseudopolycythaemia and spurious polycythaemia.[220] Patients with these syndromes are often middle-aged, slightly obese males who tend to be tense and anxious. They also show a high incidence of hypertension and thromboembolic disease. Their facial appearance may be indistinguishable from that in polycythaemia rubra vera but the spleen is not palpable. The PCV may decrease to within the normal range when the hypertension is effectively treated.[221] The aetiology of chronic apparent polycythaemia is uncertain. Many patients have a high normal red cell mass and a low normal plasma volume. The arterial oxygen saturation is normal. The neutrophil and platelet counts are also normal and the marrow is of normal cellularity.

REFERENCES

1. Bessis M. Living blood cells and their ultrastructure. Berlin: Springer, 1973: 197.
2. Brecher G, Bessis M. Blood 1972; 40: 333.
3. Heilmeyer L, Keller W, Vivell O, Betke K, Wöhler F, Keiderling W. Schweiz Med Wochenschr 1961; 91: 1203.
4. O'Hare JA, Murnaghan DJ. N Engl J Med 1982; 306: 654.
5. Gjone E, Glomset JA, Kaare NK. In: Stanbury JB, Wyngaarden JB, Fredrickson DS, eds. The metabolic basis of inherited disease. 4th ed. New York: McGraw-Hill, 1978: 589.
6. Davidson RJ, How J, Lessels S. Scand J Haematol 1977; 19: 47.
7. Sturgeon P. Blood 1970; 36: 310.
8. Herbert PN, Gotto AM, Fredrickson DS. In: Stanbury JB, Wyngaarden JB, Fredrickson DS, eds. The metabolic basis of inherited disease. 4th ed. New York: McGraw-Hill, 1978: 544.
9. Symmans WA, Shepherd CS, March WL, Oyen R, Shohet SB, Linehan BJ. Br J Haematol 1979; 42: 575.
10. Finch CA, Deubelbeiss K, Cook JD, et al. Medicine 1970; 49: 17.
11. Wickramasinghe SN. Human bone marrow. Oxford: Blackwell Scientific Publications, 1975.
12. Wickramasinghe SN, Weatherall DJ. In: Hardisty RM, Weatherall DJ, eds. Blood and its disorders. 2nd ed. Oxford: Blackwell Scientific Publications, 1982: 101.
13. Adamson J, Hillman RD. JAMA 1968; 205: 63.
14. Wallace J, Sharpey-Shafer EP. Lancet 1941; ii: 393.
15. Dacie JV. The haemolytic anaemias, part I. The congenital anaemias. 3rd ed. Edinburgh: Churchill Livingstone, 1985.
16. Dacie JV. The haemolytic anaemias, part II. The auto-immune anaemias. 2nd ed. London: Churchill, 1962.
17. Bunn HF. Semin Hematol 1972; 9: 3.
18. Mortimer PP. J Clin Pathol 1983; 36: 445.
19. Duncan JR, Potter CG, Cappelini MD, Kurtz JB, Anderson MJ, Weatherall DJ. Lancet 1983; ii: 14.
20. Kelleher JF, Luban NLC, Mortimer PP, Kamimura T. N Engl J Med 1982; 306: 654.
21. Weed RI. Arch Intern Med 1975; 135: 1316.
22. Marchesi VT. Blood 1983; 61: 1.
23. Goodman SR, Shiffer KA, Casoria LA, Eyster ME. Blood 1982; 60: 772.
24. Wolfe LC, John KM, Falcone JC, Byrne AM, Lux SE. N Engl J Med 1982; 307: 1367.
25. Dhermy D, Lecomte MC, Garbarz M, et al. J Clin Invest 1982; 70: 707.
26. Coetzer T, Zail S. Blood 1982; 59: 900.
27. Booth PB, Serjeantson S, Woodfield DG, Amato D. Vox Sang 1977; 32: 99.
28. Wiley JS, Ellory JC, Shuman MA, Shaller CS, Cooper RA. Blood 1975; 46: 337.
29. Valentine WN. Blood 1979; 54: 549.
30. Grimes AJ. Human red cell metabolism. Oxford: Blackwell Scientific Publications, 1980.
31. Luzzatto L. Clin Haematol 1975; 4: 83.
32. Bienzle U, Panich V. Clin Haematol 1981; 10: 785.
33. de Gruchy GC. Drug-induced blood disorders. Oxford: Blackwell Scientific Publications, 1975.
34. Tanaka KR, Paglia DE. Semin Hematol 1971; 8: 367.
35. Zanella A, Rebulla P, Vullo C, Izzo C, Tedesco F, Sirchia G. Br J Haematol 1978; 40: 551.
36. Beutler E. Blood 1979; 54: 1.
37. Lehmann H, Huntsman RG. Man's haemoglobins. Amsterdam: North-Holland, 1974.
38. Weatherall DJ, Clegg JB. The thalassaemia syndromes. 3rd ed. Oxford: Blackwell Scientific Publications, 1981.
39. Thompson GR. Br Med J 1963; ii: 976.
40. Koppes GM, Daly JJ, Coltman CA Jr, Butkus DE. Am J Med 1977; 63: 313.
41. Jones SR, Binder RA, Donowho EM Jr. N Engl J Med 1970; 282: 323.
42. Serjeant GR. The clinical features of sickle cell disease. Amsterdam: North-Holland, 1974.
43. Fleming AF. Sickle cell disease. Edinburgh: Churchill Livingstone, 1982.
44. Noguchi CT, Schechter AN. Blood 1981; 58: 1057.
45. Rao KRP, Patel AR, Anderson MJ, Hodgson J, Jones SE, Pattison JR. Ann Intern Med 1983; 98: 930.
46. Collins FS, Orringer EP. Am J Med 1982; 73: 814.
47. Falk RH, Hood WB Jr. Arch Intern Med 1982; 142: 1680.
48. Akinyanju OO, Ladapo F. Postgrad Med J 1979; 55: 400.
49. Bauer TW, Moore GW, Hutchins GM. Am J Med 1980; 69: 833.
50. Osegbe DN, Akinyanju OO, Amaku EO. Lancet 1981; ii: 275.
51. Charache S, Scott J, Niebyl J, Bonds D. Obstet Gynecol 1980; 55: 407.

52. Milner PF, Jones BR, Döbler J. Am J Obstet Gynecol 1980; 138: 239.
53. Tuck SM. Br J Hosp Med 1982; 28: 125.
54. Anonymous. Lancet 1983; i: 1141.
55. Smith EW, Krevans JR. Bull Johns Hopkins Hosp 1959; 104: 17.
56. Charache S, Conley CL, Waugh DF, Ugoretz RJ, Spurrell JR. J Clin Invest 1967; 46: 1795.
57. Fabry ME, Kaul DK, Raventos C, Baez S, Rieder R, Nagel RL. J Clin Invest 1981; 67: 1284.
58. Wickramasinghe SN, Akinyanju OO, Hughes M. Clin Lab Haematol 1982; 4: 373.
59. Fairbanks VF, Gilchrist GS, Brimhall B, Jereb JA, Goldstone EC. Blood 1979; 53: 109.
60. Wasi P. Clin Haematol 1981; 10: 707.
61. Wickramasinghe SN, Hughes M, Wasi P, Fucharoen S, Modell B. Br J Haematol 1981; 48: 451.
62. Carrell RW, Lehmann H. Semin Hematol 1969; 6: 116.
63. Wickramasinghe SN, Hughes M. Haematologia 1984; 17: 35.
64. Wickramasinghe SN, Hughes M, Higgs DR, Weatherall DJ. Clin Lab Haematol 1981; 3: 51.
65. Wickramasinghe SN, Hughes M, Wasi P, Fucharoen S. Br J Haematol 1981; 49: 185.
66. Wickramasinghe SN, Hughes M. Br J Haematol 1980; 46: 401.
67. Wickramasinghe SN. In: Porter R, Fitzsimons DW, eds. Ciba Foundation Symposium 37 (new series) on congenital disorders of erythropoiesis. Amsterdam: Elsevier, 1976: 221.
68. Petz LD, Garratty G. Acquired immune hemolytic anemias. Edinburgh: Churchill Livingstone, 1980.
69. Pirofsky B. Semin Hematol 1976; 13: 251.
70. Frank MM, Atkinson JP, Gadek J. Ann Rev Med 1977; 28: 291.
71. Wolach B, Heddle N, Barr RD, Zipursky A, Pai KRM, Blajchman MA. Br J Haematol 1981; 48: 425.
72. Lau P, Sererat S, Moore V, McLeish K, Alousi M. Vox Sang 1983; 44: 167.
73. Petz LD. Clin Haematol 1980; 9: 455.
74. Sirchia G, Lewis SM. Clin Haematol 1975; 4: 199.
75. Rosse WF. Blood 1982; 60: 20.
76. Dessypris EN, Clark DA, McKee LC Jr, Krantz SB. N Engl J Med 1983; 309: 690.
77. Clark DA, Butler SA, Braren V, Hartmann RC, Jenkins DE Jr. Blood 1981; 57: 83.
78. Yacoub MH, Keeling DH. Br Heart J 1968; 30: 676.
79. Marsh GW, Lewis SM. Semin Hematol 1969; 6: 133.
80. Clinicopathological Conference. Am J Med 1983; 74: 1052.
81. Paré PD, Chan-Yan C, Wass H, Hooper R, Hogg JC. Am J Med 1983; 74: 1093.
82. Anonymous. Lancet 1981; ii: 847.
83. Topley E. J Clin Pathol 1961; 14: 295.
84. Smith RP, Olson MV. Semin Hematol 1973; 10: 253.
85. Kong I, Devonshire HW, Cooper M, Sloan TP, Idle JR, Smith RL. Br J Clin Pharmacol 1982; 13: 275.
86. Mulligan I, Parfrey P, Phillips ME, Brown EA, Curtis JR. Br Med J 1982; 284: 1151.
87. Wood RW. N Engl J Med 1982; 306: 932.
88. Catterall JR, Ferguson RJ, Miller HC. Br Med J 1981; 282: 779.
89. Trowbridge AA, Green JB III, Bonnett JD, Shohet SB, Ponnappa BD, McCombs WB. Am J Clin Pathol 1981; 76: 493.
90. Reynafarje C, Ramos J. Blood 1961; 17: 562.
91. Desforges JF, Quemby F. N Engl J Med 1976; 295: 103.
92. Chugh KS, Singhal PC, Sharma BK, et al. Am J Med Sci 1977; 274: 139.
93. Schulte K-L, Kochen MM. Lancet 1981; ii: 478.
94. Donaldson GWK, McArthur M, Macpherson AIS, Richmond J. Br J Haematol 1970; 18: 45.
95. Blendis LM, Ramboer C, Williams R. Eur J Clin Invest 1970; 1: 54.
96. Eichner ER. Am J Med 1979; 66: 311.
97. Douglass CC, Twomey JJ. Ann Intern Med 1970; 72: 159.
98. Zieve L. Ann Intern Med 1958; 48: 471.
99. Smith JA, Lonergan ET, Sterling K. N Engl J Med 1964; 271: 396.
100. Cooper RA, Kimball DB, Durocher JR. N Engl J Med 1974; 290: 1279.
101. Fossaluzza V, Rossi P. Br J Haematol 1983; 55: 715.
102. Oski FA, Barness LA. J Pediatr 1967; 70: 211.
103. Gross S, Melhorn DK. J Pediatr 1974; 85: 753.
104. Jacobs HS, Amsden T. J Lab Clin Med 1974; 84: 643.
105. Bothwell TH, Charlton RW, Cook JD, Finch CA. Iron metabolism in man. Oxford: Blackwell Scientific Publications, 1980.
106. Jacobs A. ed. Clin Haematol 1982; 11/2.
107. Rajantie J, Rapola J, Siimes MA. Metabolism 1981; 30: 3.
108. Schloesser LL, Kipp MA, Wenzel FJ. J Lab Clin Med 1965; 66: 107.
109. Dallman PR, Beutler E, Finch CA. Br J Haematol 1978; 40: 179.
110. Wiener E, Saunders J, Wickramasinghe SN. Haematologica 1979; 64: 385.
111. Cartwright GE, Lee GR. Br J Haematol 1971; 21: 147.
112. Hansen NE. Scand J Haematol 1983; 31: 397.
113. Reid C, Prowse P, Gumpel M, Chanarin I. Br J Haematol 1983; 55: 174.
114. Roodman GD, Horadam VW, Wright TL. Blood 1983; 62: 406.
115. Fisher JW, Radtke HW, Rege AB. In: Dunn CDR, ed. Current concepts in erythropoiesis. Chichester: Wiley, 1983: 189.
116. Zappacosta AR, Caro J, Erslev A. Am J Med 1982; 72: 53.
117. Nunnaly RM, Levine I. Am J Med 1961; 30: 972.
118. Morgan MY, Camilo ME, Luck W, Sherlock S, Hoffbrand AV. Clin Lab Haematol 1981; 3: 35.
119. Wickramasinghe SN. Clin Lab Haematol 1981; 3: 1.
120. Dacie JV, Smith MD, White JC, Mollin DL. Br J Haematol 1959; 5: 56.
121. Mollin DL, Hoffbrand AV. In: Dyke SC, ed. Recent advances in clinical pathology, series V. Edinburgh: Churchill Livingstone, 1968: 273.
122. Bottomley SS. Clin Haematol 1982; 11: 389.
123. Wickramasinghe SN, Chalmers DG, Cooper EH. Cell Tissue Kinet 1968, 1: 43.
124. Wickramasinghe SN, Hughes M. Br J Haematol 1978; 38: 345.
125. Wickramasinghe SN, Fulker MJ, Losowsky MS, Hall R. Acta Haematol 1971; 45: 236.
126. Cheng DS, Kushner JP, Wintrobe MM. Cancer 1979; 44: 724.

127. Chanarin I. The megaloblastic anaemias. 2nd ed. Oxford: Blackwell Scientific Publications, 1979.
128. Wickramasinghe SN. Br J Haematol 1972; 22: 111.
129. Wickramasinghe SN, Bush V. Br J Haematol 1977; 35: 659.
130. Chanarin I, Deacon R, Perry J, Lumb M. Br J Haematol 1981; 47: 487.
131. Matthews JH, Wood JK. Clin Lab Haematol 1984; 6: 1.
132. Campbell M, Lofters WS, Gibbs WN. Br Med J 1982; 285: 1617.
133. Pant SH, Ashbury AK, Richardson EP. Acta Neurol Scand 1968; 44 (suppl 35).
134. Deller DJ, Witts LJ. Q J Med 1962; 31: 71.
135. Johnson HD, Hoffbrand AV. Br J Surg 1970; 57: 33.
136. McIntyre OR, Sullivan LW, Jeffries GH, Silver RH. N Engl J Med 1965; 272: 981.
137. Katz M, Mehlman CS, Allen RH. J Clin Invest 1974; 53: 1274.
138. Donaldson RM. Adv Intern Med 1970; 16: 191.
139. Brandt LJ, Bernstein LH, Wagle A. Ann Intern Med 1977; 87: 546.
140. Booth CC, MacIntyre I, Mollin DL. Q J Med 1964; 33: 401.
141. Von Bondsdorff B. Diphyllobothriasis in man. London: Academic Press, 1977.
142. Anonymous. Lancet 1977; i: 292.
143. Saarni M, Palva I, Ahrenberg P. Lancet 1977; i: 806.
144. Ben-Bassat I, Feinstein A, Ramot B. Is J Med Sci 1969; 5: 62.
145. Burman JF, Mollin DL, Sourial NA, Sladden RA. Br J Haematol 1979; 43: 27.
146. Selligman PA, Steiner LL, Allen RH. N Engl J Med 1980; 303: 1209.
147. Reynolds EH, Laundy M. Lancet 1978; ii: 682.
148. Wu A, Chanarin I, Levi AJ. Lancet 1974; i: 829.
149. Chanarin I. J Clin Pathol 1980; 33: 909.
150. Lassen HCA, Henriksen E, Neukirch F, Kristensen HS. Lancet 1956; i: 527.
151. Amess JAL, Burman JF, Rees GM, Nancekievill DG, Mollin DL. Lancet 1978; ii: 339.
152. Nunn JF, Sharer NM, Gorchein A, Jones JA, Wickramasinghe SN. Lancet 1982; i: 1379.
153. Layzer B. Lancet 1978; ii: 1227.
154. Carmel R, Bedros AA, Mace JW, Goodman SI. Blood 1980; 55: 570.
155. Carmel R, Goodman SI. Blood 1982; 59: 306.
156. Scott JM, Weir DG. Clin Haematol 1980; 9: 587.
157. Girot R, Hamet M, Perignon J-L. N Engl J Med 1983; 308: 700.
158. van der Zee SPM, Lommen EJP, Trijbels JMF, Schretlen EDAM. Acta Paediatr Scand 1970; 59: 259.
159. Haworth C, Evans DIK, Mitra J, Wickramasinghe SN. Br J Haematol 1982; 50: 549.
160. Horton L, Coburn RJ, England JM, Himsworth RL. Q J Med 1976; 45: 101.
161. Chanarin I, McFadyen IR, Kyle R. Br J Obstet Gynaecol 1974; 84: 504.
162. Freedman BJ, Penington DG. Br J Haematol 1963; 9: 425.
163. Tudhope GR. Clin Haematol 1972; 1: 475.
164. Weick JK, Hagedorn AB, Linman JW. Mayo Clin Proc 1977; 49: 110.
165. Bouroncle BA, Doan CA. Am J Med Sci 1962; 243: 697.
166. Takácsi-Nagy L, Gráf F. Clin Haematol 1975; 4: 291.
167. Di Bella NJ, Silverstein MN, Hoagland HC. Arch Intern Med 1977; 137: 380.
168. Rondeau E, Solal-Celigny P, Dhermy D, et al. Br J Haematol 1983; 53: 467.
169. Lennert K, Nagai K, Schwarze EW. Clin Haematol 1975; 4: 331.
170. Ligumski M, Polliack A, Benbassat J. Scand J Haematol 1978; 21: 81.
171. Alter BP, Potter NU, Li FP. Clin Haematol 1978; 7: 431.
172. Camitta BM, Storb R, Thomas ED. N Engl J Med 1982; 306: 645 and 712.
173. Beard MEJ. In: Porter R, Fitzsimons DW, eds. Ciba Foundation Symposium 37 (new series) on congenital disorders of erythropoiesis. Amsterdam: Elsevier, 1976: 103.
174. Steier W, van Woolen GA, Selmanowitz VJ. Blood 1972; 39: 510.
175. Schwachman H, Diamond LK, Oski FA, Kshaw K-T. J Pediatr 1964; 65: 645.
176. Shahidi NT. Br J Haematol 1979; 43: 163.
177. Champlin R, Ho W, Gale RP. N Engl J Med 1983; 308: 113.
178. Gibson J, York J, McGirr EE, Kronenberg H. Aust NZ J Med 1983; 13: 130.
179. Krantz SB. N Engl J Med 1974; 291: 345.
180. Diamond LK, Wang WC, Alter BP. Adv Pediatr 1976; 22: 349.
181. Hardisty RM. In: Porter R, Fitzsimons DW, eds. Ciba Foundation Symposium 37 (new series) on congenital disorders of erythropoiesis. Amsterdam: Elsevier, 1976: 89.
182. Nathan DG, Clarke BJ, Hillman DG, Alter BP, Housman DE. J Clin Invest 1978; 61: 489.
183. Saunders EF, Freedman MH. Br J Haematol 1978; 40: 277.
184. Mangan KF, Chikkappa G, Bieler LZ, Scharfman WB. In: Baum SJ, Ledney GD, Khan A, eds. Experimental hematology today. Basel: Karger, 1981: 161.
185. Heimpel H, Wendt F. Helv Med Acta 1968; 34: 103.
186. Lewis SM, Nelson DA, Pitcher CS. Br J Haematol 1972; 23: 113.
187. Queisser W, Spiertz E, Jost E, Heimpel H. Acta Haematol 1971; 45: 65.
188. Crookston JH, Crookston MC, Burnie KL, Francombe WH, Dacie JV, Davis JA, Lewis SM. Br J Haematol 1969; 17: 11.
189. Wickramasinghe SN, Parry TE, Hughes M. Scand J Haematol 1978; 20: 429.
190. Verwilghen RL, Tan P, De Wolf-Peeters C, Broeckhaert-van Orschoven A, Lowagie AC. Experientia 1971; 27: 1467.
191. Breton-Gorius J, Daniel MT, Clauvel JP, Dreyfus B. Nouv Rev Fr Hematol 1973; 13: 23.
192. Goudsmit R, Beckers D, De Bruijne JI, Engelfriet CP, James J, Morselt AFW, Reynierse E. Br J Haematol 1972; 23: 97.
193. Wickramasinghe SN, Goudsmit R. Br J Haematol 1979; 41: 485.
194. Wickramasinghe SN, Parry TE, Williams C, Bond AN, Hughes M, Crook S. J Clin Pathol 1982; 35: 1103.
195. Abdalla S, Weatherall DJ, Wickramasinghe SN, Hughes M. Br J Haematol 1980; 46: 171.

196. Edozien JC, Rahim-Khan MA. Clin Sci 1968; 34: 315.
197. Viart P. Proc XIIIth Int Congr Pediatr, Wien, 1971.
198. Lanzkowsky P, McKenzie D, Katz S, Hoffenberg R, Friedman R, Black E. Br J Haematol 1967; 13: 639.
199. Steckel A, Smith NJ. Am J Clin Nutr 1970; 23: 896.
200. Fondu P. Biomedicine 1973; 18: 124.
201. Khalil M, Awwad H, Hafez M. Arch Dis Child 1969; 44: 124.
202. Wickramasinghe SN, Akinyanju OO, Grange A, Litwinczuk RAC. Br J Haematol 1983; 53: 135.
203. Wickramasinghe SN, Litwinczuk RAC, Akinyanju OO, Grange A. Br J Haematol 1983; 55: 385.
204. Allen DM, Dean RFA. Trans R Soc Trop Med Hyg 1965; 59: 326.
205. Sandstead HH, Gabr MK, Azzam S, et al. Am J Clin Nutr 1965; 17: 27.
206. Pearson TC, Glass UH, Wetherley-Mein G. Scand J Haematol 1978; 21: 153.
207. Perkins J, Israels MCG, Wilkinson JF. Q J Med 1964; 33: 499.
208. Gilbert HS. Clin Haematol 1975; 4: 263.
209. Cashman J, Henkelman D, Humphries K, Eaves C, Eaves E. Blood 1983; 61: 876.
210. Thomas DJ, du Boulay GH, Marshall J, et al. Lancet 1977; ii: 161.
211. Le Blond PF, Weed RI. Clin Haematol 1975; 4: 353.
212. Lertzman M, Frome BM, Israels LG, Cherniack RM. Ann Intern Med 1964; 60: 409.
213. Burkhardt R, Frisch B, Bartl R. J Clin Pathol 1982; 35: 257.
214. Balcerzak SP, Bromberg PA. Semin Hematol 1975; 12: 353.
215. Bacon BR, Rothman SA, Ricanati ES, Rashad FA. Arch Intern Med 1980; 140: 1206.
216. Adamson JW. Semin Hematol 1975; 12: 383.
217. Jackson DV Jr, Spurr CL. N Engl J Med 1978; 298: 972.
218. Thorling EB. Scand J Haematol 1972; 17 (suppl).
219. Pearson TC, Wetherley-Mein G. Clin Lab Haematol 1979; 1: 189.
220. Weinreb NJ, Shih CF. Semin Hematol 1975; 12: 397.
221. Watts EJ, Lewis SM. Scand J Haematol 1983; 31: 241.

6

Barbara J. Bain and S.N. Wickramasinghe

Disorders affecting leucocytes

Inherited abnormalities of granulocyte morphology or
    function
  Pelger–Huët anomaly
  Hereditary hypersegmentation of neutrophil nuclei
  May–Hegglin anomaly
  Chédiak–Higashi syndrome
  Myeloperoxidase deficiency
  Alder–Reilly anomaly
  Chronic granulomatous disease
  Abnormalities of the cell membrane of neutrophils
  Other abnormalities that are probably inherited
Aquired abnormalities of granulocyte morphology
    or function
  Shifts to the left or right
  Toxic granulation of neutrophils
  Döhle bodies
  Macropolycytes
  Acquired Pelger–Huët anomaly
  Acquired myeloperoxidase deficiency
  Botryoid nuclei
  Other abnormalities
Leucopenia
  Neutropenia
    Drugs, chemicals and ionizing radiation
    Immune neutropenia
    Dialysis neutropenia
    Chronic idiopathic neutropenia
    Cyclical neutropenia
    Familial benign chronic neutropenia
    Neutropenia in healthy Blacks
    Infantile genetic agranulocytosis
    Congenital aleukia
    Other rare neutropenic syndromes
  Eosinopenia
  Basopenia
  Monocytopenia
  Lymphocytopenia
Leucocytosis
  Neutrophil leucocytosis
  Eosinophil and basophil leucocytosis
    Hypereosinophilic syndrome
  Lymphocytosis and monocytosis
    Infectious mononucleosis
Leukaemia
  Acute myeloid leukaemia
    Erythroleukaemia and erythraemic myelosis
    (di Guglielmo's syndrome)
    Acute megakaryoblastic leukaemia
    Acute myelofibrosis
  Chronic granulocytic leukaemia

  Juvenile chronic myeloid leukaemia
  Neutrophilic leukaemia
  Myelodysplastic syndromes
  Acute lymphoblastic leukaemia
  Chronic lymphocytic leukaemia
  Prolymphocytic leukaemia
  Hairy cell leukaemia
  Adult T-cell leukaemia/lymphoma
  Biphenotypic leukaemia
Leukaemoid reactions

The disorders affecting leucocytes can be considered under two headings: (1) abnormalities of their morphology or function; and (2) abnormalities of their number (or concentration) in the blood. Not infrequently, abnormalities of morphology or function are accompanied by abnormalities in number and vice versa. Many diseases are associated with changes in the concentration of one or more types of circulating leucocytes. Although such changes are often non-specific they may provide dignostic clues. Alterations in the concentration of circulating leucocytes usually represent a response of the body to diseases of various tissues other than the blood and bone marrow but may occasionally result from diseases of the haemopoietic system. The leukaemias may cause an increase or a decrease in the concentrations of mature leucocytes in the blood as well as an impairment of leucocyte function. They are discussed separately at the end of this chapter (pp. 223–267).

INHERITED ABNORMALITIES OF GRANULOCYTE MORPHOLOGY OR FUNCTION

Pelger–Huët anomaly[1, 2]

This disorder is inherited as an autosomal dominant trait and affects 1 in 1000–10 000 people. It is characterised by a marked reduction in the number of nuclear segments in neutrophil granulocytes. Heterozygotes have bilobed, spectacle-like nuclei in 50–70% of their neutrophil granulocytes (Fig. 6.1a) and round or oval unsegmented nuclei in 20–40%. The affected nuclei have abnormally coarse chromatin. There are no abnormalities in the number and only minor abnormalities in the function[3] of neutrophils. The functional abnormality is not associated with an increased tendency to infections. The condition should not be confused with the left-shift seen in a reactive neutrophil leucocytosis. Homozygotes for the Pelger–Huët anomaly are rare and show round or oval nuclei in all neutrophil granulocytes. An acquired abnormality resembling the Pelger–Huët anomaly may be seen in myelodysplastic states (see p. 242).

Hereditary hypersegmentation of neutrophil nuclei[4]

This rare condition is inherited as an autosomal dominant character. The proportion of neutrophils with five or more lobes is normally 2–3% but in these cases is usually greater than 10%. The neutrophils appear to have adequate function.

May–Hegglin anomaly[1, 5]

This is a rare disorder which is inherited as an autosomal dominant trait. It is characterized by intracytoplasmic inclusions in all types of granulocytes and in monocytes, giant hypogranular platelets, thrombocytopenia (in one third of the cases), a moderate reduction in platelet life-span and, occasionally, a mild haemorrhagic tendency. The cytoplasmic inclusions are 2–5 μm in diameter, appear greyish-blue when stained by a Romanowsky method, and are composed of rough endoplasmic reticulum. They are similar to Döhle bodies both in appearance and composition (see p. 210) but tend to be larger, more rounded and discrete, and to affect a much higher percentage of the granulocytes. Although there are minor abnormalities of neutrophil function,[3] there appears to be no increased susceptibility to infections.

Chédiak–Higashi syndrome[1, 6]

This autosomal recessive condition is characterized by the presence of a reduced number of granules and the formation of some abnormally large granules (by progressive fusion of normally-formed granules) in most granule-containing cells (Figs 6.1b, c, d). The affected cells include the neutrophils, eosinophils, lymphocytes, monocytes, melanocytes, Schwann cells of peripheral nerves, fibroblasts, vascular endothelial cells, renal tubular cells and the parenchymal cells of the adrenal and pituitary glands. Platelet granules are morphologically normal. The large granules in leucocytes vary from a pale slate-grey to a dark reddish colour (Romanowsky stain). Despite the presence of some giant melanin granules, the reduction of the total number

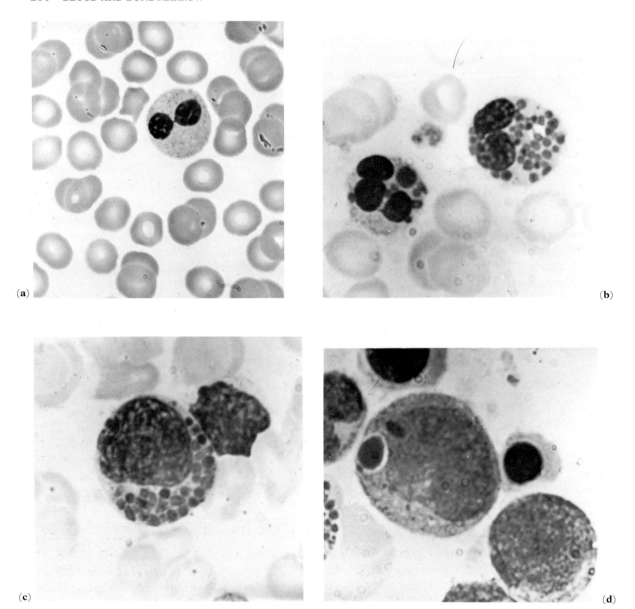

Fig. 6.1a–d Two inherited abnormalities of the morphology of neutrophils. (**a**) Peripheral blood neutrophil showing the inherited Pelger–Huët anomaly. (**b–d**) Cells from a marrow smear of a patient with the Chédiak–Higashi syndrome showing the presence of giant granules within the neutrophil series. (**b**) Two neutrophils with giant granules. (**c**) Neutrophil myelocyte with giant granules. (**d**) Neutrophil promyelocyte with two giant granules.

May–Grünwald–Giemsa stain ×940

b–d *Courtesy of Professor J.W. Stewart, Department of Haematology, Middlesex Hospital Medical School, London, UK*

of melanin granules in the skin, iris and retina gives rise to partial oculocutaneous albinism with silvery hair, photophobia and nystagmus. There is a marked reduction in circulating natural killer cells (NK cells, p. 18).[7] The leucocyte abnor-malities are associated with recurrent infections, particularly of the respiratory tract and skin, which cause death during infancy or early child-hood. The infecting organism is usually *Staphylococcus aureus* but may be *Streptococcus pyogenes*,

Haemophilus influenzae or *Streptococcus pneumoniae*. Some affected children develop a terminal lymphoma-like picture with lymphadenopathy, hepatosplenomegaly, neuropathy, pancytopenia and widespread infiltration of tissues by mononuclear cells; in one case these cells had the phenotype of T-cells and the histopathological features supported the diagnosis of T-cell lymphoma.[8]

The giant granules present in neutrophils (Fig. 6.1b) are peroxidase-positive and represent primary granules which appear to have fused together. The neutrophils have morphologically normal specific granules and increased numbers of autophagic vacuoles. They display normal phagocytic activity, defective chemotaxis, defective degranulation and delayed killing of some bacteria. It has been postulated that these defects in neutrophil function may result from an increased rate of depolymerization of tubulin,[9] the major structural protein of microtubules.

Myeloperoxidase deficiency[10, 11]

The introduction of automated differential counting based on cytochemical reactions has revealed that a deficiency of myeloperoxidase in neutrophils (but not of the peroxidase in eosinophils) is relatively common (1:2000). Most individuals with this deficiency do not have an increased susceptibility to infections, suggesting that enzymes other than myeloperoxidase play a role in the killing of bacteria by neutrophils. However, occasional myeloperoxidase-deficient patients suffer from recurrent infections due to a failure of their neutrophils to kill some bacteria and fungi. Myeloperoxidase deficiency is probably inherited as an autosomal recessive character.

Alder–Reilly anomaly[1, 12]

This anomaly consists of the presence of abnormally coarse azurophilic cytoplasmic granules in neutrophils and, sometimes, in blood lymphocytes and monocytes. In lymphocytes the individual granules may occur within vacuoles and are occasionally comma-shaped. The Alder–Reilly anomaly is found in various types of mucopolysaccharidosis including Hunter–Hurler syndrome, and Maroteaux–Lamy polydystrophic dwarfism. These syndromes, which are inherited as autosomal recessive traits, are caused by deficiencies of enzymes involved in the degradation of the carbohydrate components of mucopolysaccharides; the anomalous granules consist of the uncatabolized carbohydrate components. Only a proportion of patients with these syndromes display the anomaly in blood cells. The Alder–Reilly anomaly is easily confused with toxic granulation of the neutrophils (p. 210) but differs from the latter in that it may also affect lymphocytes and monocytes.

Chronic granulomatous disease[13, 14]

This is an inherited disorder of the ability of neutrophils and mononuclear phagocytes to kill microorganisms; it is unassociated with abnormalities in the morphology or number of these cells in the blood. It is characterized by the onset early in childhood of recurrent granulomatous and suppurative lesions of the lymph nodes, skin, liver, bone, lungs and other organs. These lesions may be caused by organisms which ordinarily are of low virulence; they usually heal slowly with appropriate antimicrobial therapy. The infecting organisms include *Staphylococcus aureus*, *Serratia marcescens*, klebsiellae, salmonellae, *Actinomyces israeli*, *Candida albicans* and *Aspergillus fumigatus*. The granulomas are composed of lymphocytes, macrophages, plasma cells, neutrophils and occasional giant cells. Hepatosplenomegaly is common. Most of the patients die in childhood (average survival, 5–7 years) but some live to adult life. The majority of cases show an X-linked inheritance. However, some show an autosomal recessive inheritance, suggesting that more than one enzyme defect may cause the same clinical syndrome.

The neutrophils, monocytes and macrophages phagocytose microorganisms normally but fail to kill them. The process of phagocytosis is not associated with the usual burst of increased respiratory activity (p. 12). The neutrophils of patients with chronic granulomatous disease fail to reduce the colourless dye nitroblue tetrazolium (NBT) to the bluish-black formazan *in vitro* following phagocytosis of dye-tagged zymosan particles. A quantitative NBT reduction test is used to detect female carriers. The X-linked form of chronic granulomatous disease is caused by an absence of cytochrome b$_{-245}$. Heterozygous female carriers have a reduced concentration of this haemoprotein in their neutrophils. In families showing an autosomal recessive inheritance, cytochrome b$_{-245}$ is present in normal amounts but for some reason is non-functional.[15]

The clinical picture of mild chronic granulomatous disease has been reported in association with a severe deficiency of glucose 6-phosphate dehydrogenase in the leucocytes[16] and that of non-X-linked chronic granulomatous disease with glutathione peroxidase deficiency.[17]

Abnormalities of the cell membrane of neutrophils

A syndrome which is caused by a deficiency of a 180 kilodalton glycoprotein in the cell membrane of the neutrophil has been described. It is characterized by delayed umbilical cord detachment, recurrent bacterial infection, marked leucocytosis, inability to form pus, defective neutrophil function (impairment of adherence, of random migration, of chemotactic migration and of the respiratory burst), a decreased natural killer cell activity (p. 18) and, usually, death during the first two years of life.[18]

Recurrent bacterial infection has also been reported in a boy with a deficiency of a 150 kilodalton membrane glycoprotein.[19]

Other abnormalities that are probably inherited

Vacuolation of neutrophil promyelocytes and more mature cells of the neutrophil series and of monocytes and occasional lymphocytes (Jordans' anomaly) has been reported in two brothers with progressive muscular dystrophy and two sisters with ichthyosis.[20]

Several congenital, familial or presumably-congenital syndromes or conditions (other than those discussed earlier in this chapter) are associated with abnormalities of neutrophil function. These include: (1) the actin dysfunction syndrome,[21] which is characterized by recurrent staphylococcal skin infections (with little pus formation), recurrent septicaemia, and both defective phagocytic activity and chemotactic motility of neutrophils, probably due to defective polymerisation of actin; (2) Job's syndrome,[22] which is characterized by recurrent infection of the nasal sinuses and lungs, cold subcutaneous staphylococcal abscesses, eczematoid rashes, high IgE levels, eosinophilia and impaired neutrophil mobility; (3) neutrophil pyruvate kinase deficiency[23] in which recurrent staphylococcal infections are caused by defective bacterial killing; and (4) the presence of a low-affinity NADPH-dependent oxidase which is associated with recurrent pulmonary aspergillosis, a prolongation of the respiratory burst, and impaired superoxide formation.[24]

A recently described congenital abnormality of neutrophils is lactoferrin deficiency.[25, 26] In this condition, recurrent infection from birth is associated with a deficiency in neutrophils of lactoferrin, vitamin B$_{12}$-binding protein and alkaline phosphatase, and impairment of neutrophil chemotaxis and adherence. The neutrophils of affected patients have bilobed nuclei, possess few or no ultrastructurally-normal specific granules and contain several elongated vesicular sacs (probably representing abnormal granules).

Abnormalities of neutrophil function are also a feature of the 'lazy leucocyte syndrome' (p. 215) and Shwachman's syndrome (p. 215).

The neutrophils in cases of Down's syndrome show a mild impairment of bacterial killing and display minor ultrastructural abnormalities of their nuclei (e.g. increased frequency of pockets and appendices).[27]

ACQUIRED ABNORMALITIES OF GRANULOCYTE MORPHOLOGY OR FUNCTION

Shifts to the left or right

In some conditions (e.g. infections) the proportion of band forms and neutrophils with only two nuclear segments may increase, and some metamyelocytes and myelocytes and a very occasional myeloblast may be seen in the blood. When this

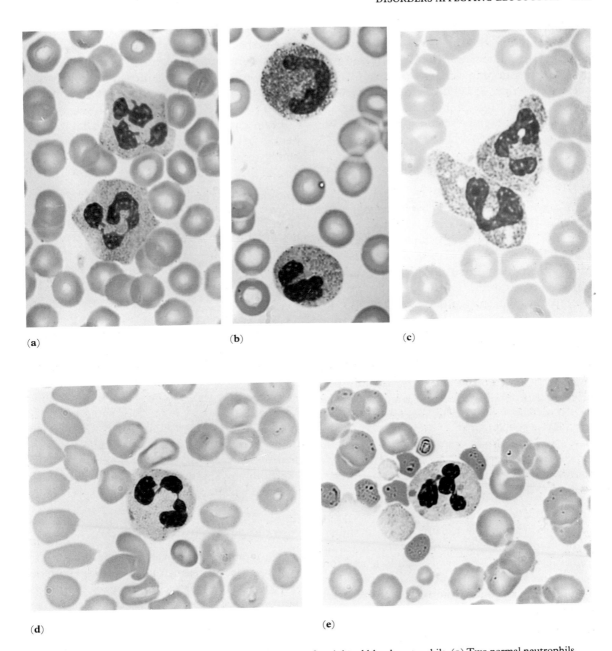

(a)   (b)   (c)

(d)   (e)

Fig. 6.2a–e Some acquired abnormalities of the morphology of peripheral blood neutrophils. (**a**) Two normal neutrophils (for comparison). (**b**) Toxic granulation in a patient with a left shift due to an infection. One of the cells is a band form (juvenile neutrophil). (**c**) Vacuolation and toxic granulation in a patient with an acute bacterial infection; one of the cells is a band form. (**d**) Neutrophil from a patient with an acute infection showing an elongated Döhle body at its periphery. (**e**) Three rounded Döhle bodies in a neutrophil from a patient with extensive burns.

May–Grünwald–Giemsa stain   × 940

happens the neutrophil series is described as showing a shift to the left.

In other conditions there is an increased proportion of neutrophils with four or five or more nuclear segments. This occurs in vitamin B_{12} or folate deficiency (see p. 170), renal disease and iron deficiency anaemia (see p. 161).

Toxic granulation of neutrophils
(Figs 6.2b, c)

'Toxic granules' are fine or coarse reddish-violet granules (Romanowsky stain) which are found scattered throughout the cytoplasm of neutrophils. They frequently occur in severe infections but are also seen in non-infective inflammatory states and in normal pregnancy. The primary granules of neutrophil promyelocytes and myelocytes are azurophilic but those of normal mature neutrophils lose this property. Toxic granules seem to result from an abnormality in the maturation of the primary granules with a consequent retention of their azurophilic property.[28] Neutrophils with toxic granulation may also show increased cytoplasmic basophilia, vacuolation or Döhle bodies.

Döhle bodies[29, 30]

These are rounded, oval or rod-shaped pale greyish-blue inclusions found within the cytoplasm of neutrophils, usually at the periphery and protruding beyond the normal contour of the cell (Figs 6.2d, e). They are 1-2 μm long and consist of stacks of rough endoplasmic reticulum. Döhle bodies are found in normal pregnancy, various infections, in patients with various neoplasms and after severe burns.

Macropolycytes

These are very large polymorphonuclear leucocytes (diameter $> 16 \mu$m) which often have hypersegmented nuclei with 6-14 nuclear segments. They may be found in the blood in vitamin B_{12} or folate deficiency and in infections, myeloproliferative disorders and drug-induced marrow damage.

The macropolycytes seen in vitamin B_{12} deficiency have tetraploid or hypotetraploid DNA contents and appear to result from nuclear segmentation in those giant metamyelocytes which are not phagocytosed by bone marrow macrophages (see p. 172).

The occurrence of macropolycytes has been reported as an inherited condition in a single family.

Acquired Pelger-Huët anomaly

Neutrophils resembling those in the inherited Pelger-Huët anomaly (see p. 205) are frequently seen in the myelodysplastic syndromes and in acute leukaemia, and rarely in chronic granulocytic leukaemia and myelofibrosis.

Acquired myeloperoxidase deficiency

An acquired myeloperoxidase deficiency may occur in acute myeloid leukaemia and myelodysplastic syndromes.

Botryoid nuclei[31, 32]

In patients with heat stroke, over 50% of the neutrophils contain increased numbers of small, moderately pyknotic nuclear segments which are clustered like grapes on a stem.

Other abnormalities

One or more acquired defects of neutrophil function have been demonstrated in a large number of conditions (usually employing in vitro techniques). Examples of such conditions are protein-energy malnutrition, severe overwhelming infections, certain specific infections (e.g. by myxoviruses[33]), extensive burns, uraemia, rheumatoid arthritis, SLE, paroxymal nocturnal haemoglobinuria, allergic reactions, alcoholism, therapy with certain drugs[34] (e.g. corticosteroids), chronic lymphocytic leukaemia, lymphocytic lymphoma, myeloma, primary acquired sideroblastic anaemia,[35] sarcoidosis,[36] cystic fibrosis,[37] morbid obesity[38] and hypophosphataemia.[39] The functional abnormalities which have been reported include impaired chemotactic motility due to an intrinsic neutrophil defect, defective adherence, impaired phagocytosis, depressed superoxide generation and bacterial killing, and impaired chemotaxis due either to an acquired deficiency of complement components (caused by intravascular complement activation) or to the presence of an inhibitory plasma factor.[36, 40] In several of the conditions listed above, the clinical significance of the reported defects of neutrophil function is uncertain.

LEUCOPENIA

The term *leucopenia* is applied to a decrease in the concentration of circulating white blood cells below the normal range. The terms *granulocytopenia, neutropenia, eosinopenia, basopenia, lymphocytopenia* and *monocytopenia* are used to describe reductions in the concentrations of circulating granulocytes, neutrophils, eosinophils, basophils, lymphocytes and monocytes correspondingly.

NEUTROPENIA

Neutropenia may arise from: (1) various disorders of bone marrow function resulting in a decreased rate of release of neutrophils from the marrow into the circulation; (2) a shift of neutrophils from the circulating to the marginated cell pools (see p. 10); (3) a reduction of the $T_{\frac{1}{2}}$ of circulating neutrophils; and (4) combinations of the above. A decrease in the rate of release of neutrophils from the marrow (i.e. a decrease of effective neutrophil granulocytopoiesis) may be caused by a reduction in the rate of production of neutrophil precursors (i.e. decreased total neutrophil granulocytopoiesis), an increased intramedullary destruction of neutrophil precursors (i.e. increased ineffective neutrophil granulocytopoiesis), or an impairment of the release of bone marrow neutrophils into the blood. A reduction of the $T_{\frac{1}{2}}$ of circulating neutrophils may be due to destruction of circulating cells (e.g. by antibodies or a hyperactive spleen) or an accelerated rate of egress of neutrophils from the blood into tissues. Because of the difficulties involved in the quantitative assessment of total, effective

and ineffective neutrophil granulocytopoiesis in humans, the mechanisms underlying the neutropenia in many clinical situations and especially in any individual patient are frequently a matter of uncertainty. When neutropenia is caused by ineffective neutrophil granulocytopoiesis due to intramedullary destruction of the most mature neutrophil precursors, or by an increased loss of circulating cells, there is a compensatory increase of total neutrophil granulocytopoiesis. In many neutropenic states the marrow contains few cells beyond the neutrophil myelocyte stage because of an accelerated release of neutrophil metamyelocytes and marrow neutrophils into the circulation.

The conditions which may be associated with a neutropenia are listed in Table 6.1. As indicated in the table, many of these are discussed elsewhere in this volume. A neutropenia may be seen in certain phases of diseases caused by a number of infectious agents. The mechanisms underlying this neutropenia, which only affects a proportion of infected patients (e.g. about 50% of patients with typhoid), are uncertain. They may include an endotoxin-induced shift of neutrophils from the circulating to the marginated cell pools, a reduced $T_{\frac{1}{2}}$ of circulating granulocytes (due either to destruction of cells within the circulation or to an accelerated rate of egress of cells from the blood) and a failure of the bone marrow to adequately increase the rate of effective granulocytopoiesis. In certain circumstances infection may be associated both with a failure to adequately increase effective granulocytopoiesis and with an exhaustion of the marrow granulocyte pool so that neutropenia is seen together with a left shift. This is particularly common in very severe bacterial infections and in bacterial infections in neonates and alcoholics (who normally have a reduced marrow granulocyte pool). The neutropenia induced by certain drugs (e.g. chlorpromazine) or found in aplastic anaemia and cyclical neutropenia is caused by decreased total granulocytopoiesis. The neutropenia found in megaloblastic anaemias and in individuals receiving some drugs (e.g. methotrexate) is caused by increased ineffective granulocytopoiesis, usually with some reduction in the $T_{\frac{1}{2}}$ of the circulating granulocytes. Finally,

Table 6.1 Causes of neutropenia

Infections
    Viral: measles, rubella, influenza, infectious hepatitis
    Bacterial: brucellosis, typhoid, paratyphoid, overwhelming
        pyogenic infections (septicaemia), miliary tuberculosis
    Rickettsial: typhus
    Protozoal: malaria, kala-azar, trypanosomiasis
    Fungal: histoplasmosis, blastomycosis

Drugs (see Table 6.2), chemicals and ionizing radiation

Hypersplenism

Leukaemia

Myelodysplastic states (preleukaemia) (p. 240)

Aplastic anaemia (p. 187) and paroxysmal nocturnal
    haemoglobinuria (p. 149)

Bone marrow infiltration (p. 183)

Myelofibrosis (p. 184)

Megaloblastic anaemia

Immune neutropenia
    Amidopyrine-induced agranulocytosis
    Systemic lupus erythematosus
    Rheumatoid arthritis
    Autoimmune neutropenia
    Neonatal alloimmune neutropenia

Dialysis neutropenia

Chronic idiopathic neutropenia

Cyclical neutropenia

Familial benign chronic neutropenia

Neutropenia in Blacks (physiological)

Infantile genetic agranulocytosis

Congenital aleukia

Other rare neutropenic syndromes

Miscellaneous conditions: hypothyroidism, hypopituitarism,
    anaphylactic shock, anorexia nervosa

the low neutrophil counts found in hypersplenism, amidopyrine-induced agranulocytosis, SLE, autoimmune neutropenia and neonatal allo-immune neutropenia are caused by a reduction of the $T_{\frac{1}{2}}$ of these cells in the blood.

Drugs, chemicals and ionizing radiation[41]

The commonest drug-induced blood dyscrasia is a neutropenia.[42] Some drugs (e.g. alkylating agents or antifolate drugs), certain chemicals (e.g. benzene) and irradiation induce a neutropenia in all individuals in a dose-dependent manner.

Other drugs produce neutropenia only in occasional individuals and this phenomenon is usually at least partly based on a genetic polymorphism of drug metabolism. Drugs of the latter category may either cause neutropenia as part of an aplastic anaemia or induce a selective neutropenia. Furthermore, several of the drugs causing aplastic anaemia in susceptible individuals (see p. 188) initially cause a neutropenia which subsequently progresses to aplastic anaemia. Drugs which may occasionally cause selective neutropenia are listed in Table 6.2. The relatively high-risk drugs

Table 6.2 Some drugs which may cause a selective neutropenia in occasional patients

Analgesic drugs
    Amidopyrine, dipyrone

Anti-arrhythmic drugs
    Procainamide, propranolol, quinidine

Antibacterial drugs
    Aminosalicylic acid, amoxycillin, ampicillin,
    benzylpenicillin, carbenicillin, chloramphenicol,
    cloxacillin, co-trimoxazole (sulphamethoxazole-
    trimethoprim), other sulphonamides, dapsone, isoniazid,
    methicillin, nafcillin, novobiocin, oxacillin, streptomycin,
    tetracycline, thiacetazone

Anticoagulant drugs
    Dicoumarol, phenindione

Anticonvulsant drugs
    Carbamazepine, ethosuximide, phenytoin, troxidone
    (trimethadione)

Antidiabetic drugs
    Carbutamide, chlorpropamide, tolbutamide

Antihistamines
    Chlorpheniramine, mebhydrolin, mepyramine,
    promethazine, trimeprazine

Anti-inflammatory drugs
    Indomethacin, oxyphenbutazone, phenylbutazone, sodium
    aurothiomalate

Antimalarial drugs
    Amodiaquine, dapsone, hydroxychloroquine, pamaquin

Antithyroid drugs
    Carbimazole, methimazole, methylthiouracil,
    propylthiouracil

Tranquillizers and antidepressants
    Amitriptyline, chlordiazepoxide, chlorpromazine,
    imipramine, meprobamate, prochlorperazine, promazine,
    trimeprazine

Miscellaneous
    Arsenicals, captopril, cimetidine, hydrochlorothiazide,
    levamisole, mercurial diuretics, methyldopa, mianserin,
    penicillamine

amongst these include amidopyrine and the anti-thyroid drugs.

Some of the drugs listed in Table 6.2 usually induce a mild to moderate neutropenia which is asymptomatic and does not progress despite continuation of the drug; others usually cause a complete or virtually complete absence of neutrophils (agranulocytosis). Agranulocytosis[43, 44, 45] results in a life-threatening clinical syndrome characterized by fever, sweating, vomiting, sore throat, dysphagia due to necrotic ulceration of the mouth and pharynx, extreme prostration and, frequently, death from overwhelming infection. At necropsy, necrotic ulcers are found in the mucous membrane of the entire alimentary tract as well as in the vagina. The prognosis is considerably improved if the offending drug is stopped and infection is adequately controlled by antibiotic therapy.

Drugs or their metabolites might induce neutropenia by one or both of two mechanisms: (1) impairment of bone marrow function; and (2) destruction of circulating neutrophils.[46] The classical example of a drug which causes agranulocytosis by a toxic effect on the marrow is chlorpromazine. This drug causes a transient and moderate neutropenia in one-third of individuals receiving it. It causes an agranulocytosis in about 1 in 1200 individuals, usually after a cumulative dose of 10–20 g over 20–30 d. Chlorpromazine appears to cause agranulocytosis by inhibiting DNA synthesis and cell proliferation in the granulocyte precursors of susceptible individuals. At the time of the agranulocytosis, the marrow shows few or no neutrophil granulocytopoietic cells. The susceptibility of occasional individuals to develop agranulocytosis following therapy with chlorpromazine or other sulphur-containing drugs such as carbimazole or metiamide may depend on their genetically determined ability to oxidize the drug to highly-reactive myelotoxic metabolites (sulphoxides) more rapidly than most individuals.[47] It is likely that many other drugs which cause neutropenia do so by directly or indirectly impairing biochemical processes within granulocytopoietic cells or by causing some form of immune destruction of these cells. The best understood example of a drug which causes agranulocytosis by destroying circulating neutrophils is amidopyrine. Individuals with amidopyrine-induced agranulocytosis give a history of previous exposure to the drug and may, after recovery from the initial agranulocytosis, show a recurrence of agranulocytosis within 12 hours of a test dose. The serum of such individuals contains an antibody which causes agglutination of neutrophils and an acute neutropenia in the presence of the drug. The agglutination is thought to be mediated by a drug-antibody complex. The marrow shows increased granulocytopoietic activity and a depletion of the more mature precursors.

Immune neutropenia

As has already been mentioned, the agranulocytosis induced by amidopyrine, and possibly also by other drugs, results from the destruction of circulating neutrophils by drug-antibody complexes. The neutropenia seen in some cases of SLE and in a disorder known as autoimmune neutropenia is caused by auto-antibodies against neutrophils. Autoimmune neutropenia[48, 49] is usually a relatively mild disease characterized by recurrent infections, particularly of the oropharynx and skin; in some cases the antineutrophil antibody has the specificity anti-NA2 (see p. 37). In the syndrome called neonatal alloimmune neutropenia,[50, 51] the fetus's neutrophils and neutrophil precursors are destroyed by the transplacental passage of maternal IgG alloantibodies formed against HLA or neutrophil-specific antigens present on fetal but not on maternal neutrophils (see p. 37). The neutropenia can be severe and may cause life-threatening neonatal infections.

In some patients with neutropenia associated with certain diseases (e.g. rheumatoid arthritis, polymyositis, polymyalgia rheumatica, preleukaemia) and also in chronic idiopathic neutropenia, the neutropenia may be caused by T-cells which are inhibitory to granulocytopoiesis.[52]

Dialysis neutropenia[53, 54]

Shortly after commencing a haemodialysis 'run', contact of plasma with dialysis membranes causes activation of complement via the alternative pathway (see p. 28). Activated complement components lead to increased neutrophil adhesiveness and aggregation, with consequent sequestration in the lungs and to a lesser extent in vessels elsewhere, and thus to a marked neutropenia. Acute cardiopulmonary failure may occur. After some hours, neutropenia is reversed and a rebound neutrophilia occurs.

Chronic idiopathic neutropenia[55, 56]

This is a benign disorder of unknown aetiology, affecting children as well as adults, in which a neutropenia develops and lasts for one or more years. There may also be a monocytosis. Recovery occurs spontaneously. Affected children, but not adults, suffer from an increased susceptibility to minor infections. There is no recognizable cause for the neutropenia such as splenomegaly or white cell antibodies. The $T_{\frac{1}{2}}$ of circulating neutrophils is normal in most but not all cases, as is the size of the marginated blood granulocyte pool. The bone marrow usually contains normal or increased numbers of CFU-GM but the formation of colony-stimulating factor (p. 50) by marrow macrophages is defective.[57] The number of proliferating neutrophil precursors in the marrow is usually normal or subnormal indicating a failure to increase granulocytopoietic activity in response to the neutropenia. The number of non-dividing precursors, particularly the juvenile neutrophils and segmented neutrophils, is reduced in about a third of the cases. In most cases, the cytokinetic basis underlying the neutropenia appears to be a high death rate both in the proliferating and non-proliferating neutrophil precursor pools (i.e. an increase of ineffective granulocytopoiesis). However, a proportion of cases show different cytokinetic disturbances (e.g. increased numbers of proliferating precursors, shortened $T_{\frac{1}{2}}$ of blood granulocytes, or an increase in the marginated granulocyte pool), suggesting that chronic idiopathic neutropenia may include a number of pathogenetically-different conditions. *In vitro* studies have shown that some cases of acquired idiopathic neutropenia have T-cells (sometimes with the phenotype of cytotoxic/suppressor cells) which inhibit the growth of autologous CFU-GM.[52]

Cyclical neutropenia[58, 59]

This is a rare disorder in which neutropenia occurs for 4–10 days at intervals of 15–35 days (average, 21 d). Most cases present in infancy or childhood with periodic bouts of fever, malaise, headache, sore throat, oral ulceration, skin infections or, occasionally, infections of the lungs and other organs. Such bouts occur during the neutropenic phases, last for a few days and recur over many years. They are sometimes accompanied by arthralgia or abdominal pain. About half the cases show a monocytosis during the neutropenic phase and some show an eosinophilia. The neutrophil count becomes nearly normal between the symptomatic periods but there is usually an increased proportion (50–80%) of juvenile (unsegmented) neutrophils. The cyclical neutropenia results from cyclical changes in neutrophil granulocytopoiesis; a severe hypoplasia of the neutrophil series precedes the onset of neutropenia. The defect probably lies in a very early progenitor cell of the granulocyte-monocyte series or an abnormality of feedback regulation of granulocytopoiesis. Cyclical neutropenia has been transferred by bone marrow transplantation to a histocompatible sibling with acute lymphoblastic leukaemia.[60] In some cases the condition is inherited as a dominant trait with high penetrance and variable expression. Individual patients have benefited from therapy with testosterone, prednisone or lithium or from plasmaphaeresis.

Familial benign chronic neutropenia[61]

This disorder, which is inherited as an autosomal dominant trait, is characterized by chronic neutropenia, sometimes associated with monocytosis and hypergammaglobulinaemia and, occasionally, with moderate eosinophilia. Some cases have only a mild or moderate neutropenia and are asymptomatic. Others have a more severe neutropenia and suffer from periodontal disease and recurrent boils from infancy. However, even these cases run a relatively benign course. The bone marrow is normocellular and usually shows few neutrophil precursors beyond the myelocyte stage.

Neutropenia in healthy Blacks

Ethnic variations in the normal neutrophil count are mentioned on page 12.

Infantile genetic agranulocytosis[62]

This condition is inherited as an autosomal recessive trait. Affected patients suffer from very severe neutropenia (bordering on complete agranulocytosis) and recurrent infections (e.g. boils and carbuncles). They usually die from overwhelming sepsis during infancy but may occasionally survive (with antibiotic therapy) to the second decade. Some cases have an absolute monocytosis and eosinophilia and may develop hypergammaglobulinaemia. The bone marrow shows normal, increased or decreased cellularity of the neutrophil series, with an absence of cells beyond the promyelocyte/myelocyte stage. The neutrophils and their precursors show prominent vacuolation. Only rare neutrophil colonies are formed when marrow is cultured on soft agar and electron-microscopic studies of such colonies show gross abnormalities of maturation (asynchronous nucleo-cytoplasmic maturation, convoluted nuclei, paucity of granules). Cells in monocyte and eosinophil colonies mature normally.[63] The neutropenia appears to result from an intrinsic defect in an early progenitor cell which causes ineffectiveness of neutrophil granulocytopoiesis. Some cases convert to a leukaemia.

Congenital aleukia (reticular dysgenesis)[64]

In this rare disorder, no granulocytes, monocytes or lymphocytes are present in the blood and there are no lymphocytes in the thymus. There are also no peripheral lymphoid tissues. The bone marrow shows erythropoiesis and megakaryocytopoiesis but no lymphopoiesis, monocytopoiesis or granulocytopoiesis. Affected individuals die of infection shortly after birth.

Other rare neutropenic syndromes

Neutropenia has been described as a feature of a number of other rare syndromes usually affecting one or a very few cases. In Shwachman's syndrome,[65, 66] which is inherited as an autosomal recessive trait, neutropenia is associated with frequent infections, malabsorption due to congenital pancreatic hypoplasia, metaphyseal chondrodysplasia, thrombocytopenia and defective neutrophil motility.

In the syndrome of 'cartilage-hair hypoplasia',[67] the neutropenia is associated with dwarfism, abnormally fine and sparse hair, hyperextensible joints and lymphopenia.

In a few patients, neutropenia has been associated with hypogammaglobulinaemia[68] (sometimes with elevated IgM levels), as a familial or non-familial characteristic.

Neutropenia is also a feature of two disorders of neutrophil function, the 'lazy leucocyte syndrome'[69] (in which recurrent mouth and ear infections are associated with an impairment of the release of neutrophils from the marrow, normal neutrophil morphology, and an impaired response to chemotactic stimuli) and the Chédiak-Higashi syndrome (p. 205).

The term congenital dysgranulopoietic neutropenia has been used to describe a disorder affecting six unrelated children who had recurrent severe bacterial infections since birth, marked neutropenia, impaired neutrophil migration, normal numbers of CFU-C in the bone marrow, normal or slightly increased colony-stimulating activity in the serum, and prominent morphological and ultrastructural abnormalities in cells at and after the neutrophil promyelocyte/myelocyte stage.[70] The abnormalities of the cells included numerous autophagic vacuoles, abnormally electron-lucent primary granules, myelinization of primary granules, granule fusion, absence or marked decrease of secondary granules, and maturation of the cytoplasm ahead of the nucleus.[70]

EOSINOPENIA[71]

A transient eosinopenia develops after the administration of corticotrophin or corticosteroids, or in response to severe exercise, the administration of adrenaline, emotional stress, trauma and most acute viral and bacterial infections. In the case of corticosteroid therapy, the eosinopenia appears to result both from an impairment of the release of eosinophils from the marrow and the increased margination (or sequestration) of blood eosinophils. An eosinopenia may also be seen in Cushing's syndrome, acromegaly, SLE and aplastic anaemia.

BASOPENIA[72]

A basophil granulocytopenia (basopenia) may be found in acute hypersensitivity reactions, hyperthyroidism and pregnancy as well as in response to injections of corticosteroids or corticotrophin.

The blood basophil count falls on the day of ovulation.

MONOCYTOPENIA

A monocytopenia is seen in cases of aplastic anaemia, particularly when there is a marked neutropenia.[73] It is characteristic of 'hairy cell' leukaemia (see p. 260). Monocytopenia also occurs after the administration of corticosteroids.[74]

LYMPHOCYTOPENIA[75]

Temporary lymphocytopenia (lymphopenia) develops after the administration of corticosteroids. In addition, lymphocytopenia, probably due to elevated plasma cortisol levels, is seen following surgery or trauma and in many acute illnesses, including most infections and heart failure. Other causes of lymphocytopenia include uraemia, SLE, carcinoma, Hodgkin's disease, malaria, anorexia nervosa and some immune deficiency syndromes including the acquired immunodeficiency syndrome (AIDS) and immune deficiency secondary to radiotherapy or treatment with immunosuppressive drugs (e.g. after organ transplantation or cytotoxic chemotherapy).

LEUCOCYTOSIS

An increase in the concentration of circulating leucocytes above the normal range for the age of an individual is termed leucocytosis. This can be due to an increase in one or more of the five types of leucocytes normally present in blood or to the appearance of immature leucocytes in the circulation, or both. Increases in the neutrophils, eosinophils, basophils, monocytes or lymphocytes are described as neutrophil leucocytosis (neutrophilia), eosinophil leucocytosis (eosinophilia), basophil leucocytosis (basophilia), monocytosis and lymphocytosis, respectively.

NEUTROPHIL LEUCOCYTOSIS

Neutrophil leucocytosis may be generated by one or more of the following mechanisms: (1) a shift of cells from the marginated to the circulating blood neutrophil pools (see p. 10); (2) an increased rate of entry of neutrophils into the blood; (3) a prolonged $T_{\frac{1}{2}}$ of neutrophils in the circulation; and (4) a decreased rate of egress of neutrophils from the blood into the tissues.

Some of the causes of a neutrophil leucocytosis are listed in Table 6.3. The high neutrophil counts seen after exercise and electric shocks, in emotional states, and in patients with vomiting, convulsions or paroxysmal tachycardia, are caused by a shift of cells from the marginated to the circulating pool. The neutrophil leucocytosis seen in most other conditions results from an increased rate of release of neutrophils from the marrow into the blood. This occurs acutely as a result of the emptying of the marrow granulocyte pool into the blood and more chronically in association with an increased rate of production of marrow granulocytes. The first of these mechanisms is responsible for the initial acute neutrophilia in response to bacterial endotoxins, corticosteroids and etiocholanolone. The second operates when there is a sustained neutrophil leucocytosis as in conditions such as infections, inflammation and malignant disease. In some patients with carcinoma or sarcoma the increased neutrophil granulocytopoiesis appears to result from the production by the tumour cells of proteins which stimulate the growth of CFU-GM.[76, 77] The high neutrophil leucocyte counts in the chronic myeloproliferative disorders result partly from increased production of leucocytes in

Table 6.3 Causes of neutrophil leucocytosis

Physiological

Neonates (p. 11)

Exercise, emotion

Pregnancy

Parturition

Lactation

Pathological

Certain acute infections
Bacterial: various pyogenic cocci, *Escherichia coli*, *Pseudomonas aeruginosa*, *Corynebacterium diphtheriae*, *Francisella tularensis*
Spirochaetal: syphilis, Weil's disease
Rickettsial: typhus
Chlamydial: psittacosis
Viral: rabies, poliomyelitis, smallpox, herpes zoster, chickenpox
Mycotic: actinomycosis, coccidioidomycosis
Parasitic: liver fluke

Acute inflammation not caused by infections
Surgical operations, burns, infarcts, hepatic necrosis, crush injuries, rheumatoid arthritis, rheumatic fever, vasculitis, myositis, pancreatitis, hypersensitivity reactions, etc.

Metabolic
Uraemia, diabetic acidosis, gout, acute thyrotoxicosis

Acute haemorrhage

Acute haemolysis

Chronic myeloproliferative disorders
Chronic granulocytic leukaemia, polycythaemia rubra vera, myelofibrosis

Malignant disease
Carcinoma, lymphoma, etc.

Drugs
Adrenaline, corticosteroids, lithium

Miscellaneous
Convulsions, paroxysmal tachycardia, electric shock, vomiting, after splenectomy, post-neutropenic rebound neutrophilia

the marrow and partly from an abnormally long survival time ($T_{\frac{1}{2}}$) of these cells in the blood. The neutrophil leucocytosis seen in patients on long-term corticosteroid therapy is associated with a normal rate of release of neutrophils from the marrow into the blood and a decreased rate of egress from the blood into the tissues.

The commonest cause of neutrophil leucocytosis is an acute infection with a pyogenic organism. However, neutrophil leucocytosis also occurs in infections with certain non-pyogenic organisms (e.g. in poliomyelitis, herpes zoster, typhus). Tuberculosis does not usually cause a neutrophil leucocytosis but may do so when there

is rapid local spread of tubercle bacilli, as for example in tuberculous meningitis. In acute infections involving the organisms listed in Table 6.3, the neutrophil counts are usually in the range $10\text{--}30 \times 10^9/l$ (but may be $>80 \times 10^9/l$) and the eosinophil and basophil counts are reduced. Severe infections may be accompanied by a shift to the left and the development of toxic granulation and Döhle bodies within neutrophils. Young children may respond to acute infections with a lymphocytosis rather than a neutrophil leucocytosis.

EOSINOPHIL LEUCOCYTOSIS[71]

An eosinophilia may occur in many conditions, several of which are listed in Table 6.4. It is most commonly caused by allergic disorders in non-tropical areas and by parasitic infestations (Fig. 6.3) in tropical areas. In the case of parasitic infestations the highest eosinophil counts are found with metazoan parasites which invade tissues or the blood. A tropical syndrome characterized by eosinophilia, lymph node enlargement and pulmonary symptoms has been described under the name tropical eosinophilia: although microfilariae are absent from the blood, this syndrome is caused by occult filariasis, the microfilariae being destroyed in the tissues by an immune mechanism.

Very high eosinophil counts are also seen in the hypereosinophilic syndrome (see below).

The eosinophilia associated with malignant tumours may be caused by a tumour-derived glycoprotein which stimulates eosinophil granulocytopoiesis.[78] Tumours may also elaborate a factor chemotactic for eosinophils which resembles eosinophil chemotactic factor for anaphylaxis (ECF-A).[79]

Hypereosinophilic syndrome[80, 81]

The hypereosinophilic syndrome (HES) is an acquired condition, the cause of which is unknown. It is characterized by hypereosinophilia and tissue damage, particularly cardiac damage, which is attributable to secretory products of eosinophils. The majority of patients are males. The

Table 6.4 Causes of eosinophil leucocytosis

Parasitic infestations

   Metazoan infestations: strongyloidiasis, ascariasis,
   toxocariasis, ancylostomiasis (hookworm infestation),
   trichinosis, filariasis (Fig. 6.3), schistosomiasis,
   echinococcosis (hydatid cyst), cysticercosis

   Arthropod infestations: scabies

Allergic disorders
   Bronchial asthma, hay fever, allergic vasculitis, Stevens–
   Johnson syndrome, drug sensitivity

Graft-versus-host reaction

Skin diseases
   Pemphigus, pemphigoid, eczema, psoriasis, herpes
   gestationis, subcutaneous angioblastic hyperplasia with
   eosinophilia

Post-infection rebound eosinophilia

'Pulmonary' eosinophilia
   Löffler's syndrome (pulmonary infiltration with
   eosinophilia), tropical pulmonary eosinophilia

Hypereosinophilic syndrome (p. 217)

Leukaemias and chronic myeloproliferative disorders
   Chronic granulocytic leukaemia, polycythaemia rubra
   vera, acute lymphoblastic leukaemia, eosinophilic
   leukaemia

Thrombocytopenia with absent radii (p. 276)

Certain disorders of neutrophils
   Job's syndrome, infantile genetic agranulocytosis, familial
   benign chronic neutropenia

Malignant diseases
   Mycosis fungoides, Hodgkin's disease, other lymphomas,
   angioimmunoblastic lymphadenopathy, carcinoma (usually
   with metastasis), multiple myeloma, heavy chain disease

Immune deficiency syndromes
   Wiskott–Aldrich syndrome, etc.

Familial eosinophilia

Miscellaneous
   Polyarteritis nodosa, ulcerative colitis, Crohn's disease,
   eosinophilic gastroenteritis, Goodpasture's syndrome,
   pancreatitis, chronic active hepatitis, rheumatoid arthritis,
   scarlet fever, acute infectious lymphocytosis,
   coccidioidomycosis, pneumocystis pneumonia, after
   splenectomy, after irradiation of intra-abdominal tumours

Idiopathic

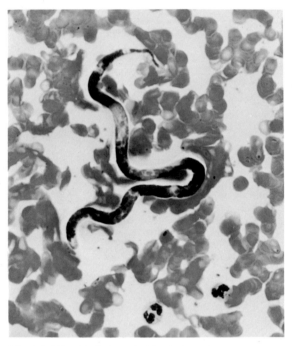

Fig. 6.3 Microfilaria from the blood of a patient with loiasis.
May–Grünwald–Giemsa stain   × 94

absolute eosinophil count ranges from 3–4 ×
10^9/l up to 100–300 × 10^9/l. Eosinophils are frequently vacuolated and extensively degranulated
(Fig. 6.4a, b). Both hypersegmented and non-
segmented forms are seen and some cells may
have doughnut-shaped nuclei (Fig. 6.4b). Eosinophil receptors for the Fc segment of IgG may
be increased. Neutrophils of patients with HES
may show aberrant staining, the granules being
larger and often more basophilic than those of
normal neutrophils (Fig. 6.4c). Anaemia and
thrombocytopenia may occur. The bone marrow
shows an increase of eosinophils and eosinophil
myelocytes; bone marrow cells show less degranulation and vacuolation than those in the peripheral blood.

   Cardiac damage consequent on hypereosinophilia (Löffler's endocarditis) is characteristic of
the idiopathic hypereosinophilic syndrome, but
not confined to it.[82] In the acute phase there is
necrosis of myocardium, particularly subendocardial myocardium, with an infiltrate which may
consist predominantly of eosinophils, or of
plasma cells and lymphocytes. Other cardiac
lesions include mural thrombosis with underlying eosinophil infiltration, pericarditis and arteritis. Valves may show fibrosis or formation of
vegetations. The mural thrombi may give rise to
single or multiple emboli. In the chronic phase
subendocardial fibrosis occurs, initially with a
surrounding zone of inflammation; chordae be-

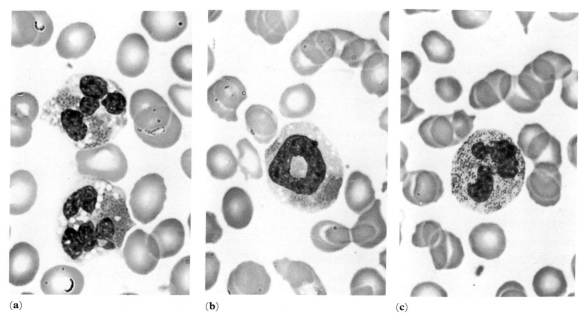

(a)   (b)   (c)

Fig. 6.4a,b,c Blood film from a patient with the hypereosinophilic syndrome. (**a**) Two abnormal eosinophil granulocytes which are vacuolated and partially degranulated and which show increased nuclear segmentation. (**b**) Partially degranulated eosinophil granulocyte with a ring-shaped nucleus. (**c**) Neutrophil granulocyte with abnormally large, basophilic granules (the granules are smaller than those of a basophil granulocyte).

May–Grünwald–Giemsa stain   × 940

come shortened, valves, particularly the mitral and tricuspid, become incompetent and a restrictive cardiomyopathy and arrhythmias develop. Endomyocardial biopsy may be used to confirm the diagnosis.

Other features of the hypereosinophilic syndrome may include fever, night sweats, weight loss, hepatomegaly, splenomegaly and lymphadenopathy (with eosinophil infiltration), vasculitis (including retinal and choroidal vasculitis), pulmonary fibrosis, and damage to the central and peripheral nervous system. Vasculitic lesions are often associated with thrombosis and increased plasma levels of β thromboglobulin and platelet factor 4, which suggest activation of platelets. Levels of fibrinogen and factor-VIII-related-antigen are increased, probably as a reaction to tissue damage. Choroidal and retinal vasculitis may be demonstrated by fluorescein angiography, which shows haemorrhage, microaneurysms, attenuation of vessels and areas of avascularity. Neurological lesions (mononeuritis multiplex, peripheral neuritis) are common; they may be a consequence of embolism, vasculitis,

thrombosis, haemorrhage, or damage from products secreted by eosinophils. Diarrhoea due to eosinophilic gastroenteritis may occur.

The relationship between the hypereosinophilic syndrome and eosinophilic leukaemia is problematic. Some patients in whom there is no apparent cause for a hypereosinophilic syndrome are subsequently found to have a cytogenetic abnormality and some undergo a blastic transformation. Some develop tumours composed of myeloblasts and eosinophils. Whether the majority of patients with HES have 'leukaemia' or a related myeloproliferative disorder of an eosinophil stem cell, or whether they have a reactive eosinophilia to an unknown stimulus is uncertain. Tissue damage similar to that seen in idiopathic hypereosinophilic syndrome also occurs when eosinophilia is secondary to a demonstrable cause such as Hodgkin's disease, non-Hodgkin's lymphoma or acute lymphoblastic leukaemia.[83] The relationship of Löffler's eosinophilic endocarditis and Davies's tropical endomyocardial fibrosis is also uncertain, despite the histological similarity of the latter to the end-stage of the former.

BASOPHIL LEUCOCYTOSIS[72]

A basophil leucocytosis may occur in hypersensitivity reactions, hypothyroidism, ulcerative colitis, smallpox, chickenpox, polycythaemia rubra vera and chronic granulocytic leukaemia (see p. 235). In the case of chronic granulocytic leukaemia, a considerable increase in both immature and mature basophils may precede transformation of the disease to a more malignant phase.

LYMPHOCYTOSIS AND MONOCYTOSIS

The various causes of lymphocytosis and monocytosis are listed in Tables 6.5 and 6.6. The two

Table 6.5 Causes of lymphocytosis

Physiological
  Infants and young children (p. 11)

Certain viral infections
  Acute infectious lymphocytosis, infectious mononucleosis, cytomegalovirus infection, infectious hepatitis, chickenpox, smallpox, measles, rubella, mumps, influenza

Certain bacterial infections
  Pertussis, brucellosis, tuberculosis, secondary and congenital syphilis

Bacterial infections in infants and young children

Chronic lymphocytic leukaemia

Lymphomas, Waldenström's macroglobulinaemia and heavy chain disease

Post-splenectomy

chronic infections, tuberculosis and brucellosis, may be associated with an increase in either or both cell types. The only acute bacterial infection which is frequently associated with a lymphocytosis is whooping cough (pertussis); in some children with this disorder the lymphocyte count may exceed $50 \times 10^9/l$. A lymphocytosis may be found in several viral infections. In infectious mononucleosis the high lymphocyte counts are accompanied by large, atypical lymphocytes. Changes very similar to those of infectious mononucleosis may be seen in cytomegalovirus infection, and similar but lesser changes may be seen in toxoplasmosis, malaria, infectious hepatitis

Table 6.6 Causes of monocytosis[84]

Physiological
  Infants (p. 11)

Certain bacterial infections
  Tuberculosis, brucellosis, syphilis, subacute bacterial endocarditis, typhoid, recovery from many acute infections

Certain protozoal infections
  Leishmaniasis (visceral and cutaneous), malaria, trypanosomiasis (Fig. 6.5)

Certain rickettsial infections
  Typhus, Rocky Mountain spotted fever

Myelodysplastic syndromes (p. 240)

Monocytic and myelomonocytic leukaemias (Table 6.9)

Chronic granulocytic leukaemia, polycythaemia rubra vera, myelofibrosis

Malignant diseases
  Hodgkin's disease, other lymphomas, carcinoma, multiple myeloma

Miscellaneous
  Recovery from neutropenia, ulcerative colitis, sarcoidosis, regional enteritis, collagen disease, post-splenectomy, cirrhosis

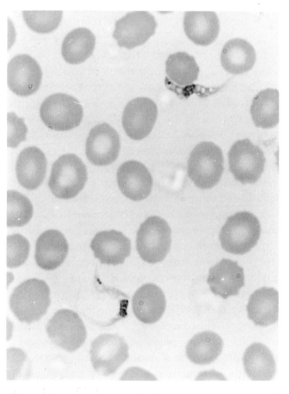

Fig. 6.5 Photomicrograph of two trypanosomes in the blood smear of a patient with African trypanosomiasis.
May–Grünwald–Giemsa stain   × 940

and other viral infections, as a sequel of immunization, and as part of a reaction to drugs.

Infectious mononucleosis

Infectious mononucleosis is a clinical syndrome due to an acute self-limiting primary infection by the Epstein–Barr virus (EBV). The most typical features of the syndrome are fever, pharyngitis, the presence of increased numbers of highly atypical lymphocytes ('mononuclear cells') in the peripheral blood, and the production of hetero-phile antibodies (antibodies developed following exposure to antigens from one species which recognize antigens in a different species). The EB virus proliferates in the nasopharynx and also in-fects the B-lymphocyte (which has specific recep-tors for EBV), establishing a long-term carrier state.

Clinical features

Primary infections in children are often asymp-tomatic or clinically mild. Typical acute infec-tious mononucleosis most commonly occurs when primary infections occur in adolescents and young adults, though small numbers of typical cases are seen in younger and older persons. Fever and malaise are usual. Acute tonsillitis and pharyngitis may be severe, sometimes with the formation of a pseudomembrane resembling that of diphtheria. Cervical lymph nodes are com-monly enlarged and lymphadenopathy may be generalized (hence the synonym 'glandular fever'). Splenomegaly is common, with sponta-neous splenic rupture a rare complication. Hepatic enlargement and jaundice occur in a minority. Other clinical features are multiple but less common. They include oedema of the eye-lids, rash and arthritis and the clinical manifes-tation of pericarditis, meningitis, encephalitis, mononeuritis and transverse myelitis.

Peripheral blood

The lymphocytes are increased in number and many are so atypical that, in Romanowsky-stained blood smears, they are barely recogniz-able as lymphocytes (hence 'atypical mono-

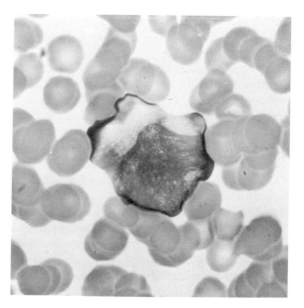

Fig. 6.6 Atypical lymphocyte in the blood film of a patient with infectious mononucleosis. In addition to the features mentioned in the text, this cell showed increased basophilia at the periphery of the cytoplasm, another commonly found atypical feature.

May–Grünwald–Giemsa stain   × 940

nucleosis') (Fig. 6.6). Atypical features include large size, irregular shape, increased cytoplasmic basophilia, diffuse chromatin pattern, prominent nucleoli and a scalloped margin at points of contact with other cells. The atypical lympho-cytes are not the virus-infected B-lymphocytes, but are T-lymphocytes. These T-lymphocytes may contain tartrate-resistant acid phosphatase (the same isoenzyme as is found in hairy cell leu-kaemia) and may show block-positivity when stained by the periodic acid-Schiff (PAS) method. Studies employing monoclonal anti-bodies have shown that the majority of atypical cells have the phenotype of cytotoxic/suppressor T-cells. The eosinophil count is reduced. Neutrophil alkaline phosphatase tends to be low. Haematological complications include auto-immune haemolytic anaemia due to a cold anti-body with anti-i specificity, thrombocytopenia due to peripheral destruction of platelets, and rarely granulocytopenia or aplastic anaemia, the latter occurring several weeks after infectious mononucleosis. Another rare complication is severe pancytopenia secondary to haemophagocytosis. Disseminated intravascular coagulation has been observed in association with the haemophagocytic syndrome.

Serological features. Infectious mononucleosis is accompanied by the development of multiple antibodies which may be categorized as: (1) virus-specific antibodies; (2) heterophile antibodies; and (3) autoimmune antibodies.

The most characteristic heterophile antibody (which is the basis of the Paul Bunnell test and other simpler screening tests for infectious mononucleosis) is an agglutinin of sheep or horse red blood cells which is adsorbed by ox red cells but not by guinea-pig kidney. Agglutinins of rhesus monkey, goat and camel erythrocytes and haemolysins of ox red cells may also occur. Antibodies may also develop against bacteria, and against viruses other than EBV.

Autoantibodies which may develop in infectious mononucleosis include anti-i and less often anti-I, anti-IgG (rheumatoid factor), antinuclear factor and the antibodies responsible for a positive Wassermann reaction.

A presumptive diagnosis of infectious mononucleosis may be made when typical clinical and haematological features are associated with the presence of a heterophile antibody. A definitive diagnosis requires serological evidence of a primary EBV infection.

Bone marrow

The marrow aspirate is infiltrated with atypical pleomorphic lymphocytes. There are focal accumulations of lymphocytes, and granulomas composed of lymphocytes, histiocytes and epithelioid cells. The granulomas tend to be smaller than those in tuberculosis and sarcoidosis and giant cells are infrequent.[85]

When infectious mononucleosis is associated with a haemophagocytic syndrome (p. 82), the bone marrow shows increased numbers of promonocytes and phagocytic histiocytes which are cytologically more mature than the cells of malignant histiocytosis. Bone marrow aplasia is a rare complication.[86]

Lymph nodes

The lymph nodes show marked hyperplasia with some obscuring of nodal architecture. Early in the infection there is predominantly expansion of the paracortical zone and other T-cell dependent areas. A 'pepper and salt' or 'moth-eaten' appearance of the interfollicular zone is produced by a mixture of small lymphocytes, immunoblasts, plasma cells, eosinophils, neutrophils, epithelioid histiocytes and mast cells. Some pyknotic cells and small necrotic foci occur. The subcapsular and trabecular sinuses contain histiocytes, large lymphocytes, plasma cells and PAS-positive proteinaceous fluid. The presence of pleomorphic lymphocytes in the subcapsular sinus is particularly characteristic of infectious mononucleosis. The capsule and the hilar and pericapsular connective tissue may show small lymphoid aggregates. Vascular proliferation and swelling of endothelial cells are prominent in the interfollicular area. Later in the infection the paracortex regresses and follicular hyperplasia becomes prominent. Cells resembling but not identical to mononuclear Hodgkin's cells and Reed-Sternberg cells may be seen and, occasionally, haemophagocytic histiocytes may be prominent in lymph nodes.

Liver and spleen

The liver is enlarged and pale. The sinusoids and portal tracts are infiltrated by pleomorphic lymphoid cells. Limiting plates are intact. There is random focal necrosis of hepatocytes, including single cell necrosis, with anucleate liver cells forming acidophilic bodies and being shed into sinusoids. The mitotic index of hepatocytes is increased. Kupffer cells are swollen and proliferate.

The red pulp of the spleen is heavily infiltrated by atypical lymphocytes which also infiltrate the splenic capsule and the subendothelial connective tissue of splenic blood vessels.

Other organs

Other less common pathological manifestations may be due either to lymphoid infiltration or immunologically-mediated phenomena. Infiltration by atypical lymphocytes may be seen in the heart, pericardium, lungs, adrenals, kidneys and other organs. Atypical lymphocytes are also present in serous exudates. Pathological lesions consequent on the immune response include those due to immune complexes and autoantibodies as well as less clearly-defined mechanisms. Lesions due to immune complexes include cutaneous vasculitis and proliferative glomerulonephritis; complement and immunoglobulins may be detected in the skin and kidneys, respectively, and there may be circulating immune complexes and cryoglobulins, and reduction of serum complement levels. Immune complexes could also be responsible for arthralgia and arthritis. Neurological lesions which may develop include mononeuritis, optic neuritis, Guillain–Barré syndrome, transverse myelitis and encephalitis. The pathogenesis of such lesions is uncertain. Histological features include perivascular lymphocyte infiltration, demyelination, oedema, necrosis, haemorrhage and production of foam cells.

Atypical manifestations of EBV infection

Patients with defective immunity may have an atypical outcome following primary EBV infection. Duncan's syndrome is an X-linked recessive condition in which there is a specific inability to deal with the EB virus. In this syndrome primary EBV infection may be fatal due to unrestrained infectious mononucleosis, or may be followed by acquired agammaglobulinaemia, aplastic anaemia, agranulocytosis or B-cell lymphoma (immunoblastic sarcoma or lymphoma resembling Burkitt's lymphoma).[87] Prolonged disease with primary EBV infection may reflect a lesser degree of immunological inadequacy.

Patients who are immunosuppressed following renal transplantation and who are carriers of EBV may develop lymphoma-like polyclonal proliferations of B-lymphocytes carrying the viral genome; in some cases evolution to a monoclonal lymphoma may occur.[88] An immunosuppressed recipient of a bone marrow transplant also developed a monoclonal immunoblastic sarcoma of donor cell origin which carried EBV DNA,[89] and a patient with ataxia-telangiectasia developed an apparent lymphoma (clonality not studied) with EBV DNA in tumour tissue.[90] The tumour cells of a central nervous system lymphoma in a patient who appeared to be immunologically normal were found to contain the EB viral genome.[91] It is important that apparent lymphomas in transplant recipients, sufferers from the acquired immunodeficiency syndrome and other patients should be studied for monoclonality and for presence of EBV DNA.

LEUKAEMIA[92]

The leukaemias are a group of disorders characterized by a malignant proliferation of leucocyte precursors in which the proliferating cells and their progeny have the potential to circulate in the peripheral blood and infiltrate tissues. The leukaemias result from clonal proliferations, i.e. the leukaemic cell population is derived from a single cell. The leukaemias may be broadly divided into myeloid and lymphoid and further into acute and chronic forms. A myeloid leukaemia is one in which the cell which gives rise to the malignant clone is a precursor of granulocytes and/or monocytes or a multipotent precursor of granulocytes, monocytes, erythrocytes and megakaryocytes. A lymphoid leukaemia is one in which the cell which gives rise to the malignant clone is a precursor of B- or T-lymphocytes. The term lymphocytic is best restricted to those leukaemias within the lymphoid category in which the leukaemic cell resembles a mature lymphocyte. Classification of a leukaemia as acute or chronic depends on the natural history of the disease; patients with untreated acute leukaemias usually die within weeks or months whereas patients with untreated chronic leukaemias usually survive for longer periods. Uncommonly, leukaemia may be mixed myeloid and lymphoid, suggesting an origin from a common pluripotent precursor cell (see p. 226).

As it is often impossible to establish the tissue of origin of a clone of malignant cells after widespread dissemination, the generally accepted difference between leukaemia and lymphoma is that in the former the predominant pathological manifestations are usually in the bone marrow and peripheral blood, whereas in the latter the pre-dominant manifestations are in extramedullary tissues. Malignant change in cells of the same phenotype may in one patient cause a leukaemia and in another a lymphoma (e.g. both chronic lymphocytic leukaemia and diffuse well-differentiated lymphocytic lymphoma arise from malignant proliferation of mature B-lymphocytes). In the majority of lymphomas the malignant cell is a lymphocyte or lymphocyte precursor, but in a minority the malignant clone is derived from another constituent of lymphoid tissue; for example, a true histiocytic 'lymphoma' is derived from a histiocyte (macrophage). The distinction between leukaemia and lymphoma is not always clear-cut as patients presenting with lymphoma may subsequently progress to a leukaemic phase (e.g. the leukaemic phase of follicular lymphoma or 'lymphosarcoma cell leukaemia'). Others presenting with typical leukaemia may subsequently have marked proliferation of leukaemic cells in extramedullary tissues and their disease may thus simulate a lymphoma (e.g. Richter's syndrome in chronic lymphocytic leukaemia).

A categorization of leukaemias and lymphomas according to the cell of origin is shown in Table 6.7.

Monoclonal antibodies prepared by the hybridization technique[93] are of considerable use in classifying leukaemias, particularly lymphoid leukaemias. Some of the commonly used antibodies are shown in Table 6.8.

ACUTE MYELOID LEUKAEMIA (AML)

Definition

The acute myeloid leukaemias are a group of related diseases resulting from the malignant pro-

Table 6.7 Classification of acute and chronic leukaemias and related disorders

Myeloid leukaemia (and related disorders)	Lymphoid leukaemias/lymphomas (and related disorders)	
	B-cell & precursors of B cells	T-cell & precursors of T cells
Acute myeloid leukaemias 　Acute myeloblastic leukaemia (M1, M2) 　Acute promyelocytic leukaemia (M3) 　Acute myelomonocytic leukaemia (M4) 　Acute monocytic leukaemia (M5) 　Acute erythroleukaemia (M6) 　Acute megakaryocytic leukaemia 　Acute myelofibrosis	Acute lymphoblastic leukaemia 　c-ALL 　pre B-ALL 　B-ALL	Acute lymphoblastic leukaemia—T-ALL T-lymphoblastic lymphoma Chronic lymphocytic leukaemia (minority)
Chronic granulocytic (myeloid) leukaemia (CGL)	Lymphoid blast crisis of CGL	Prolymphocytic leukaemia (minority)
Juvenile myeloid leukaemia	Chronic lymphocytic leukaemia (majority)	Hairy cell leukaemia (the small minority)
Myeloid blast crisis of CGL	Prolymphocytic leukaemia (majority)	
Chronic myelomonocytic leukaemia		T-cell lymphomas 　T-zone lymphoma 　Some diffuse lymphomas
Chronic monocytic leukaemia	Hairy cell leukaemia (the large majority)	Immunoblastic sarcoma
Erythraemic myelosis (di Guglielmo's syndrome)	B-cell lymphomas 　Follicular lymphoma	Adult T-cell leukaemia-lymphoma
Neutrophilic leukaemia	Some diffuse lymphomas 　Burkitt's lymphoma	Mycosis fungoides and Sézary syndrome
Eosinophilic leukaemia	Immunoblastic sarcoma 　Plasmacytoid lymphoma★	
Systemic mastocytosis	Waldenstrom's macroglobulinaemia★	
Malignant histiocytosis	Multiple myeloma★	
	Solitary plasmacytoma★	
	Heavy chain diseases★	
Biphenotypic (lymphoid/myeloid) leukaemia		

★ See chapter 8

Table 6.8 Monoclonal antibodies used in the classification of leukaemias and lymphomas[94, 95, 96, 97]

	Antibody	Specificity
T-cell markers	OKT6 (NA1/34; Leu 6)	Common (stage II) thymocyte; Langerhans cell[98]
	OKT11 (T11; OKT17; Leu 5; Lyt 3; 9.6)	E-rosette receptor
	OKT3 (Leu 4; UCHT1)	Pan-T plus mature (stage III) thymocyte
	OKT4 (T4; Leu 3a; Leu 3b; 9.3; 3A1)	'Helper' subset and common (stage II) thymocyte
	OKT8 (OKT5; Leu 2a; Leu 2b; T8a; UCHT4)	'Suppressor' subset and common thymocyte
	T101 (Leu 1; Lyt 2; 10.2)	Pan-T; pan-thymocyte; B-CLL; B-PLL; centrocytic lymphoma[99]
	OKT1 (A50)	Pan-T; B-CLL; B-PLL; B-cell lymphomas[100]
	OKT10	Pan-thymocyte; cALL; plasma cells; multiple myeloma cells; AML
	OKT9 (T16, 5E9)	Transferrin receptor on immature (stage I) thymocytes and other rapidly dividing cells
B-cell markers	J5 (24.1; BA-3; CALL 1)	cALL; cALL + ve haemopoietic precursors; centrocytic-centroblastic lymphoma;[99] certain non-haemopoietic cells
	DA2 (HLA-DR; OKIal; Q5/13; FMC4; I2)	Ia-like antigen (non-polymorphic HLA-DR antigen); B-cells and precursors; Langerhans cells; interdigitating cells of lymph nodes
	BA-1	B-cells and precursors; granulocytes
	BA-2	Precursors of B-cells
	B-1	Some B-cells and precursors (appears later in B-cell development than BA-1)
	B-2	Mature B-cells
	P1 153/3	B-cells and precursors; neural tissue
Natural killer cells	HNK-1 (Leu 7); Leu 11	Natural killer (NK) cells and killer (K) cells; Leu 11 identifies a smaller but more potent subset than Leu 7
Pan-leucocyte[101]	T-200; 2D1; L3B12; T29/33; F10-89-4; PD7/26; 2B/11	All leucocytes (common leucocyte antigen)
Granulocytic	MY1 (MY5, MY6, MY18, MY24); FMC10-13; D5	Granulocytes
	M1/N1	Granulocytes; neural tissue
	3C4	Granulocytes; duct epithelium
Granulocytic/ Monocytic	Leu-M1 (MMA); Mac 1; MY7; MY8; VIM-D5	Granulocytes and monocytes
	OKM1 (Mol)	Granulocytes and monocytes; some NK cells
Monocytic	Mo2; D5 D6; 63D3; 61D3; MY4	Monocytes
	TA1	Monocytes; T-cells and thymocytes; centroblastic-centrocytic lymphoma[99]
	OKM	Monocytes; dendritic reticulum cells[102]
Erythroid	R18 (L1CR, LON, R10)	Antiglycophorin A
	R6A	Antimembrane-band-3
Platelet[103]/ Megakaryocyte	An 51	Antiplatelet glycoprotein I
	C2, C8	Antiplatelet glycoprotein IIa
	C15, C17	Antiplatelet glycoprotein IIIa

The OK series of monoclonal antibodies are produced by Ortho Pharmaceutical Corporation, Raritan, New Jersey, the Leu series, HLA-DR and T-200 by Becton-Dickinson & Co., Mountain View, California, and J5, 12 and some others by Coulter Electronics, Hialeah, Florida, USA.

liferation of precursors of granulocytes, monocytes, erythrocytes or megakaryocytes and
characterized by the presence of increased
numbers of blast cells in the marrow. If untreated, the leukaemia causes death within weeks
or months. More than one cell line may be
overtly involved in the leukaemic process, e.g.
granulocytic and erythroid, or granulocytic and
megakaryocytic. Cytogenetic evidence and the
study of isoenzymes of G6PD indicate that some
or all of the erythroid cells belong to the leukaemic clone, even when they are morphologically
normal.

Incidence

The incidence of acute myeloid leukaemia rises
steeply with age. In young adults the overall incidence of all types of acute leukaemia is of the
order of two cases per 100 000 population per
year whereas in the elderly (over 65 years) (in
whom acute leukaemias are commonly myeloid
in type) it is of the order of 10–20 cases per
100 000 per year.[104] The incidence is higher in
males than females.

Classification

The minimum requirements for the diagnosis of
acute myeloid leukaemia are that blasts exceed
30% of the nucleated bone marrow cells, and
blasts plus promyelocytes exceed 50%.[105] The
acute myeloid leukaemias have been classified by
a French-American-British (FAB) cooperative
group into six categories, M1 to M6, based on
the degree and direction of differentiation of the
leukaemic cells (Table 6.9).[106, 107] Acute megakaryoblastic leukaemia is not as yet included in
the FAB classification.

Aetiology

In many cases of AML no aetiological factors
are yet identifiable. In some cases, the condition
follows damage to stem cells by irradiation,
cytotoxic drugs, benzene or other chemicals.
Irradiation and cytotoxic drugs appear to be
synergistic in their leukaemogenic effect. AML
may develop in patients with pre-existing bone
marrow disease who have not been exposed to irradiation or cytotoxic drugs. This happens in poly-

Table 6.9 FAB classification of acute myeloid leukaemias[106, 107]

Category		Haematological features
M1	Myeloblastic leukaemia without maturation	Blasts have some azurophilic granules, Auer rods or both, or >3% of blasts in the marrow are myeloperoxidase-positive. Further maturation of blasts not seen
M2	Myeloblastic leukaemia with maturation	Maturation to or beyond the promyelocyte stage and >50% of bone marrow cells are myeloblasts plus promyelocytes (Fig. 6.7)
M3	Hypergranular promyelocytic leukaemia	The majority of bone marrow cells are hypergranular promyelocytes which may have bundles (faggots) of Auer rods (Fig. 6.8)
M3 Variant	Variant promyelocytic leukaemia[107]	Cells with bilobed, multilobed or reniform nuclei with small numbers of typical hypergranular promyelocytes
M4	Myelomonocytic leukaemia	Granulocytic and monocytic differentiation with promonocytes plus monocytes >20% in peripheral blood and/or bone marrow (Fig. 6.9)
M5	Monocytic (monoblastic) leukaemia (a) poorly differentiated (b) differentiated	Granulocytopoietic cells in bone marrow <20% of nucleated cells (a) monoblasts predominate in bone marrow (Fig. 6.10) (b) monoblasts, promonocytes and monocytes are present; promonocytes predominate in bone marrow
M6	Erythroleukaemia	Bone marrow erythropoietic component >50% of nucleated cells or >30% of nucleated cells plus >10% of erythropoietic cells morphologically very abnormal (multiple nuclei, lobulated nuclei, megaloblastic changes, giant erythroblasts) (Fig. 6.11)

cythaemia rubra vera, idiopathic myelofibrosis, paroxysmal nocturnal haemoglobinuria and congenital, drug-induced and idiopathic aplastic anaemia. The incidence of AML is also increased in patients with certain congenital chromosome abnormalities (eg. Down's syndrome, Bloom's syndrome). Activation of oncogenes may be important in the development of AML. The translocation t(8;21) (see below) may be associated with the activation of the cellular oncogene c-mos.[108]

Cytogenetics

Non-random chromosomal abnormalities are common in AML and studies employing new techniques suggest that they may actually be present in all cases.[109] Some cytogenetic abnormalities are uniquely associated with specific subclasses of AML. Thus a translocation between chromosomes 15 and 17, t(15q+; 17q−) is associated with M3; t(8q−; 21q+) is associated with M2 and an inversion in chromosome 16, inv (16) (p13 q22), is associated with M4 with abnormal eosinophils.[110] Rearrangements of chromosome 11 with a breakpoint at q23 are common in M4 and M5 but not restricted to them.[111] The association of specific chromosome defects with particular morphological types of acute leukaemia suggests that the development of a specific karyotypic abnormality may be a factor in the aetiology of the leukaemia. The frequency of different chromosomal abnormalities is related also to the age of the patient and whether the leukaemia has arisen *de novo* or is secondary to chemotherapy. Thus trisomy 8 is equally common in children and adults but trisomy 19 is much commoner in children.[111] Monosomy of 5, monosomy of 7 and deletion of part of 5 (i.e. 5q−) are characteristic of dysmyelopoietic syndromes and secondary leukaemias, and are much less common in children.[111] The variation of chromosome pattern with age suggests the operation of different aetiological factors in different age groups. An association between specific chromosomal abnormalities and aetiological factors is also indicated by the finding that −5, 5q−, −7, 7q− are commoner in patients with AML who have been occupationally ex-

posed to chemicals, including solvents, insecticides and petroleum products, than in those who have not been so exposed.[112]

Pathogenesis

AML results from a progressive expansion of a single clone of myeloid cells with absent or imperfect differentiation. The proportion of blast cells in the DNA synthesis phase of the cell cycle is usually normal or reduced, and the generation time of the blast cells is normal or prolonged. Despite this, the size of the leukaemic cell renewal system increases steadily. The clinical and laboratory manifestations of the acute myeloid leukaemias result from: (1) replacement of normal bone marrow by leukaemic cells with consequent pancytopenia and haemorrhagic and infective manifestations; and (2) expansion of the mass of leukaemic cells, which in turn may cause: (a) tissue infiltration; (b) metabolic complications including hyperuricaemia and less often hypercalcaemia and hypophosphataemia; (c) tissue damage induced by lysozyme released from leukaemic cells; (d) leucostatic lesions (i.e. obstruction of small vessels and hyperviscosity) when the white cell count is very high; and (e) disseminated intravascular coagulation (DIC) due to release of thromboplastins from leukaemic cells (DIC is particularly common with acute promyelocytic leukaemia [M3] but may occur with any of the acute myeloid leukaemias).

Pathology

Peripheral blood

Anaemia, neutropenia and thrombocytopenia are common. In many patients primitive leukaemic cells (which are morphologically similar to those found in the marrow) are present in the peripheral blood. Depending on the subclassification of the leukaemia these may be myeloblasts, monoblasts or promyelocytes. Leukaemic myeloblasts may contain small numbers of azurophilic granules and/or azurophilic cytoplasmic rods (Auer rods) (Fig. 6.7) which are thought to result from fusion of primary granules (possibly within autophagic vacuoles). Myeloblasts have small

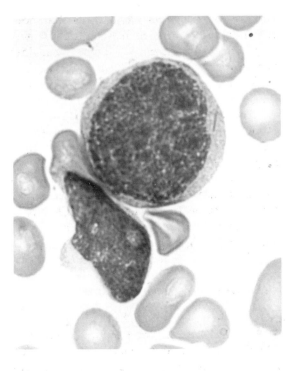

Fig. 6.7 Bone marrow smear from a patient with acute myeloblastic leukaemia, category M2. Two myeloblasts are shown, one of which contains an Auer rod.

May–Grünwald–Giemsa stain ×1880

nucleoli and a fine chromatin pattern (Figs 6.7, 6.9 and 6.11). The promyelocytes of the M3 category often have a bilobed or reniform nucleus and cytoplasm which is crowded with large granules (staining pink, red or purple with Romanowsky stains) (Fig. 6.8) and bundles, or 'faggots', of Auer rods. Leukaemic monoblasts have voluminous cytoplasm and a nucleus which is sometimes folded or lobulated and contains one or more large vesicular nucleoli (Fig. 6.10). Myelocytes and metamyelocytes are uncommon; when there are only blasts and neutrophils in the peripheral

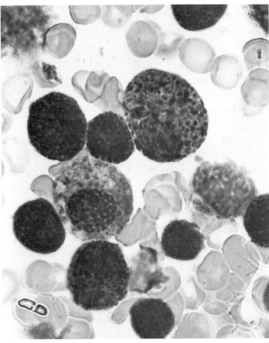

(a)

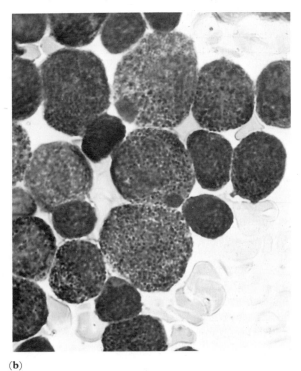

(b)

Fig. 6.8a,b Photomicrographs of a bone marrow smear from a patient with acute promyelocytic leukaemia (AML, category M3). Hypergranular promyelocytes are seen, including two cells (in **b**) each of which has a block-shaped giant granule. In some cells, the granules are so numerous that the nucleus is obscured.

May–Grünwald–Giemsa stain ×940

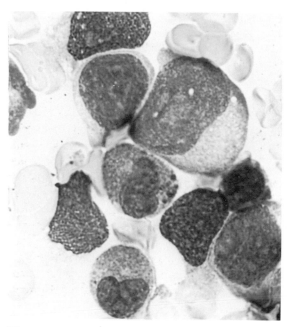

Fig. 6.9 Bone marrow smear from a patient with acute myelomonocytic leukaemia (AML, category M4). The two cells at the top are a monoblast (large in size with voluminous cytoplasm and a nucleus containing a large nucleolus) and a myeloblast (smaller with less cytoplasm and small nucleolus). Two neutrophil myelocytes are also seen.

May–Grünwald–Giemsa stain   × 940

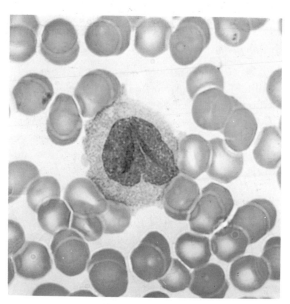

Fig. 6.10 A monoblast from the peripheral blood film of a patient with acute monoblastic leukaemia (AML, category M5). This cell is large and has a lobulated but immature-looking nucleus and voluminous cytoplasm.

May–Grünwald–Giemsa stain   × 940

blood, the term 'hiatus leukaemicus' has been used to emphasize the absence of cells of intermediate maturity. Morphological abnormalities of neutrophils (hypogranularity and the acquired Pelger–Huët anomaly) may be present (see Fig. 6.18b), providing evidence that the neutrophils are derived from the leukaemic clone. Nucleated red blood cells may be present in the peripheral blood, particularly in M6 but also in the other categories. A minority of patients have no primitive cells in the peripheral blood; such cases have been described as suffering from 'aleukaemic' or 'subleukaemic leukaemia' but are essentially no different from other patients with circulating primitive cells.

Bone marrow

In the majority of cases the bone marrow is markedly hypercellular due to the presence of leukaemic cells; there is a concomitant decrease of normal cells though an increase of macrophages, plasma cells, lymphocytes or mast cells may be seen. There may be an increased proportion of small mononucleate and binucleate micro-megakaryocytes (see p. 274). Dyserythropoiesis (see p. 77) is characteristic of M6 (Fig. 6.11) but may also be seen in other categories. In the M4 category, monocytic differentiation may be much less apparent in the bone marrow than in the peripheral blood. In a minority of cases, particularly in the elderly, the bone marrow is normocellular or hypocellular despite the presence of leukaemic cells. Trephine biopsies of some early cases have been reported to show islets of blast cells scattered within marrow tissue more or less depleted of haemopoietic cells.[113] Such clusters of myeloblasts and monoblasts are primarily peritrabecular and around arterioles and arterial capillaries. Erythroblasts and megakaryoblasts tend to be associated with sinusoids. With disease progression there are sheets of blast cells (Fig. 6.12) with residual foci of haemopoietic cells.[113] Patchy bone marrow necrosis may be seen; necrosis may affect bone as well as haemopoietic tissue (see also p. 94). Trephine biopsy commonly shows an increased quantity of reticulin. In a minority there is also an increased

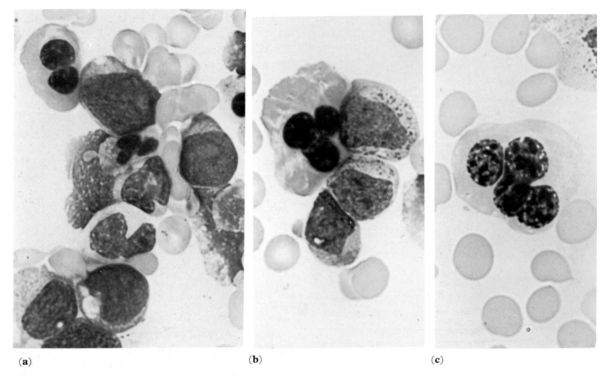

(a) (b) (c)

Fig. 6.11a,b,c Marrow cells from a patient with erythroleukaemia (AML, category M6). Three multinucleate erythroblasts, three agranular myeloblasts and two granule-containing blast cells are shown.

May–Grünwald–Giemsa stain × 940

quantity of collagen; this is a reactive change which is reversed if remission occurs. Both reticulin and collagen deposition are more common in acute megakaryoblastic leukaemia than in M1 to M6 and when this is pronounced the clinical presentation may be that of acute myelofibrosis (see p. 235).

Liver

Leukaemic cells infiltrate the portal tracts and the interlobular septa and form linear infiltrates through the lobules. Hepatic enlargement (apparently due to an increase in size of parenchymal cells) may be seen in the absence of a significant degree of infiltration.[114]

Spleen

Leukaemic cells characteristically infiltrate the red pulp, compressing the white pulp.

Lymph nodes

Leukaemic cells initially infiltrate the hilum, interfollicular zone, marginal sinus, capsule and perinodal fat. Later the entire node is infiltrated with complete loss of normal architecture. Nodes usually remain discrete. Lymph node enlargement is more common in acute monocytic leukaemia than in acute myeloblastic leukaemia.

Cutaneous lesions

Skin infiltration is characteristically around the skin appendages. Nodules and plaques of a blue or violaceous hue may be formed. Skin involvement is more characteristic of acute leukaemias with rather than without a monocytic element. Non-infiltrative skin lesions may also be seen, e.g. pyoderma gangrenosum, acute febrile neutrophilic dermatosis (Sweet's syndrome), erythema nodosum and erythema multiforme. Pyo-

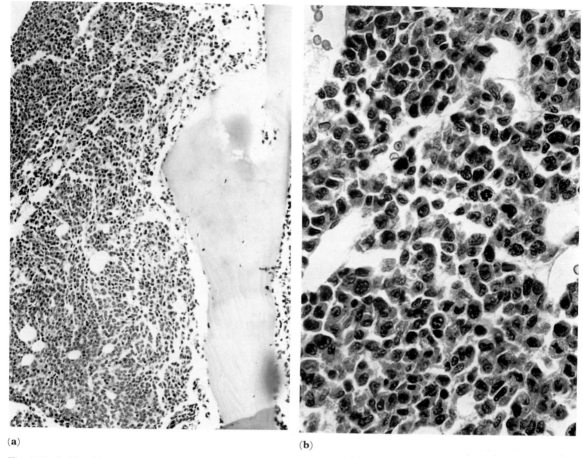

(a)   (b)

Fig. 6.12a,b Trephine biopsy of bone marrow from a patient with acute myeloid leukaemia. (a) There is marked hypercellularity of the marrow with replacement of fat cells and normal haemopoietic cells by a uniform population of large cells. (b) Higher power view demonstrating the presence of nucleoli in some of the large cells. Several mitotic figures are seen.

Haematoxylin–eosin   (a) × 94; (b) × 375

derma gangrenosum in association with leukaemia may be atypical, being bullous and more superficial than the classic disease.[115] Both pyoderma gangrenosum and Sweet's syndrome may occur in the preleukaemic phase of acute myeloid leukaemia.[116]

Gum hypertrophy

Gum hypertrophy due to infiltration of leukaemic cells is characteristic of acute leukaemias with a monocytic element (Fig. 6.13). It does not usually occur in edentulous patients, suggesting that the leukaemic monocytes may be responding to chemotactic stimuli.

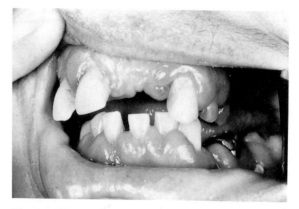

Fig. 6.13 Swelling of gums due to infiltration by leukaemic cells in a case of acute monoblastic leukaemia.

Lung

Leukaemic infiltration of the lung is most often seen in acute leukaemias with a monocytic element—M4 and M5.[117] Infiltration is peribronchial, peribronchiolar and in alveolar septa.

Kidneys

Kidneys may show interstitial medullary and cortical infiltration. There may also be irregular confluent infiltrates in the cortex and outer pyramids. Increase of renal size is common in the absence of significant infiltration.[114] In M4 and M5 leukaemia, lysozymuria may be associated with proximal tubular damage, which is characterized by cytoplasmic degeneration and the formation of granular casts.

The eye

Infiltrative and non-infiltrative lesions of the eye may be detected clinically or pathologically. Infiltration is most commonly of the choroid, the sclera and episclera. Infiltration of the ciliary body and iris is less common. Infiltration of the iris is readily detectable clinically; it results in alteration of iris colour, leukaemic nodule formation, poorly-reacting pupils, synechiae, keratic precipitates, hypopyon and hyphaema. Infiltration of the trabeculae and canal of Schlemm may cause secondary glaucoma. Retinal changes include tortuous veins, pale blood vessels, 'sheathing' of vessels by white streaks, and haemorrhages and exudates. Leukaemic infiltrates in the retina are found particularly in the posterior part of the eyes and are usually associated with haemorrhage. A haemorrhage with a central white spot is characteristic of leukaemia but not pathognomonic. White areas within haemorrhages may be either leukaemic infiltrates or the result of vascular impairment, with ischaemia causing swelling and degeneration of nerve fibres; in fact, this appearance was first described by Roth in 1872 in septic retinitis rather than in leukaemia. Haemorrhages may be flame-shaped or circular. Subretinal haemorrhage may cause retinal detachment and preretinal haemorrhage may involve the vitreous. The soft exudates seen

in the retina in leukaemia are non-infiltrative, being ischaemic infarcts at the terminal bifurcation of precapillary arterioles.[118] Retinal haemorrhages are more common in, but not confined to, leukaemic patients with severe anaemia or thrombocytopenia. Infiltration of the optic nerve head may produce the same ophthalmoscopic appearance as papilloedema; the retrobulbar part of the optic nerve may also be infiltrated.

Infiltration of other tissues

Other tissues which may be infiltrated include the pericardium and myocardium, brain (perivascular cuffing and extension into surrounding brain) and meninges. Infiltration of the tonsils (Fig. 6.14) is particularly characteristic of acute leukaemia with monocytic differentiation.

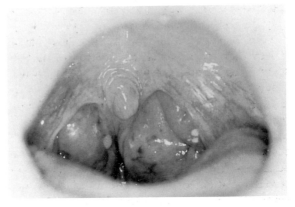

Fig. 6.14 Infiltration of the tonsils in a patient with acute myeloid leukaemia.
Courtesy of Dr Helen Dodsworth

Leucostatic lesions

This term is used to describe functional or pathological abnormalities caused by hyperviscosity of blood due to a very high WBC or by obstruction of small blood vessels by leukaemic cells. Leucostatic lesions usually cause impairment of brain and pulmonary function. Priapism may occur in acute myeloid leukaemia and is likely to be consequent on obstruction of vascular channels by leukaemic cells.

Granulocytic sarcoma

Leukaemic cells not only infiltrate diffusely in many tissues but may also proliferate in one site causing tumour formation. Such tumours are designated chloromas (indicating the green coloration which is not infrequently seen because of the presence of peroxidase in the leukaemic cells), myeloblastomas or granulocytic sarcomas. (A diffuse green colour is also occasionally seen in the bone marrow and other tissues which are diffusely infiltrated by leukaemic cells.) Common sites of occurrence of granulocytic sarcomas are the skin, subcutaneous tissue, breasts, ovaries, lymph nodes, dura, orbits (causing proptosis and paresis of ocular muscles), skull (subperiosteally), sternum, ribs and proximal long bones. Almost any site may be involved.

Granulocytic sarcomas may be single or multiple. They may develop during the course of the disease, or be the presenting feature; they may precede other evidence of leukaemia by months or even years.[119] A green coloration of the cut surface may suggest the nature of this tumour; the colour fades on exposure to light but may be restored by application of weak hydrochloric acid. Histologically, an admixture of eosinophils with the primitive cells may suggest the diagnosis. The diagnosis may be confirmed by the demonstration of peroxidase or chloroacetate esterase activity in myeloblasts. Granulocytic sarcomas are commonly misdiagnosed as lymphoma, carcinoma or eosinophilic granuloma.

Monocytic sarcoma

Extramedullary tumour formation may also occur in myelomonocytic and monocytic leukaemia (M4 and M5). In pure monocytic tumours a green coloration is unlikely to be present since cells of the monocyte series have a low peroxidase activity. Eosinophils are not present and the tumour cells lack chloroacetate esterase activity. If the diagnosis is suspected it may be confirmed by the demonstration of α_1-antitrypsin or of lysozyme activity in the tumour cells. Extramedullary tumour formation appears to be commoner in acute monocytic leukaemia than in acute myeloblastic leukaemia. Misdiagnosis as anaplastic carcinoma or large cell lymphoma is common.

Haemorrhagic and thrombotic manifestations

Haemorrhagic manifestations are common (Fig. 6.15) being usually secondary to an impairment of platelet production and function. Haemorrhage is more common in M3 than in the other

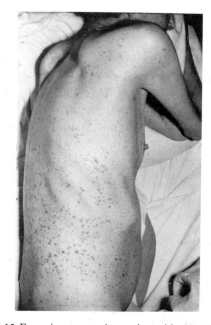

Fig. 6.15 Extensive purpura in a patient with severe thrombocytopenia due to acute myeloid leukaemia.

acute myeloid leukaemias; this is attributable to the consumption of platelets and coagulation factors which commonly occurs in M3 (due to DIC). Thrombotic lesions may be seen in acute promyelocytic leukaemia (M3)[120] but they are often inconspicuous since there is activation of fibrinolysis as well as of coagulation.

Treatment

Acute myeloid leukaemia requires aggressive treatment with combination chemotherapy. Reversible bone marrow aplasia occurs after such treatment. Complete remission rates are now well in excess of 50% and median survival is greater than 1 year. Results are continuing to improve and it is now reasonable to contemplate treating AML with curative intent. Immunotherapy and prophylactic treatment of the CNS (to prevent a recurrence localized to the CNS) do not substantially improve the outlook. Allogeneic bone marrow transplantation during the first remission or for refractory AML is an experimental form of treatment.

Erythroleukaemia, erythraemic myelosis, di Guglielmo's syndrome

Definition. These names all indicate a proliferation of malignant erythroid precursors associated with a variable degree of proliferation of malignant granulocytic precursors (Fig. 6.11). These terms have not been used consistently but, in general, erythroleukaemia may be taken as synonymous with the M6 category of acute myeloid leukaemia. Erythraemic myelosis and di Guglielmo's syndrome are usually regarded as synonymous and indicate a more chronic condition in which the myeloblastic element is less prominent. Erythraemic myelosis may become more acute and evolve into erythroleukaemia (M6) or myeloblastic or myelomonocytic leukaemia (M2 or M4).

Aetiology

Erythroleukaemia and erythraemic myelosis may arise *de novo* or may follow paroxysmal nocturnal haemoglobinuria, polycythaemia rubra vera or (rarely) chronic granulocytic leukaemia or the use of cytotoxic chemotherapy.

Pathogenesis

These are clonal disorders with the abnormal erythroid cells and myeloblasts being derived from a single malignant clone. A high proportion of the red cell precursors show dyserythropoietic changes (p. 77) and erythropoiesis is frequently megaloblastic. Synthesis of globin chains or of haem may be defective. Glycogen may accumulate within erythroblasts causing a positive reaction with the periodic acid-Schiff stain. Anaemia results from a combination of increased ineffective erythropoiesis and a shortening of the red cell life-span. Megakaryocytes may be bizarre and there may be ineffective thrombocytopoiesis.

Pathology

Infiltration by malignant cells of the erythroid and granulocytic series may cause splenomegaly and, less often, hepatomegaly and may involve the skin.

Acute megakaryoblastic leukaemia

This is a variant of acute myeloid leukaemia. The malignant cells in the bone marrow and blood vary in their state of maturity from megakaryoblasts, which are morphologically undifferentiated, to micromegakaryocytes which may bud platelets (see Fig. 6.17 on p. 239). The platelet count may be high in patients with more differentiated cells. Megakaryoblasts are round, have a high nucleocytoplasmic ratio and are agranular. They may show cytoplasmic protrusions or 'blebs'. 'Bare nuclei' of megakaryocytes may circulate in the peripheral blood. Micromegakaryocytes and megakaryoblasts with some degree of cytoplasmic maturation stain positively by the periodic acid-Schiff reaction, and give positive reactions for non-specific esterase (fluoride-sensitive) and acid phosphatase. They are negative for terminal deoxynucleotidyl transferase (TdT) activity. Cells which appear as undifferentiated blasts in smears stained by a Romanowsky method may be identified as megakaryoblasts by the demonstration of: (1) characteristic platelet granules or platelet demarcation membranes by electron microscopy; (2) platelet peroxidase (in the nuclear envelope and endoplasmic reticulum) by ultrastructural cytochemistry;[121] and (3) a positive reaction with heteroantisera against factor-VIII-related-antigen and with monoclonal antisera which recognize antigens of platelets and megakaryocytes. Megakaryocytic leukaemia commonly presents as acute myelofibrosis (see below), a presentation which may be related to the stimulation of fibroblasts by platelet-derived-growth-factor produced by megakaryoblasts or megakaryocytes. In those patients who do not have overt myelofibrosis, reticulin deposition is often marked. Acute megakaryoblastic leukaemia may be particularly frequent in Down's syndrome,[122, 123] and has been associated with acquired defects of chromosome 21 (ring 21, trisomy and quadrosomy 21).[123]

Acute myelofibrosis (malignant myelosclerosis)[124]

Acute myelofibrosis is a rapidly progressive condition in which increased quantities of reticulin and collagen are deposited in the bone marrow in response to an underlying myeloid malignancy. Acute myelofibrosis may follow cytotoxic chemotherapy,[125] and is most closely associated with acute megakaryoblastic leukaemia[121] or with acute myeloid leukaemia in which megakaryoblast and megakaryocyte proliferation is prominent. Patients with acute myelofibrosis may also have agranular neutrophils, the acquired Pelger-Huët anomaly,[125, 126] sideroblastic anaemia[127] and increased myeloblasts,[125, 128, 129] suggesting that the target cell in the malignant transformation is often a progenitor of all three myeloid cell lines. Cytogenetic evidence indicates that the proliferating fibroblasts are not part of the clone of malignant cells.[130, 131] Acute myelofibrosis is in some ways similar to chronic idiopathic myelofibrosis (see p. 184) and in some ways dissimilar. Hepatomegaly and splenomegaly are uncommon. Anaemia and neutropenia are usual. The platelet count may be high or low and large dysplastic platelets may be seen. Morphological abnormalities of red cells are slight in comparison with those of chronic myelofibrosis. Agranular blasts (which can often be characterized as megakaryoblasts) may be present in the peripheral blood, usually in modest numbers. Attempts at bone marrow aspiration result in a 'dry tap'. Trephine biopsy shows increased reticulin and collagen and an increase of blast cells and megakaryocytes. Megakaryocytes may be atypical; for example there may be micromegakaryocytes and large megakaryocytes with bizarre hyperchromatic or hyperlobulated nuclei, and mitotic figures may be increased. The erythroid and granulocytic series may share in the hyperplasia or be suppressed. Osteosclerosis may occur.[132] The myelofibrosis may result from the stimulation of fibroblasts by a growth factor produced by megakaryocytes and megakaryoblasts. The prognosis of acute myelofibrosis is generally poor. If remission of the leukaemic process occurs, then the fibrosis regresses.[126]

CHRONIC GRANULOCYTIC LEUKAEMIA

Definition

Chronic granulocytic leukaemia (CGL) or chronic myeloid leukaemia (CML) is a disease in which there is a malignant proliferation of a common precursor of the three granulocytic lines (neutrophil-monocyte-macrophage, eosinophil and basophil lines), the erythroid line and the megakaryocyte line. It is likely that in some or all cases the malignant clonogenic cell is a pluripotent cell which is also a potential precursor of lymphocytes. The disorder is usually characterized by an insidious onset, progressive splenomegaly and an increase in the circulating white cell count, often to values greater than $200 \times 10^9/l$, most of the white cells being neutrophils and neutrophil myelocytes (Fig. 6.16). Chronic granulocytic leukaemia is initially a disease of relatively low-grade malignancy but undergoes inevitable evolution into a more malignant form after a period varying from days to many years from diagnosis.

Incidence

CGL is a rare disease. In one large survey the annual incidence was 1.4 new cases per 100 000 of population[133] and in another 1.1 cases per 100 000 males and 0.7 cases per 100 000 females (median incidence over a decade adjusted to the age distribution of the 'European standard population').[104]

Aetiology

In the majority of cases of CGL no aetiological factors are yet identifiable. The incidence is increased following irradiation and exposure to benzene. The development of chronic granulocytic leukaemia is preceded by the appearance of the Philadelphia (Ph[1]) chromosome, which consists of a chromosome 22 which has lost part of its long arm, usually by reciprocal translocation with chromosome 9; this translocation is designated t(9q+; 22q−). Studies in identical twins and serial studies of subjects exposed to atomic explosions have shown that the Ph[1] chromosome

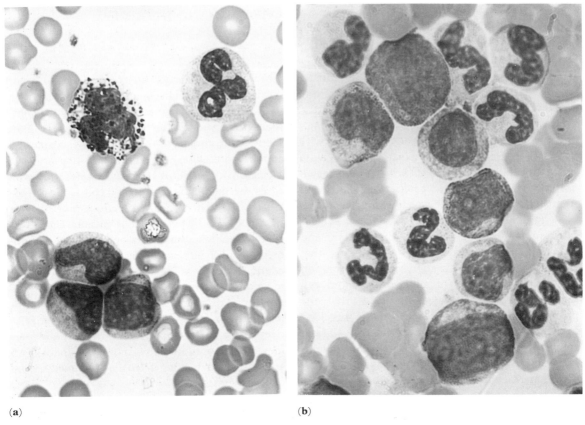

(a)   (b)

Fig. 6.16a,b Two photomicrographs of parts of the peripheral blood film of a patient with chronic granulocytic leukaemia. (**a**) Basophil granulocyte, neutrophil granulocyte and three neutrophil myelocytes. (**b**) Neutrophil granulocytes, band forms, neutrophil myelocytes and neutrophil promyelocytes.

May–Grünwald–Giemsa stain   × 940

is an acquired abnormality. The formation of the Ph[1] chromosome involves translocation of a cellular gene termed c-abl (which is structurally related to the murine Abelson-leukaemia-virus transforming gene, v-abl) from chromosome 9 to chromosome 22; it has been hypothesized that c-abl may be an oncogene which is activated by the transfer.[134]

Pathogenesis

The clone of cells bearing the Ph[1] chromosome expands progressively at the expense of other marrow cells so that by the time of clinical presentation virtually 100% of bone marrow cells are Ph[1]-positive (though at least some patients have a small number of residual cells with normal chromosomes). Granulocytopoietic hyperplasia and megakaryocytic hyperplasia are usual, but there is little or no erythroid hyperplasia even though the erythroid cells also belong to the malignant clone. The rate of release of granulocytes from the marrow (i.e. the rate of effective granulocytopoiesis) is increased despite a decreased proportion of CFU-C and myeloblasts in the DNA synthesis phase of the cell cycle. Cytokinetic studies in CGL have also shown that the time taken for a stem cell to develop into mature neutrophils is prolonged and that there is probably a substantial degree of ineffective granulocytopoiesis. The $T_{\frac{1}{2}}$ of the mature granulocytes in the circulation is two to four times, and of immature plus mature granulocytes five to ten times, longer than that of normal granulocytes. The clinical manifestations of CGL result from: (1) an increasing number of leukaemic cells; and

(2) anaemia. The expanding mass of leukaemic cells causes splenomegaly, bone pain and increased metabolic rate, with low-grade fever, malaise and weight loss. The anaemia is mainly caused by a failure of the marrow to increase the rate of effective erythropoiesis in the face of some reduction of red cell life-span. The granulocytes retain adequate function so that infection is not a feature of CGL. Response to physiological stimuli is retained to some extent; for example, the WBC and neutrophil alkaline phosphatase score may rise during pregnancy and fall after delivery. Cyclical variation in the neutrophil count (with a long periodicity of 30–110 days) is occasionally seen.

Pathology (chronic phase)

Peripheral blood

The WBC is moderately to markedly increased with the most marked increase being in neutrophil granulocytes, metamyelocytes and myelocytes (Fig. 6.16). More primitive cells appear in the blood in similar proportion to their relative frequency in normal bone marrow. The absolute basophil count is almost invariably increased (Fig. 6.16a) and the absolute eosinophil count is commonly so.[135] The monocyte count is increased but not proportionately to the neutrophil count. Anaemia is common but not invariable; nucleated red blood cells may appear in the peripheral blood but red cell morphology is relatively normal. The platelet count may be normal, high or low; megakaryocytes, particularly micromegakaryocytes, may be seen in the peripheral blood. Cytochemical stains show the neutrophil alkaline phosphatase score to be usually (but not invariably) reduced, a useful feature in distinguishing CGL from a leukaemoid reaction (see p. 267).

Bone marrow

The bone marrow is intensely hypercellular due to hyperplasia of the three granulocyte lines (see Fig. 3.28b on p. 68). The myeloid:erythroid ratio is usually 20-30:1. Megakaryocytes are increased and tend to be small and of low ploidy. The increased turnover of myeloid cells leads to

the formation of pseudo-Gaucher cells (containing glycolipids, haemosiderin and cellular debris) (see p. 88) and also 'sea-blue histiocytes' (see p. 88). Plasma cells and mast cells may be increased. Trephine biopsy[136, 137] shows the spatial distribution of various types of haemopoietic cells to be the same as normal, with erythropoiesis and megakaryocytopoiesis being perisinusoidal and granulocytopoiesis being peritrabecular and around arterioles and arterial capillaries. There is marked granulocytopoietic hyperplasia and there may be a ten-fold increase in arterial capillaries. In addition, there are prominent histiocytes containing basophilic crystalloid material in close proximity to aggregates of eosinophils, basophils and mast cells. Mast cells and plasma cells may be scattered or perivascular. There may be lymphoid infiltration, lymphoid nodule formation and focal osteolysis. Osteoporosis may occur and may be attributable to diversion of capillary blood supply. Reticulin formation is increased. Occasionally extensive collagen formation occurs; fibrosis correlates with megakaryocytosis. Myelofibrosis present at diagnosis does not have the same bad prognostic significance as that which develops during the course of the disease. Osteosclerosis may occur in association with myelofibrosis. Rarely, there may be necrosis of bone and bone marrow (see p. 94 and Figs 4.15 and 4.16).

Spleen

The splenic pulp is infiltrated by cells of the granulocyte series, with follicular compression. The ratio of myeloblasts to promyelocytes plus myelocytes is higher than in the bone marrow and the mitotic index of myeloblasts is lower.[138] Fibrosis, haemosiderosis and splenic infarction may occur.

Liver

There is infiltration of the portal tracts with linear infiltrates radiating into the lobules. The liver has a higher ratio of myeloblasts to myelocytes plus promyelocytes than the bone marrow. The mitotic index of myeloblasts is similar to that in marrow.[138]

Hypertrophy of hepatic parenchymal cells may occur. Symptomatic portal hypertension may develop and is attributable to increased resistance from sinusoidal infiltration and increased blood flow as a consequence of splenomegaly.

Eye

Haemorrhages and exudates are common. Retinal veins are tortuous and blood within retinal vessels may appear paler than normal. Microaneurysms are not uncommon[139, 140] and neovascularization may occur.[139] The optic disc may become blurred. Exudative retinal detachment three months prior to acute transformation has been described.[141]

Leucostasis

Blood viscosity is increased, particularly when the WBC exceeds 500×10^9/l. Hyperviscosity may cause headache, dizziness, tinnitus, deafness, ataxia, papilloedema and coma. Priapism is also related to a high WBC and is presumably due to obstruction of cavernous veins by leucocytes. A particularly high WBC may also be associated with peripheral vascular insufficiency with ischaemic necrosis of digits. Cardiorespiratory failure with angina pectoris may be caused by pulmonary leucostasis. Engorgement and a creamy-pink colour of retinal veins may be noted when the WBC is very high. Retinal haemorrhages and exudates may also occur but are related to the anaemia and thrombocytopenia rather than a high WBC.

Non-infiltrative manifestations

The incidence of peptic ulcer appears to be increased; hyperhistaminaemia has been suspected as a cause. Hyperuricaemia, gout and uric acid stones may occur secondary to increased nucleic acid turnover. Pulmonary alveolar proteinosis has been described in five patients with CGL.[142]

Pathology (acute-phase transformation or metamorphosis)

New clones of cells which emerge from the Ph^1-positive clone may be more malignant than the parent clone and lead to an accelerated phase of the disease and often to blastic transformation (i.e. the formation of increasing numbers of blast cells). A new clone of cells may be recognized by the appearance of extra chromosome abnormalities and by an alteration of behaviour on bone marrow culture. Eventually a new clone arises with sufficient growth advantage to largely replace the parent clone. Acute phase transformation may occur initially at an extramedullary site with later spread to blood and bone marrow or may occur in the bone marrow with spread to the peripheral blood and other sites. Thus a patient may have a rapidly-growing tumour of myeloid cells (myeloblastoma, chloroma or granulocytic sarcoma) at an extramedullary site, while the peripheral blood and bone marrow still show the findings of the chronic phase. Similarly, bone marrow trephine biopsies early in intramedullary transformation may show focal proliferation of myeloblasts while chronic-phase findings persist in other parts of the section and in the blood. Common sites of extramedullary transformation are the skin, subcutaneous tissues (including the breasts), orbit, meninges, lymph nodes, spleen and bones. Other sites include the liver, joints, heart, extradural space (causing spinal cord compression) and bowel (with ulceration causing melaena). Hypercalcaemia may occur, particularly in association with lytic bone lesions. In blastic transformation the blasts are often identifiable as myeloblasts but in about a third of patients they have the morphology of lymphoblasts and the cell marker phenotype of either common acute lymphoblastic leukaemia (cALL) or pre-B-ALL (positive for the cALL antigen, high levels of terminal deoxynucleotidyl transferase, rearrangement of heavy and light chain genes indicating commitment to the B-cell line, and in the cases identified as having the pre-B phenotype, cytoplasmic μ chains). Patients with a lymphoblastic transformation may respond to vincristine and prednisone and their prognosis is better than that of patients with myeloblastic

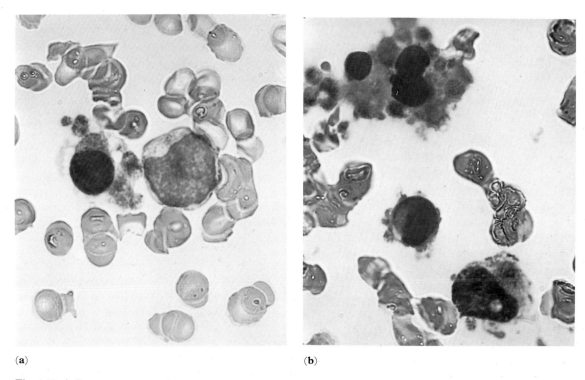

(a)   (b)

Fig. 6.17a,b Bone marrow smear from a patient with megakaryoblastic transformation of chronic granulocytic leukaemia. (a) A megakaryoblast (on the right) and a micromegakaryocyte which is budding platelets. (b) Several micromegakaryocytes which are budding dysplastic platelets: the micromegakaryocyte in the centre has very little cytoplasm.

May–Grünwald–Giemsa stain   × 940

transformation. Mixed myeloid/lymphoblastic transformations may occur.

Myeloid transformations often result in the accumulation in the bone marrow and blood (in the case of intramedullary transformation) of increasing numbers of myeloblasts or sometimes of promyelocytes, megakaryoblasts[143] (Fig. 6.17), monoblasts,[144] erythroblasts,[145] basophil or mast cell precursors, or combinations of these cell types. Uncommonly, marked basophilia may be associated with hyperhistaminaemia and clinical features resembling systemic mastocytosis. Myelofibrosis may be particularly common in association with megakaryoblastic transformation. Some patients present in typical chronic phase but undergo transformation within days or weeks of presentation; others present already in transformation, but with basophilia, splenomegaly and other features of CGL; yet others present as AML before the marrow has been completely replaced by the Ph[1]-positive clone and without any

indication other than the Ph[1] chromosome of the prospensity to develop CGL. The relationship between CGL and Ph[1]-positive-ALL is complex. Typical CGL may undergo a lymphoblastic transformation and Ph[1]-positive but otherwise typical ALL may remit, only to be followed by CGL. Intermediate states also exist; patients who present with ALL may be noted to have basophilia, neutrophilia or morphological abnormalities of neutrophils suggesting that they are Ph[1]-positive. Ph[1]-positive patients whose ALL remits may subsequently undergo myeloblastic transformation. These relationships between CGL and Ph[1]-positive ALL suggest that the malignant clonogenic cell may, at least in some patients, be a premyeloid, prelymphoid pluripotent stem cell with the potential to manifest itself as CGL, Ph[1]-positive ALL, ALL converting to CGL, and CGL transforming to ALL. Mixed myeloid/lymphoid transformations give further evidence that the clonogenic cell is pluripotent.

Treatment

The treatment of CGL is unsatisfactory. During the chronic phase, control of the disease process is readily achieved with alkylating agents (e.g. busulphan) or other cytostatic drugs. Such therapy does not lead to the reappearance of Ph[1]-negative cells and the effect on life expectancy is modest; the median survival of treated patients is about 3.5 years. As essentially all of the bone marrow cells remain Ph[1]-positive, the use of the term 'remission' is not appropriate in CGL. Intensive chemotherapy similar to that used for acute myeloid leukaemia will allow reappearance of Ph[1]-negative cells in a considerable proportion of patients, but comparison with conventionally-managed patients shows no clear improvement in survival. Routine splenectomy has been shown to be of no benefit in prolonging the chronic stage or ameliorating the effects of acute transformation. The majority of transformed patients die in 1–2 months. The prognosis of acute transformation is best in those patients (approximately 20%) who respond to the type of chemotherapy used in ALL (vincristine and prednisone); some patients also revert to a chronic phase with chemotherapy of the type used in AML (see p. 233). Better methods of treatment of CGL are clearly needed. One experimental mode of treatment is syngeneic (identical twin) or allogeneic (histocompatible sibling) bone marrow transplantation during the chronic phase. Such treatment will only be of significant benefit if patients are rendered totally Ph[1]-negative prior to transplantation.

JUVENILE CHRONIC MYELOID LEUKAEMIA

Juvenile chronic myeloid leukaemia is a rare condition occurring in infants. Clinical features include hepatomegaly, splenomegaly, lymphadenopathy and skin rash. Neutrophils, eosinophils, basophils and monocytes may all be increased. The neutrophil alkaline phosphatase is low. The haemoglobin F level is characteristically high and the erythrocytes may show other features of fetal erythrocytes such as reduced levels of carbonicanhydrase and reduced expression of I antigen. The Ph[1] chromosome is not present. Prognosis is poor.

NEUTROPHILIC LEUKAEMIA

Neutrophilic leukaemia is a rare condition occurring mainly in the middle aged and elderly. Clinical features include splenomegaly and, usually, hepatomegaly. The peripheral blood shows a neutrophil leucocytosis with very few immature cells (WBC, 30–100 $\times$ 10^9/l). The haemoglobin concentration may be normal or moderately reduced and the platelet count is usually normal. In contrast to chronic granulocytic leukaemia, the neutrophil alkaline phosphatase score is increased and the Ph[1] chromosome is not present. Survival is similar to that in chronic granulocytic leukaemia.

MYELODYSPLASTIC SYNDROMES (DYSMYELOPOIETIC SYNDROMES, PRELEUKAEMIA)

Definition

Certain multilineage maturation defects of myeloid cells may precede acute myeloid leukaemia. Patients displaying such maturation defects are commonly described as having preleukaemia, but as it is not possible to predict which of these patients will eventually develop AML the terms dysmyelopoietic syndrome or myelodysplastic syndrome may be preferred. Myelodysplasia may arise *de novo* (primary myelodysplastic syndrome) or may be secondary to an agent (such as cytotoxic chemotherapy and/or irradiation) which damages stem cells. In the myelodysplastic syndromes, haemopoiesis is not only dysplastic (i.e. shows morphological evidence of disturbed maturation), but is also ineffective (see p. 211). Usually erythropoiesis, granulocytopoiesis and thrombocytopoiesis are all abnormal; in some cases dysplasia appears to be restricted to one or two cell lines.

Classification

Several distinct entities with somewhat different natural histories are included under the overall designation of myelodysplastic syndrome. Primary acquired sideroblastic anaemia (see p. 165) and chronic myelomonocytic leukaemia are sometimes considered as a form of myelodysplas-

Table 6.10 Classification of myelodysplastic syndromes[105]

Syndrome	Peripheral blood	Bone marrow
Refractory anaemia*	Anaemia and reticulocytopenia; blasts <1%	Blasts <5%; ringed sideroblasts <15% of nucleated cells
Refractory anaemia with ringed sideroblasts†, or idiopathic acquired sideroblastic anaemia (see p. 165)	Anaemia and reticulocytopenia	Blasts <5%; ringed sideroblasts >15% of nucleated cells
Refractory anaemia with excess of blasts (RAEB)	Anaemia and reticulocytopenia; blasts <5%	Blasts 5–20%
Chronic myelomonocytic leukaemia	Monocyte count >1.0 × 10⁹/1; granulocyte count often increased; blasts <5%	Blasts <20%; promonocytes may be increased
Refractory anaemia in transformation	Blasts >5% or Auer rods present	Blasts 20–30% or Auer rods present

* Some patients who have refractory neutropenia and/or refractory thrombocytopenia without anaemia are classified with this group; the designation refractory cytopenia may therefore be preferred

† A ringed sideroblast is defined as an erythroblast with six or more Prussian-blue-positive granules along a third or more of the circumference of the nucleus

tic syndrome and sometimes as separate diseases. The French-American-British (FAB) cooperative group have classified the myelodysplastic syndromes as shown in Table 6.10.[105] It is not always possible to relate publications by other groups to this classification. Certain diseases, including aplastic anaemia and paroxysmal nocturnal haemoglobinuria, are recognized as being preleukaemic but are not usually classified with the myelodysplastic syndromes.

Incidence

The myelodysplastic syndromes are most commonly seen in elderly patients, predominantly males, or in persons of any age who have been exposed to cytotoxic chemotherapy, radiotherapy or both. Some myelodysplastic syndromes have been recognized in children.

Aetiology

Myelodysplastic syndromes may follow exposure to agents which damage DNA (i.e. alkylating agents, irradiation). Myelodysplastic states leading to AML have been seen following chemotherapy for carcinoma of the lung, carcinoma of the ovary, and multiple myeloma, and chemotherapy with or without radiotherapy for Hodgkin's disease and non-Hodgkin's lym-

phoma. Dysmyelopoiesis followed by acute myeloid leukaemia has also been observed following cytotoxic chemotherapy for non-malignant conditions. The aetiology of myelodysplastic states which arise *de novo* is unknown.

Cytogenetics

Non-random chromosomal abnormalities are frequently present in bone marrow cells. Monosomy 5, monosomy 7, 5q- and 7q- are most characteristic, and 20q- and trisomy 8 are also found. In patients with chromosomal abnormalities, residual cytogenetically normal cells are sometimes but not always present.[146] Monosomy 7 is associated with preleukaemia in children[147] and 5q- is particularly associated with refractory anaemia with excess of blasts (RAEB) (Table 6.10).

Pathogenesis

It is likely that in dysmyelopoietic syndromes normal haemopoietic cells are largely replaced by a population of dysplastic cells derived from an abnormal multipotent stem cell. The abnormal clone may be stable for some years, as is commonly the case in primary idiopathic sideroblastic anaemia. In others haemopoiesis may become increasingly ineffective. Clonal evolution (which may be marked by the appearance of additional cytogenetic defects[148]) may lead to acute myeloid leukaemia.

Clinical features

These result from anaemia and from the reduced number and function of neutrophils and platelets. Splenomegaly occurs in less than half the patients with chronic myelomonocytic leukaemia and is uncommon in other myelodysplastic states.

Pathology

Peripheral blood[105, 149]

Anaemia may be normocytic and normochromic, or macrocytic and normochromic. Macrocytosis is most common in primary acquired sideroblastic anaemia, but may occur in any of the categories. A minor population of cells may be hypochromic. Basophilic stippling, poikilocytes (including ovalocytes) and occasional circulating nucleated red blood cells may be seen. The absolute reticulocyte count is low or normal despite the anaemia. Acquired HbH disease has occurred. Acquired deficiencies of pyruvate kinase,[150] 2,3-diphosphogliceromutase and phosphokinase have been reported[148] as has an acquired G6PD variant with increased activity.[151] Haemoglobin F and the percentage of F-cells (p. 124) are often increased.[152] In chronic myelomonocytic leukaemia the neutrophil count is usually elevated and in primary acquired sideroblastic anaemia it is often normal. In other myelodysplastic syndromes neutropenia is characteristic. Neutrophils are often hypogranular with nuclei resembling those seen in the inherited Pelger-Huët anomaly (Fig. 6.18). Cytochemical studies may show neutrophils to be lacking in peroxidase,[153] chloroacetate esterase[154] or alkaline phosphatase[155, 156] and neutrophil function may be impaired.[153] Neutrophil abnormalities are not usual in primary acquired sideroblastic anaemia. Monocytosis is an essential feature of chronic myelomonocytic leukaemia, but may also occur in other myelodysplastic syndromes. In primary acquired sideroblastic anaemia the platelet count is usually normal or somewhat elevated. In other

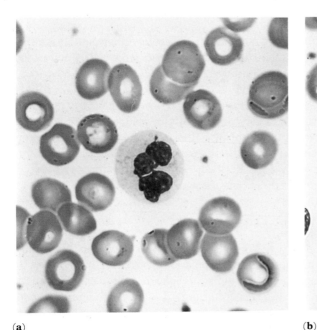

(a)

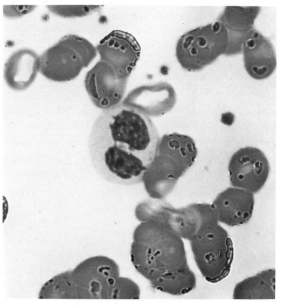

(b)

Fig. 6.18a,b Peripheral blood neutrophils from a patient with a myelodysplastic syndrome. (a) Hypogranular neutrophil. (b) Hypogranular neutrophil with the acquired Pelger-Huët anomaly.
May–Grünwald–Giemsa stain   × 940

myelodysplastic syndromes, thrombocytopenia is usual though thrombocytosis occasionally occurs. Platelets may have a deficiency of platelet peroxidase,[157] abnormal granules (e.g. giant granules, or absent or decreased granules),[158] and poor function.[158] Abnormally large platelets (megathrombocytes or macroplatelets) are common. Abnormal and immature megakaryocytes may circulate in the peripheral blood.[105] Serum lysozyme may be elevated, particularly in chronic myelomonocytic leukaemia.

Bone marrow

The bone marrow is usually hypercellular or normocellular. Hypocellularity may occur in secondary myelodysplasia and may be accompanied by some fibrosis. Hypercellularity is usual in chronic myelomonocytic leukaemia. Dyserythropoietic features include multinuclearity, abnormal nuclear shape, nuclear fragmentation, megaloblastosis, vacuolation of cytoplasm, heavily granulated sideroblasts and ringed sideroblasts. The presence of ringed sideroblasts is essential for the diagnosis of primary acquired sideroblastic anaemia but ringed sideroblasts are also often found, albeit usually in smaller numbers, in other myelodysplastic states, particularly when induced by chemotherapy or radiotherapy.[105] Erythroblasts may constitute from more than 60% to fewer than 5% of nucleated bone marrow cells. Erythroid hyperplasia is characteristic of primary acquired sideroblastic anaemia. Dysgranulopoietic features include a lack or reduction of primary or secondary granules, giant primary granules, hyper- and hyposegmentation of nuclei, bizarre nuclear shapes, and persistence of cytoplasmic basophilia in more mature cells. Myeloblasts may be increased and Auer rods may be present. Auer rods have been interpreted as indicating transformation to a more aggressive phase;[105] others have found them not to be related to disease course.[159] In chronic myelomonocytic leukaemia the bone marrow often appears more 'acute' than the peripheral blood; promyelocytes are often prominent in addition to cells of the monocyte series. Various abnormalities of megakaryocytes may occur in the myelodysplastic syndromes: these include micromegakaryo-

cytes, large mononuclear megakaryocytes and megakaryocytes with multiple small separate nuclei.[105] Megakaryocyte numbers may be reduced. Lymphocytes, plasma cells and mast cells are increased and the marrow may show oedema and endothelial degeneration. There may be increased quantities of reticulin. In vitro culture of bone marrow gives varying results. Granulocyte-macrophage colonies (formed by CFU-GM) may be increased, normal, decreased or absent, or colonies may be replaced by clusters.[160] An increased colony count is characteristic of chronic myelomonocytic leukaemia. In a study of 10 cases of preleukaemia (refractory anaemia, RAEB, and one case of primary sideroblastic anaemia), erythroid colonies were found to be generally abnormal, BFU-E being either markedly decreased or grossly defective in proliferative and differentiation capacities.[161]

Disease progression

Many patients with myelodysplasia die of haemorrhage or infection without developing AML. If AML does develop the prognosis is considerably worse than in AML developing de novo. The prognosis of cases of myelodysplastic syndrome can be related to the type of syndrome; RAEB 'in transformation' has a worse prognosis than RAEB or refractory anaemia. Patients with a primary acquired sideroblastic anaemia have a low percentage of blasts, are less likely to develop acute leukaemia, and have a better prognosis. Patients with a marked increase of reticulin may form a subgroup with a rapidly progressive disease. Patients with cytogenetic abnormalities have a worse prognosis[148] as do those with a post-therapy (secondary) myelodysplastic syndrome[148]. Other specific features which have been found to worsen prognosis are: a high percentage of bone marrow blasts, neutropenia, thrombocytopenia, monocytopenia, the presence of circulating blasts and the presence in the bone marrow of reduced numbers of CFU-GM.[162] In culture conditions permitting the growth of CFU-GM, the finding of an increase of clusters[162, 163] or absent growth is predictive of transformation to acute leukaemia.

Treatment

The treatment of primary acquired sideroblastic anaemia is mentioned on page 166. Treatment of other myelodysplastic syndromes is generally ineffective. Androgens and corticosteroids are of no benefit. Cytotoxic chemotherapy has occasionally been of value.

ACUTE LYMPHOBLASTIC LEUKAEMIA

Definition

Acute lymphoblastic leukaemia (ALL) is a disease characterized by a malignant proliferation of lymphoblasts; if untreated, it causes death in weeks or months.

Incidence

Acute lymphoblastic leukaemia is a rare condition with a peak incidence at the age of 3 years. In an Australian study the incidence of new cases was one per 100 000 of population per year,[164] whereas in several European surveys the total incidence of all types of acute leukaemia in children was about 4–4.5 cases per 100 000 males per year with a somewhat lower rate in females.[104] In Caucasian children, the great majority of cases of acute leukaemia are cases of acute lymphoblastic leukaemia. The incidence of ALL in Black children both in Africa and the USA is considerably lower than in White children with the consequence that in some areas of Africa up to 50% of children with acute leukaemia have AML.

Classification

The lymphoblasts of acute lymphoblastic leukaemia are characteristically uniform in shape with a high nucleus:cytoplasm ratio and agranular cytoplasm. Differences in the morphological features of the leukaemic blast cells between patients allow further classification. One such classification, the FAB (French-British-American)[106] classification, is:

ALL$_1$ (typical childhood ALL). The blasts are relatively small with a fine chromatin

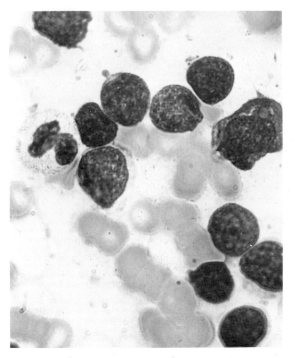

Fig. 6.19 Bone marrow smear from a patient with ALL$_1$. The blasts are uniform in appearance but vary in size from that of a small lymphocyte to larger than that of a neutrophil. The nucleus and the cell are regular in outline. The nucleocytoplasmic ratio is high.

May–Grünwald–Giemsa stain   × 940

pattern, small nucleoli and scanty cytoplasm (Fig. 6.19).

ALL$_2$. The blasts are larger and more heterogeneous in size and shape (Fig. 6.20).

ALL$_3$. The blasts are morphologically the same as those of Burkitt's lymphoma. Cells are large, with moderately abundant basophilic cytoplasm. Cytoplasmic vacuolation is common (Fig. 6.21).

ALL may also be classified on the basis of antigenic differences between leukaemic cells demonstrable by immunological techniques (using heteroantisera or monoclonal antibodies). This approach divides ALL into five main classes, the characteristics of which are shown in Table 6.11, together with their relative frequency in childhood cases. The blast cells of 15–20% of cases of childhood ALL have the same phenotype as thymocytes; such children are, therefore, said to suffer from T-ALL. In 80% of these cases, the cells

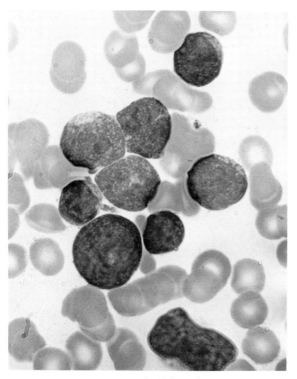

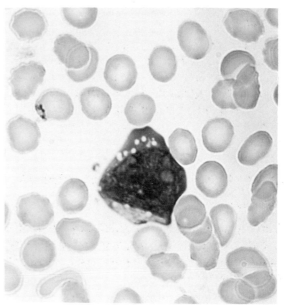

Fig. 6.21 Lymphoblast from the bone marrow smear of a patient with ALL₃. The blast cell resembles the cells of Burkitt's lymphoma, the cytoplasm being vacuolated and strongly basophilic.

May–Grünwald–Giemsa stain   × 940

Fig. 6.20 Bone marrow smear from a patient with ALL₂. The blast cells are more pleomorphic and larger in size that those of ALL₁. Some nuclei are cleft. The cells did not form rosettes with sheep red blood cells (E-rosettes) but were shown by monoclonal antibodies to be pre-T-cells.

May–Grünwald–Giemsa stain   × 940

have the phenotype of the stage I or immature thymocyte and in the remaining 20% the phenotype of the stage II or common thymocyte.[94] The blast cells of cases of T-ALL usually have the morphological features of ALL₂. It is likely that the leukaemic cells of cases belonging to the four categories of non-T ALL all have phenotypes of normal B-cells or their precursors. In a minority of cases, the cells have SmIg, the marker of mature B-cells, and display the morphological features of ALL₂ or ALL₃; such cases are classified as having B-ALL. In a significant number of cases, the leukaemic cells can be identified as pre-B-cells by the presence of cytoplasmic μ heavy chains; such cases are, therefore, placed in the category pre-B ALL. The majority of cases fall into the category of common ALL (cALL); in some cases the blast cells demonstrate rearrangement of heavy chain and sometimes light

chain genes (a characteristic of an early B-cell precursor), and the phenotype of these cells is therefore considered to be that of a cell committed to the B-cell lineage.[94] cALL may thus be designated pre-pre-B ALL or early pre-B ALL. The sharing of markers between unclassified ALL on the one hand, and cALL, pre-B-ALL and B-ALL on the other, makes it likely that the cells of unclassified ALL also have the phenotype of a B-cell precursor (or possibly a common precursor of B- and T-cells). The leukaemic cells in cases of unclassified ALL, pre-B-ALL and cALL have the morphological features of ALL₁ or ALL₂.

Approximately 25% of adults and 1–4% of children with ALL are found to have the Ph¹ chromosome (see p. 235);[165] this chromosomal abnormality may be present in unclassified ALL, cALL or pre-B-ALL. In adults, T-ALL and cALL make up a lower proportion of ALL than in children, and unclassified ALL and B-ALL (which may be a leukaemic phase of a non-Hodgkin's lymphoma) account for a higher proportion.

Table 6.11 Cytoplasmic and surface markers in acute lymphoblastic leukaemia

	Unclassified ALL	Common ALL	pre-B ALL	B-ALL	T-ALL
% of all childhood cases of ALL	8	50	20	1–2	15–20
Immunoglobulin	−	−	Cyμ	SmIg	−
Ia antigen	+	+	+	+	−
TdT	+	+	+	−	+
BA-1	+/−	+/−	+	+	−
BA-2	+	usually +	usually +	usually +	−
B1	−	+	+	+	−
CALLA	−	+	+	<10% of cells +	−
Other markers				C3bR +; FcR +	Thymic antigens +; ERFC +/−; acid phosphatase (focal) +

Ia antigen = Ia-like (HLA-DR) antigen
TdT = terminal deoxynucleotidyl transferase
BA-1, BA-2 and B1 = monoclonal antibodies reacting with cells of B-cell lineage
CALLA = cALL antigen recognized by monoclonal antibodies (J5, BA-3) or heteroantisera
Cyμ = cytoplasmic μ chain
SmIg = surface membrane immunoglobulin
C3bR = receptor for activated C3
FcR = receptor for Fc fragment of Ig
Thymic antigens = antigens characteristic of thymocytes ± T-cells (recognized by monoclonal antibodies or heteroantisera)
ERFC = cells forming rosettes with sheep red blood cells

Aetiology

In the majority of cases of ALL no aetiological factors are yet identifiable. The incidence is increased following irradiation and in the presence of certain congenital chromosome defects (e.g. in Down's syndrome and ataxia telangiectasia).

Cytogenetics

Non-random chromosomal abnormalities are common in ALL. 6q- may be found in both cALL and T-ALL with the breakpoint in the region of the cellular oncogene, c-myb[166]. As mentioned above, the Philadelphia chromosome is found in some cases of ALL.

Pathogenesis

In ALL there is progressive expansion of a single clone of cells, which fail to differentiate normally. The proportion of cells in the DNA synthesis phase of the cell cycle varies markedly but is, on average, less in leukaemic lymphoblasts than in normal lymphoblasts. This indicates that in many cases of ALL, the fraction of the leukaemic blast cell population that is actively proliferating (i.e. progressing through the cell cycle) is low and/or the cell cycle time is prolonged, when compared with normal lymphoblasts. The clinical and laboratory features of ALL result from: (1) progressive replacement of normal marrow by leukaemic cells causing pancytopenia and infective and haemorrhagic complications; and (2) infiltration of tissues by leukaemic cells. In addition, complications of treatment may lead to pathological processes.

Pathology

The clinical, laboratory and pathological features of T-ALL differ in some respects from those of cALL. Sufferers from T-ALL are more likely to be male, have a higher average WBC, and are more likely to have marked thymic enlargement or to present with a localized tumour. Some patients with T-ALL may present with a lymphoma-like clinical picture characterized by a thymic mass with or without lymphadenopathy but with little or no evidence of bone marrow infiltration (less than 25% of blasts in the marrow).[167, 168] Such patients are usually designated as having T-lymphoblastic lymphoma, but with the recognition that T-ALL and T-lymphoblastic lymphoma are two phases of the one disease. In comparison with T-ALL a greater proportion of patients presenting as T-lymphoblastic lymphoma have malignant cells with a more mature phenotype.[94, 167] Patients with pre-B ALL may be more likely than those with cALL to present with localized tumours.[169] Cases of ALL₃ are more likely than cases of other types of ALL to have bone lesions; these may include jaw tumours.[170]

Peripheral blood

Anaemia, thrombocytopenia and neutropenia are common. Except in some patients who are found to have the Philadelphia chromosome (see p. 235), the red cells and the granulocytes are morphologically normal. A marked eosinophilia is sometimes seen in patients with ALL. A minority of patients are aleukaemic, but the majority have leukaemic lymphoblasts in the peripheral blood, conforming to the morphology of ALL₁, ALL₂ or ALL₃ (see p. 244). In most patients with T-ALL a minority of the leukaemic cells have a markedly hyperchromatic convoluted nucleus (which may be more apparent in conventional histological sections or the thin sections used for electron microscopy than in blood or marrow smears). T-lymphoblasts may also show radial segmentation.[171] Although lymphoblasts characteristically have agranular cytoplasm, rare patients have granular blasts.[172]

The lymphoblasts of ALL show a negative reaction with cytochemical stains for myeloperoxidase (Fig. 6.22a) and chloroacetate esterase. They also almost always stain negatively with Sudan black B but rare exceptions occur.[173] In most cases of ALL, the cytoplasm of at least a few leukaemic lymphoblasts stains positively with the periodic acid-Schiff (PAS) reaction; the positi-

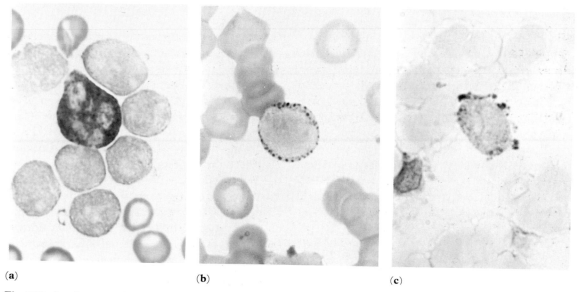

(a)   (b)   (c)

Fig. 6.22a,b,c Some cytochemical reactions of the blast cells in a marrow smear of a patient with acute lymphoblastic leukaemia. (a) Peroxidase reaction: the neutrophil shows a positive reaction and the surrounding lymphoblasts a negative reaction. (b,c) PAS reaction: the cytoplasm of the blast cell in b shows coarse granules, and that in c shows both coarse granules and blocks of PAS-positive material.

× 940

vity is characteristically in solid blocks or coarse granules and the rest of the cytoplasm is entirely PAS-negative (Fig. 6.22b, c). This contrasts with the findings in AML where most of the blasts are PAS-negative and some may show diffuse cytoplasmic staining, sometimes together with fine PAS-positive granules and, very rarely, with coarse granules or block-positivity. The blast cells of the great majority of cases of T-ALL give a strongly positive reaction for acid phosphatase which is localized to one region of the cytoplasm (corresponding to the Golgi apparatus). In patients with ALL$_3$ the cytoplasmic vacuoles of the leukaemic cells stain with lipid stains such as oil red 0.[170]

In the majority of cases of ALL, the leukaemic lymphoblasts have a high level of terminal deoxynucleotidyl transferase (TdT), which may be detected by a biochemical assay or by immunofluorescence. TdT cannot be detected in the blast cells of most cases of acute myeloid leukaemia, but is present at moderately high levels in about 5%. Ia-like antigen is detectable in the blast cells of B-ALL and pre-B-ALL (and usually in AML) but is not detectable in T-ALL.

Bone marrow and bones

The bone marrow is extensively infiltrated by lymphoblasts and is intensely hypercellular. Areas of bone marrow infarction may occur. Local proliferation of leukaemic cells may lead to osteolytic lesions and periosteal new bone formation. X-rays may also show translucent transverse metaphyseal bands. In contrast to AML, trephine biopsy in ALL shows that early infiltration is diffuse.[136] In a minority of patients, transient aplastic anaemia (with remission occurring spontaneously, or after corticosteroids) precedes the development of ALL by several months.[174, 175]

Liver[92]

The portal tracts may be infiltrated and lymphoblasts may be seen in lymphatics.

Spleen[92]

Macroscopically, follicles may be barely visible, minimally enlarged or very prominent. Microscopically, lymphoblasts are seen within follicles and in arteries, arterioles, and subintimal lymphatics of trabecular veins. Spontaneous rupture of the infiltrated spleen is a rare complication.[176]

Lymph nodes[92]

Early infiltration may be seen in the marginal and medullary sinuses.

Other lymphoid organs

Tonsils and other oropharyngeal lymphoid tissue may be infiltrated. Infiltration of Peyer's patches may be followed by necrosis and ulceration. About half of the patients with T-ALL have an anterior mediastinal mass due to leukaemic infiltration of the thymus.

Other organs[92]

Infiltration of the orbit may cause exophthalmos. Meningeal infiltration is rare at presentation but commonly develops during the course of the illness if prophylactic measures are not applied. In addition to a diffuse infiltrate in the subarachnoid space there may be focal or pseudonodular infiltration which is subdural, dural or epidural. The calvarium and soft tissues of the scalp may be infiltrated. The brain may show plugging of intracerebral vessels by leukaemic cells, perivascular cuffing with leukaemic cells, and infiltration of adjacent brain tissue.

Rarely hypothalamic infiltration may lead to increased appetite, obesity and behavioural change and vasopressin-responsive diabetes insipidus.[177] Testicular infiltration is common during the course of the illness. Renal infiltration may be diffuse or localized, often mainly in the cortex and outer pyramids; rarely, a nodular proliferation of leukaemic cells may be detected by ultrasonography.[178] The kidneys may also be enlarged due to hyperplasia rather than infiltration.[179] Infiltration may also occur in the lungs (particularly peribronchially), pericardium, breasts, uterus,[180] prostate[181] and lacrimal and salivary glands. Ocular infiltration may involve the iris (with hyphaema or hypopyon, and secondary glaucoma), the choroid, the retina and the optic nerve.[182]

Residual leukaemic cells during apparent complete remission

Autopsies or multiple biopsies in patients who appear to be in complete remission may show foci of leukaemic cells in the testes, bone marrow, liver, central nervous system and kidneys. Patients remaining in peripheral blood and bone marrow remission may have leukaemic relapse at similar sites—testes, ovaries, meninges, hypothalamus, kidneys. Splenomegaly during remission does not necessarily indicate relapse; splenectomy may reveal no evidence of leukaemia.[183]

Treatment

Treatment of ALL includes chemotherapy with antineoplastic drugs (e.g. vincristine, prednisolone, methotrexate, mercaptopurine, colaspase [L-asparaginase], cyclophosphamide), together with radiotherapy and intrathecal methotrexate for prophylaxis of CNS disease. With modern treatment, many patients with ALL may be cured, i.e. their survival curves plateau and parallel those for normal people. Treatment may, however, have adverse consequences.

Treatment-related pathological processes

Infective complications

These include bacterial, viral, fungal and protozoal infections. Bacterial infections are common during remission induction. Susceptibility to serious viral infections persists during remission and is a consequence of immunosuppression. Varicella infection may cause fulminating varicella pneumonia and meningoencephalitis. The measles virus may cause inclusion–body encephalitis and giant cell pneumonitis. Multifocal leucoencephalopathy may occur, consequent on activation of the papova virus.[184] Herpes simplex may cause encephalitis, interstitial pneumonitis and disseminated infection. Cytomegalovirus may cause a morbilliform rash, chorioretinitis, hepatitis and splenomegaly. Toxoplasmosis may cause lymphadenopathy or a disseminated infection with or without a necrotizing encephalitis preferentially affecting the grey matter.[185] Other infections include those caused by Pneumocystis carinii, cryptococcus and mycoplasma. In areas where hepatitis B infection is endemic, chronic liver disease associated with hepatitis B infection is very common in children who have been treated for ALL;[186] viral antigen may be demonstrated in the liver in the absence of any serological evidence of infection.

Long-term effects of CNS prophylaxis

Some degree of cerebral atrophy with dilation of the subarachnoid space and ventricles may occur following cranial irradiation. This correlates with a minor impairment of intellectual development. Patients who have required high-dose intrathecal or systemic methotrexate in addition to cranial irradiation may develop severe neurological damage with a subacute necrotizing demyelinating leucoencephalopathy and dystrophic calcification, including calcification of the walls of small blood vessels; rarely such changes have followed conventional dosage.[187] A small proportion of children given higher than usual radiation doses (e.g. >2500 rads in $2\frac{1}{2}$ weeks) have developed clinical features of growth hormone deficiency; others have a subclinical deficiency.[188]

Gonadal damage

Gonadal damage may be caused by chemotherapy, particularly with cyclophosphamide and high doses of cytarabine.[188] Boys who have received prepubertal chemotherapy have a 50% reduction in the percentage of seminiferous tubules containing recognizable spermatogonia but show normal Leydig cell function. If the testes are irradiated for leukaemic infiltration, there is impairment of Leydig cell function also. Combination chemotherapy for ALL may cause ovarian dysfunction with impaired follicular maturation and increased levels of FSH but recovery usually occurs, allowing normal puberty.

Other treatment-related pathological processes

During treatment, fatty change in the liver is common. Periportal fibrosis and even cirrhosis may be a consequence of long-term methotrexate therapy.[187] Osteoporosis may result from therapy with methotrexate[187] or corticosteroids.

CHRONIC LYMPHOCYTIC LEUKAEMIA

Definition

Chronic lymphocytic leukaemia (CLL) is a disease caused by a monoclonal proliferation of lymphoid cells and is characterized by a progressive increase in circulating mature lymphocytes. In the great majority of cases the malignant clone consists of B-lymphocytes (B-CLL). In a minority of cases (approximately 2%)[189] the clone consists of T-lymphocytes (T-CLL). The clinical and pathological features of T-CLL are somewhat different from those of B-CLL and are discussed separately on page 255.

Prevalence

In a Norwegian survey, the incidence was 2.6 cases per 100 000 males and 1.3 cases per 100 000 females per year (median incidence for a decade adjusted to age distribution of European standard population).[104] In the USA the prevalence was estimated at 2.4 per 100 000.[133]

Aetiology

The cause of CLL is unknown. Several families have been observed with a high incidence of CLL; in some of these an inherited abnormality of a G group chromosome was also found. CLL is uncommon in Japanese, but T-cell leukaemia-lymphoma associated with a retrovirus (HTLV I, see p. 264) has been observed particularly in this racial group.

Cytogenetics

The availability of mitogens for B-lymphocytes (phorbol esters, bacterial lipopolysaccharide) has allowed the demonstration of non-random chromosome abnormalities in a significant percentage of patients; these abnormalities include 14q+ translocations, trisomy 3 and aberrations of chromosome 6. In one patient a translocation t(2;14) had breakpoints close to the genes for the κ light chain on chromosome 2 and heavy chains on chromosome 14 with expression of $\mu\kappa$ and $\delta\kappa$ on the malignant cells; this is analogous to the much more commonly described translocations in Burkitt's lymphoma with breakpoints near the κ or λ genes[190] and expression of the equivalent light chain type. It is possible that such translocations may lead to activation of oncogenes with consequent malignant proliferation. The target cell in the malignant transformation of CLL may be a cell of the same phenotype as a cell which has been demonstrated in small numbers in normal tonsils and lymph nodes.[191]

Pathogenesis

The clinical manifestations of CLL are due to a progressive increase in the mass of leukaemic cells, a reduction of humoral and cellular immunity and, sometimes, superimposed autoimmune phenomena. Proliferation of leukaemic cells causes lymphadenopathy, splenomegaly and hepatomegaly as well as cytopenias due to replacement of normal bone marrow. The proliferation of a malignant clone of B-lymphocytes is associated with a reduction in the number of normal B-lymphocytes and consequently hypogammaglobulinaemia and poor primary and secondary antibody responses. This impairment of humoral immunity results in a susceptibility to pneumococcal and other pyogenic bacterial infections. A minority of patients have a serum paraprotein. In B-CLL the absolute number of T-lymphocytes is increased. There is a consistent increase of T-cells of suppressor phenotype and a reduction of cells with helper phenotype[192] which may explain the impairment of cell-mediated immunity and the consequent susceptibility to mycoses and to viral infections. The commonest autoimmune phenomena are the development of autoimmune haemolytic anaemia (AIHA) and autoimmune thrombocytopenic purpura.

Staging

Several systems of staging have been devised to divide patients into prognostic groups. The most commonly used is that of Rai.[193]

Stage 0: Increased lymphocytes in peripheral blood and bone marrow; no organomegaly

Stage 1: Lymphadenopathy

Stage 2: Hepatomegaly or splenomegaly $\pm$ lymphadenopathy

Stage 3: Anaemia (Hb < 11 g/dl) $\pm$ other manifestations

Stage 4: Thrombocytopenia (platelets < 100 $\times$ 10^9/l) $\pm$ other manifestations.

Pathology

Peripheral blood

A prerequisite for the diagnosis of CLL is an increased peripheral blood lymphocyte count. The lymphocytes are relatively mature and uniform in appearance. They are also mechanically fragile and, therefore, form 'smear cells' or 'smudge cells' during the spreading of blood films (Fig. 6.23). The cells of B-CLL are smaller than normal B-lymphocytes[194] but with advancing disease an increasing proportion of cells which are larger than normal B-cells may appear.[195] Immunological studies show that the lymphocytes of most cases of B-CLL have small amounts of surface membrane immunoglobulin (SmIg) of one light chain type. The heavy chains of SmIg may be restricted to one type, μ (SmIg = IgM), or may be both δ and μ (SmIg = IgD and IgM); if IgD and IgM are both present they are of the same idiotype. The lymphocytes of B-CLL form rosettes on incubation with mouse red blood cells (mouse-rosette-forming cells, MRFC). In one study 18% of patients with B-CLL had no detectable SmIg on their lymphocytes, but were identified as having B-CLL because of the presence of a high proportion of MRFC.[165] In contrast to the findings in CLL, patients with prolymphocytic leukaemia or with follicular lymphoma in a leukaemic phase have monoclonal B-lymphocytes with larger amounts of SmIg (i.e. staining more intensely with the appropriate fluorescein-labelled anti-

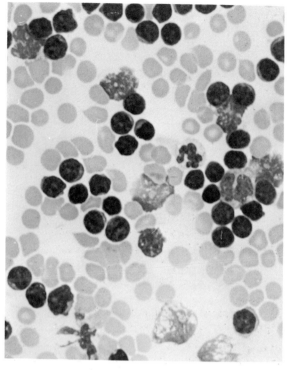

Fig. 6.23 Peripheral blood smear of a patient with chronic lymphocytic leukaemia showing many mature small lymphocytes with scanty cytoplasm and hyperchromatic nuclei. There are also several smear cells.

May–Grünwald–Giemsa stain   × 940

body) and have a lower percentage of MRFC. B-CLL cells have a consistent pattern of reactions with monoclonal antibodies; positive reactions are seen with various antibodies directed against B-cells (BA-1, B1, P1 153/3) as well as with a group of antibodies which react with T-cells but not with normal B-cells (OKT1, Leu-1, T101).[94] CLL cells also have receptors for C3 and the Fc fragment of Ig. A comparison of important markers in B- and T-CLL is shown in Table 6.12. Some patients without lymphocytosis have the other pathological lesions characteristic of CLL that are described below; the designation of diffuse, well-differentiated lymphocytic lymphoma is then appropriate.[196] A mild normocytic normochromic anaemia is usual in CLL but neutropenia and thrombocytopenia are found at presentation only in a minority of cases. Generalized hypogammaglobulinaemia is often present. A minority of patients have a monoclonal protein

Table 6.12 Cytoplasmic and surface markers in chronic lymphocytic leukaemia of B-cell or T-cell lineage

	B-CLL	T-CLL
SmIg	usually + (weak)	−
MRFC	+	−
ERFC	−	+
OKT1	+	+
OKT3	−	+
OKT4	−	−/+
OKT8	−	−/+
BA-1, B1, P1 153/3	+	−
Ia antigen	+	−/+
Acid phosphatase	−/+*	+ (strong)
ANAE	−/+*	weak or −

* Positive cells are more mature on ultrastructural examination

SmIg = surface membrane immunoglobulin
MRFC = mouse rosette forming cells
ERFC = sheep rosette forming cells
OKT1, OKT3, OKT4, OKT8 = monoclonal antibodies reacting with some or all thymocytes and T-cells
BA-1, B1, P1 153/3 = monoclonal antibodies reacting with cells of B-cell lineage
Ia = Ia-like antigen
ANAE = α-naphthylacetate esterase

in the serum, which is of the same idiotype as that on the surface of the leukaemic cells. Monoclonal light chain excretion (Bence Jones proteinuria) is occasionally observed.[197]

Bone marrow

The bone marrow aspirate shows a hypercellular marrow which is heavily infiltrated by relatively small, mature lymphocytes. Normal myeloid cells are reduced. Mast cells may be increased.[198] Histological studies of aspirated bone marrow fragments or of a trephine biopsy allow a more accurate assessment of the extent of infiltration (Figs 6.24 and 6.25). There is some correlation of clinical stage with the nature and degree of infiltration.[199, 200] It has been observed that in Rai stages 0, 1 and 2, infiltration is usually either interstitial (with preservation of architecture), nodular, or mixed interstitial and nodular and that in stages 3 and 4 it is diffuse (with loss of architecture), or diffuse and nodular.[199] A nodular infiltrate has been found to be more common in the early stages and an interstitial or diffuse infiltrate in the later stages; a nodular infiltrate is said to be associated with a better prognosis, regardless of stage.[201] With disease progression the histological pattern may change from nodular to diffuse and with disease regression the reverse may be observed.[202] Occasionally, treatment may lead to the return of the biopsy appearance to normal.

Lymph nodes

Lymph nodes are generally, but not always, enlarged. Lymphadenopathy is symmetrical, with involvement of many node groups. Histologically, lymph nodes are diffusely infiltrated by small lymphocytes with round nuclei and clumped chromatin. In a minority of patients (less than 10%) the infiltrate also contains some plasma cells. Mitotic figures are rare. In about 50% of patients, lymph nodes contain cells which are less mature than those in the peripheral blood and bone marrow.[203] Such cells may range from medium-sized lymphocytes with nucleoli to large blast-like cells with vesicular nuclei and prominent nucleoli. The mitotic index is higher in lymph nodes containing less mature cells. When proliferation of less mature cells is focal, a pseudonodular pattern is produced; in contradistinction to follicular lymphoma, peripheral compression of reticulin fibres does not occur.[203] In a minority of cases pleomorphic and polyploid cells may be seen. A moderate degree of immaturity may not indicate a worse prognosis; a marked degree of immaturity is a late development.[203]

Liver

The liver is commonly enlarged. Infiltration is detected microscopically in the great majority of cases; it is predominantly periportal and to a lesser extent sinusoidal. Hepatic fibrosis is seen in about 40% of autopsies, with pseudolobule formation and bile duct proliferation; in approximately 10% there is fully developed cirrhosis which has no other apparent cause.[204]

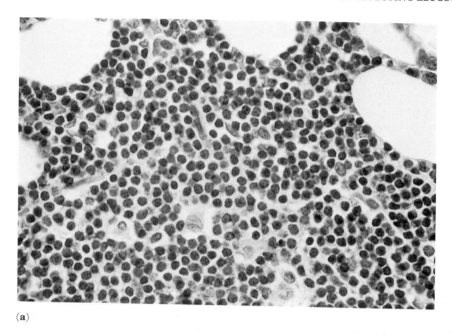

(a)

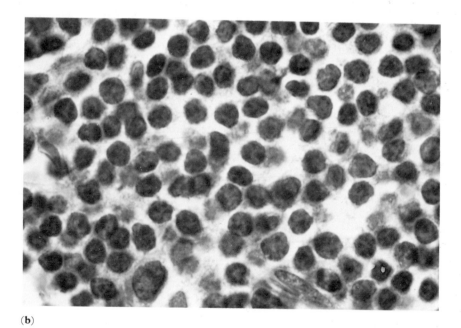

(b)

Fig. 6.24a,b Section of an aspirated bone marrow particle from a case of chronic lymphocytic leukaemia. The majority of the cells have a uniform appearance and consist of small lymphocytes with round hyperchromatic nuclei and scanty cytoplasm.

Haematoxylin–eosin   (**a**) × 375; (**b**) × 940

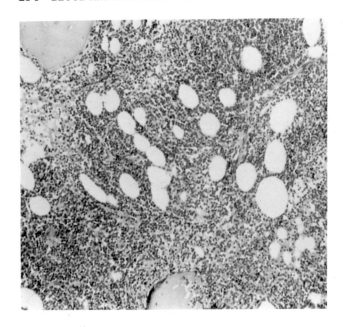

Fig. 6.25 Trephine biopsy of bone marrow from a patient with chronic lymphocytic leukaemia. The marrow is hypercellular due to diffuse infiltration by a uniform population of small lymphocytes.

Haematoxylin–eosin   × 940

Spleen

The spleen is clinically enlarged in the majority of patients. In a small minority of patients the disease appears to be largely confined to the spleen.[205] Infiltration is diffuse in the red pulp and more compact in the white pulp. With disease progression, white pulp infiltrates coalesce into large masses which compress the red pulp.[206]

Other lymphoid organs

The tonsils and adenoids may be infiltrated. The thymus is rarely enlarged. Gastrointestinal lymphoid tissues may be infiltrated.

Skin

Skin lesions may be infiltrative (plaques, ulcers, tumours and exfoliative erythroderma) or non-specific and non-infiltrative (urticaria, increased pigmentation).

Eye

Infiltration of the eye is less common in CLL than in CGL or the acute leukaemias. Infiltration of the iris, with hyphaema, and secondary glaucoma[207] and glaucoma probably attributable to infiltration of the limbus[208] have been reported. Microaneurysms may be seen in the retina but less commonly than in CGL.[140]

Other organs

Lytic bone lesions, pathological fractures and hypercalcaemia are rare. Corticosteroid-related osteoporosis may be seen. Urolithiasis is found in approximately 8% of patients at autopsy.[209] Renal infiltration is common on microscopy, occurring particularly in the subcapsular cortex and along the vasa recta at the corticomedullary junction. Fibrosis is usually associated with tubular atrophy and glomerular sclerosis.[204] Uraemia related to the leukaemia is found in approximately 3% of patients, being secondary to infiltration, stone formation or the compression of ureters by enlarged lymph nodes. Prostatic infiltration may cause acute urinary retention.[210] Pulmonary infiltration is mainly septal, perivascular and peribronchial: radiological abnormalities (diffuse, miliary or nodular) are uncommon. Infiltration of the pleura may cause pleural effusion. In an autopsy series adrenal infiltration was seen in 70% and pancreatic infiltration in 37%. Adrenal infiltration was confined to the medulla. Pancreatic infiltration was associated with prominent fibrosis.[204] Infiltration of the pituitary gland and hypothalamus may cause diabetes insipidus. A rare manifestation is Mikulicz's syndrome due to infiltration of the cornea, sclera, lacrymal glands and salivary glands. The pericardium, myocardium and endocardium may be infiltrated, with associated fibrosis, in a minority.[204, 211] Osteolytic lesions are rare; these may cause hypercalcaemia or pathological fractures.[212, 213].

Leukaemic meningeal infiltration is rare, and the few cases reported have generally not been unequivocally demonstrated to be B-CLL.[214, 215] The presence of neurological symptoms and increased lymphocytes in the cerebrospinal fluid may be due to occult cryptococcal infection rather that CNS infiltration; immunological typing of lymphocytes will help in the distinction by demonstrating monoclonal B-cells when leukaemic infiltration is present.

Amyloidosis

This is a rare concomitant of CLL.[197]

Infective complications

Bacteria which are of low pathogenicity in normal people (e.g. *Staphylococcus epidermidis* [*Staph. albus*]) may cause serious infections. There is a marked susceptibility to pneumococcal infection, both pneumonia and meningitis. Recurrent pneumococcal infections may occur. Fungal infections which occur include candidosis and cryptococcosis. Viruses to which CLL patients are particularly susceptible include herpes simplex, herpes zoster and vaccinia.

Prolymphocytic transformation and Richter's syndrome

Chronic lymphocytic leukaemia uncommonly terminates either in prolymphocytic transformation or in Richter's syndrome (blastic transformation); more commonly death occurs from complications of the disease without cytological change, or from intercurrent disease. Both prolymphocytic transformation and Richter's syndrome result from a further change occurring within the malignant clone; the light and heavy chain type present in the chronic phase is also detectable in the prolymphocytes or blast cells of the more acute phase. In both conditions there are residual typical CLL cells together with the less well-differentiated cells. Prolymphocytic transformation is associated with resistance to standard therapy and a steady increase of the number of prolymphocytes in the blood.[216] There is conflicting evidence as to whether morphological alteration is accompanied by an alteration of cell markers. Some workers have observed no alteration of the quantity of SmIg or of the ability to form M-rosettes,[216] whereas others have found an increase in the quantity of SmIg.[217] Histologically, foci of prolymphocytes in lymph nodes may produce a pseudofollicular appearance.[217] In the bone marrow, prolymphocytes may be present as aggregates or as a diffuse infiltrate either admixed with small lymphocytes or largely replacing them. Splenic infiltration may be nodular or diffuse, involving both the red pulp and the white pulp. Liver infiltration is predominantly around the portal triads and in sinusoids. Infiltrates of large lymphoid cells may also be seen in the lungs, adrenal glands, kidneys and gastrointestinal tract.[217] In Richter's syndrome, transformation (with emergence of a more malignant clone) occurs in one site with spread to other sites. The disease becomes more aggressive, with fever, night sweats, weight loss, rapid growth of tumour tissue at one or more sites and pronounced clinical deterioration. The peripheral blood may show either a persisting CLL picture, or lymphopenia or increasing lymphocytosis with blast cells. The bone marrow is rarely involved by the more malignant cells at transformation but usually is at autopsy. Histologically the disease, which Richter called 'generalized reticular cell sarcoma', resembles large cell lymphoma or immunoblastic sarcoma; the lymphoma cells may be pleomorphic with multinucleated giant cells; cells resembling Reed–Sternberg cells may be present and sometimes lead to a misdiagnosis of lymphocyte-depleted Hodgkin's disease.[218, 219, 220]

T-CLL

T-CLL results from a malignant proliferation of cells with the phenotype of mature T-cells. T-

CLL is morphologically, clinically and immunologically heterogeneous. Unless monoclonality can be demonstrated by cytogenetic studies, it may be difficult to distinguish T-CLL from chronic T-cell lymphocytosis. The latter condition is of uncertain significance but may be an immunoregulatory disorder rather than a malignant condition. T-CLL tends to present at a younger age than B-CLL.[221] The WBC is relatively low. Bone marrow infiltration is moderate in comparison with B-CLL but marked when related to the WBC.[222] There is less lymphadenopathy than in B-CLL; skin infiltration (Fig. 6.26), hepatomegaly and splenomegaly are more prominent.[223, 224] In contrast to mycosis fungoides, skin infiltrates are dermal, without epidermal extension.[222] Bone marrow infiltration may be diffuse or focal. Splenic infiltration is in the red pulp.[225] Leukaemic meningeal infiltration, which is rare in B-CLL, appears to be more common in T-CLL.[215] The malignant cells lack SmIg and do not form rosettes with mouse red blood cells. They do form rosettes with sheep red blood cells and give positive reactions with monoclonal antibodies directed at T-lymphocytes (OKT1/Leu 1 [weak], OKT3/Leu 4); they are usually of suppressor-cytotoxic phenotype (OKT5,8/Leu 2 +), or less often helper phenotype (OKT4/Leu 3+), but may show neither set of markers or both.[94] Morphologically, the cells are not always distinguishable from those of B-CLL (Fig. 6.27) but may show convoluted nuclei, abundant cytoplasm and prominent azurophilic granules. The cells of T-CLL are usually strongly positive for acid phosphatase and negative or weakly-positive for α-naphthyl acetate esterase and may be positive for the Ia antigen. In contrast to cells of T-ALL, TdT is not elevated. On electron microscopy, parallel tubular arrays

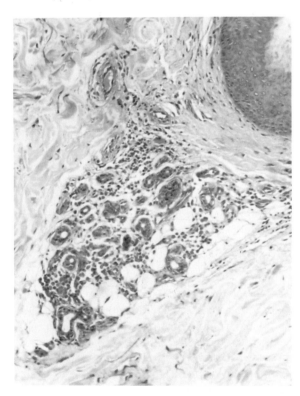

Fig. 6.26 Skin biopsy of a patient with T-CLL whose peripheral blood film is shown in Figure 6.27. There is a lymphocytic infiltrate around the sweat glands in the dermis.

Haematoxylin–eosin   × 94

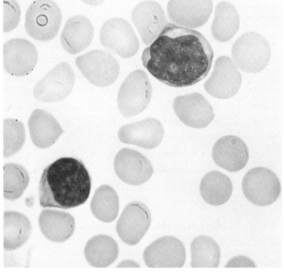

Fig. 6.27 Peripheral blood smear of a patient with T-CLL, showing a mature small lymphocyte with considerable quantities of condensed chromatin and a somewhat less mature lymphocyte with a nucleolus and a more diffuse chromatin pattern. In this case, the majority of the cells were mature small lymphocytes which were morphologically similar to those of B-CLL, but which lacked surface membrane immunoglobulin and formed rosettes with sheep red blood cells.

May-Grünwald-Giemsa stain   × 940

within lysosomes are characteristic but not pathognomonic; these may correspond to the prominent azurophilic granules seen under the light microscope.[226] Immunoglobulin levels are usually normal or high (polyclonal hypergammaglobulinaemia) but hypogammaglobulinaemia may occur, as a result of the suppression of immunoglobulin synthesis by the T-cells.[227] Neutropenia,[222, 228] pure red cell aplasia,[222, 227] and megaloblastic anaemia[221] may also be due to effects of the T-lymphocytes on other cell lines. The clinical course of T-CLL may be more aggressive than that of B-CLL. Intraclonal evolution to a large-cell lymphoma may occur.

It has been suggested[225] that there may be clinical and pathological differences between T4-positive and T8-positive T-CLL, with the former having higher lymphocyte counts, small agranular lymphocytes, more infiltration of bone marrow and other organs, and a worse prognosis, while the latter has large lymphocytes with prominent azurophilic granules and on electron microscopy parallel tubular arrays,[229] and is more likely to show neutropenia.

PROLYMPHOCYTIC LEUKAEMIA

Definition

Prolymphocytic leukaemia (PLL) is a disease caused by a monoclonal proliferation of cells which are more mature than the lymphoblasts of ALL but less mature than the lymphocytes of CLL. The majority are of B-cell origin (B-PLL, 82%) and a minority of T-cell origin (T-PLL, 18%).[230]

Prevalence

PLL is commonest in the elderly; there is a male preponderance both in B-PLL and T-PLL.

Aetiology

The aetiology of this disease is unknown. Cytogenetic abnormalities are common.

Pathogenesis

Clinical features are consequent on a considerable degree of splenomegaly, with hypersplenism leading to pancytopenia, and on the proliferation of leukaemic cells which may cause fatigue, weight loss, and other systemic symptoms. Cases of B-PLL characteristically have marked splenomegaly and little lymph node enlargement while cases of T-PLL may have lymphadenopathy, hepatomegaly and skin infiltrates in addition to marked splenomegaly. The prognosis of T-PLL is considerably worse than that of B-PLL.[231]

Pathology

Peripheral blood

The WBC is characteristically very high; it is usually greater than $100 \times 10^9/1$ and may be as high as $1000 \times 10^9/1$. The majority of the cells are larger than the lymphocytes of CLL, with more abundant cytoplasm, a less condensed chromatin pattern and a prominent nucleolus. Such cells are called prolymphocytes (Fig. 6.28). They are less

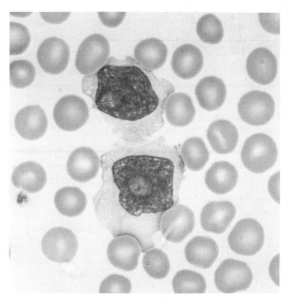

Fig. 6.28 Peripheral blood smear of a patient with prolymphocytic leukaemia (PLL), showing two typical prolymphocytes. When compared with CLL cells, PLL cells are larger and have a more diffuse chromatin pattern, a more prominent nucleolus and more abundant cytoplasm.

May–Grünwald–Giemsa stain   × 940

mechanically fragile than the lymphocytes of CLL and, therefore, are not prone to form smear cells. The morphological features of the leukaemic cells of cases of B-PLL and T-PLL are very similar, both on light and electron microscopy,[232] though the cells of T-PLL sometimes have an irregular nucleus.[189] Anaemia, neutropenia and thrombocytopenia are usual. On electron microscopy PLL cells appear more active than CLL cells with more prominent mitochondria and rough endoplasmic reticulum; the nucleolus is usually very large. The leukaemic cells of patients with B-PLL have heavy monoclonal SmIg, which is usually IgM but in some patients is IgM plus IgD or IgD or IgG alone. The percentage of MRFC is lower in PLL than in CLL. PLL cells are positive for the Ia antigen and react positively with monoclonal antibodies directed against B-cells, such as B1. In addition, B-PLL cells share with B-CLL cells a reactivity with monoclonal antisera which otherwise react only with T-cells (OKT1, Leu 1, T101).[94] The monoclonal antibody FMC7 which reacts with cells of a minority of patients with B-CLL usually reacts with the cells of patients with B-PLL. T-PLL cells form E-rosettes. They also usually stain positively for acid phosphatase but in contrast to T-CLL cells the reaction may be weak. T-PLL cells show a strong dot positivity when stained for α-naphthyl acetate esterase, whereas T-CLL cells stain weakly or not at all.[230] When investigated with monoclonal antibodies and heteroantisera, the cells of most cases of T-PLL show a helper phenotype (OKT3+, OKT4+, OKT8−); those of some cases display a suppressor/cytotoxic phenotype (OKT3+, OKT4−, OKT8+, anti-Tγ1+),[231] and those of other patients cannot be categorized as showing either of these phenotypes. A patient has been described whose PLL cells had both B- and T-markers. Erythrophagocytosis by PLL cells has been described;[233] this is a non-specific phenomenon which is occasionally observed with malignant cells.

Cytogenetics

Marker chromosomes are common; a specific chromosome abnormality t(6;12) is characteristic of B-PLL[234] and 14q+ and 6q− are also common.

Bone marrow

The bone marrow is heavily infiltrated with leukaemic cells; the infiltrate is partly nodular and partly diffuse[235] (Fig. 6.29). In contrast to the paratrabecular distribution of malignant cells in many lymphomas, the infiltration in PLL is concentrated in the centre of the intertrabecular space.[206]

Lymph nodes

Lymphadenopathy may be minimal or clinically undetectable. Microscopically, infiltration is preferentially in the mantles of the follicles or in the paracortical region and medullary cords.[206] With more advanced disease, lymph nodes may be heavily infiltrated by prolymphocytes, though with some preservation of architecture and with a vague nodularity.[206]

Spleen

Splenomegaly is usually striking, with the spleen weighing up to 3 kg or more. Occasionally the spleen is impalpable. Infiltration is usually of both the red and white pulp. In all patients there is heavy, diffuse infiltration of the red pulp and occasionally the infiltrate is confined to the red pulp. In the white pulp, infiltration is more compact and dense and is preferentially around the arterioles. With progressive disease, expanding white pulp infiltrates compress the red pulp.[206] Cytological differences from CLL are most readily detected in the red pulp where prolymphocytes appear larger, have nucleoli and often have notched nuclei.

Liver

Hepatomegaly is slight. Microscopically there is heavy infiltration of the portal tracts and a lesser degree of infiltration of sinusoids.[206]

Therapy

Cases of PLL may benefit from chemotherapy but the leukaemic cells are more resistant than

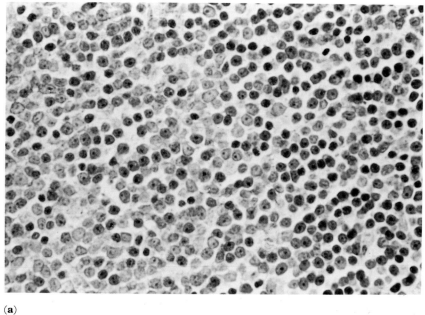

(a)

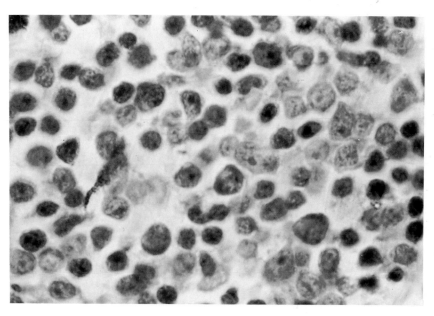

(b)

Fig. 6.29a,b Trephine biopsy of bone marrow from a patient with prolymphocytic leukaemia (PLL) showing marked diffuse infiltration with leukaemia cells. When compared with CLL cells, many of the PLL cells are larger and have a more diffuse chromatin pattern and more prominent nucleoli.

Haematoxylin-eosin   (**a**) × 375; (**b**) × 940

those of CLL. Occasional complete remissions have occurred with aggressive chemotherapy. Splenic irradiation, splenectomy and leucaphaeresis may be of benefit.

HAIRY CELL LEUKAEMIA (LEUKAEMIC RETICULOENDOTHELIOSIS)

Definition

Hairy cell leukaemia (HCL) results from a monoclonal proliferation of a lymphoid cell of unusual phenotype characterized by distinctive morphology and cytochemistry.[236] In the great majority of cases the malignant cell appears to be a B-cell but in a minority it is a T-cell. The cell of origin may be a splenic cell.[237]

Prevalence

The disease is most common in the middle-aged, with a median age of presentation in the sixth decade and a marked male preponderance.[238, 239]

Aetiology

The aetiology is unknown. A single patient with T-cell hairy cell leukaemia has been reported to have serum antibodies to a human T-cell leukaemia-lymphoma virus and this patient's cultured T-lymphocytes expressed viral antigen (see p. 264).[240] Whether these observations are coincidental or relevant to aetiology is uncertain.

Pathogenesis

Hairy cells show a predilection to infiltrate and proliferate in the bone marrow and the spleen with relative sparing of lymph nodes. Bone marrow infiltration leads to chronic bone marrow failure, pancytopenia being usual. Splenomegaly secondary to splenic infiltration may aggravate the cytopenia. Clinical presentation usually results from constitutional symptoms, bleeding associated with thrombocytopenia, or symptomatic splenomegaly.

Pathology

Peripheral blood

The majority of patients have hairy cells in the peripheral blood but such cells may be quite infrequent. Hairy cells are larger (diameter 10–20 μm) and have more abundant pale-blue cytoplasm (Romanowsky stain) than normal lymphocytes. Characteristically they have thread-like cytoplasmic processes extending outwards from the cell surface (Figs 6.30 and 6.31). The nucleus is usually round or oval with a fine chromatin pattern; less often it is convoluted, indented or shaped like a dumb-bell. On electron microscopy, the most characteristic finding is the ribosomal-lamellar complex which is found in about half the cases (Fig. 6.32) and which is also seen in a minority of patients with CLL and in some non-haemopoietic tissues.[241] Pyroninophilic rod-shaped inclusions which correspond to ribosomal-lamellar complexes may be seen on light microscopy.[242] Anaemia is common and is usually due to bone marrow infiltration and the effects of splenomegaly (see p. 156). Uncommonly, autoimmune haemolytic anaemia occurs. Neutropenia, thrombocytopenia and monocytopenia are usual. Neutrophil alkaline phosphatase activity is usually increased. Macrocytosis and dyserythropoiesis may occur. Platelet function may be abnormal, probably as a consequence of an *in vivo* release reaction causing an acquired storage pool defect.[243] Hairy cells appear to be B-lymphocytes in the great majority of cases, but some of their characteristics are unusual. They are phagocytic both for bacteria and latex particles and they are capable of adhering to glass. Small amounts of endogenously produced SmIg are present; Fc and C receptors may also be present. HCL cells may form rosettes with mouse red blood cells but the percentage of rosetting cells is smaller in HCL than in CLL. Hairy cells give positive reactions with monoclonal antibodies against B-lymphocytes but not in general with those against T-lymphocytes or monocytes/macrophages.[244] An exception to the latter is positivity with monoclonal antibody OKM-1, which otherwise is known only to react with cells of the monocyte and granulocyte lineages.[245] Hairy cells show acid phosphatase activity which is tartrate-

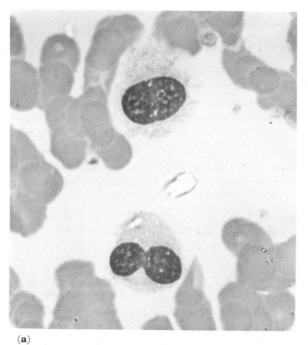

(a)

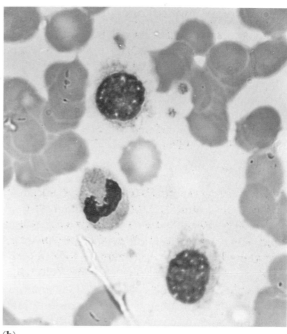

(b)

Fig. 6.30a,b Four hairy cells and a neutrophil from the bone marrow smear of a patient with hairy cell leukaemia. The hairy cells are larger than CLL cells and have a more open nuclear chromatin pattern and more abundant cytoplasm which often has characteristic hair-like surface projections. The nuclei of hairy cells may be round, oval or dumb-bell-shaped.

May–Grünwald–Giemsa stain   × 940

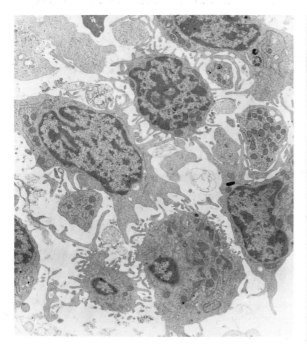

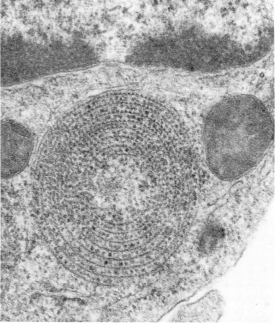

Fig. 6.31 Electron micrograph of hairy cells from the bone marrow of a patient with hairy cell leukaemia. The leukaemic cells have numerous fine ('hair-like') cytoplasmic processes projecting from the cell surface.

Uranyl acetate and lead citrate   × 5025

Fig. 6.32 Electron micrograph of part of a hairy cell showing a ribosomal lamellar complex.

Uranyl acetate and lead citrate   × 49 300

resistant (isoenzyme 5 of acid phosphatase); this activity is highly characteristic but neither pathognomonic nor invariably present. Several examples of patients with T-cell HCL have also been described[246, 247] as have patients whose cells showed both T and B characteristics.[248] A polyclonal increase of immunoglobulins is seen in about a half of the patients with HCL.[239]

Bone marrow[239, 249]

Bone marrow aspiration is usually difficult and a 'dry tap' is common. If this occurs diagnosis may be aided by making imprints from a trephine biopsy for cytological and cytochemical studies. Histological sections of bone marrow trephine biopsies show an infiltrate of hairy cells (Fig. 6.33). The infiltrating cells form small multiple patches (25% of cases), large confluent infiltrates (50% of cases) or completely replace the marrow (25% of cases).[239] The infiltration shows no specific topographic pattern. In some patients the marrow is hypoplastic, with only small numbers of hairy cells, and aplastic anaemia is simulated.[250] Hairy cells appear relatively uniform with a wide rim of water-clear or finely-reticulated cytoplasm so that the nuclei appear widely spaced. Nuclei may be round, oval, indented or convoluted, with stippled chromatin and no obvious nucleoli. In some cases there are foci containing fusiform cells which resemble proliferating fibroblasts.[249] Reticulin fibres are increased in infiltrated areas. Sinusoids are sometimes disintegrated, with oedema of the marrow and extravasation of erythrocytes.[239]

Bone

Osteoporosis is found in about a third of patients.[239] Osteosclerosis occurs but is uncommon,[239] as are osteolytic lesions and pathological fractures.[251]

Spleen

Splenomegaly is usual, but not invariable, and is moderate to marked. Infiltration is characteristically of the red pulp, sparing the follicles and T-cell zones. Pulp cords are engorged and sinuses are distended by hairy cells; endothelial cell destruction leads to the formation of pseudosinuses lined by hairy cells.[252, 253] Gradually the infiltrate encroaches on the white pulp as well. Hairy cells may accumulate in the subendothelial lymphatics of trabecular veins and narrow the venous lumen. Plasma cells and phagocytic macrophages may be increased in numbers with haemophagocytosis by the latter possibly contributing to the pancytopenia. Splenic infarction and rupture may occur. Splenic red cell pooling occurs in excess of that seen in myeloproliferative or other lymphoproliferative disorders with a comparable degree of splenomegaly.[254]

Liver

Hepatomegaly is present in about a half of the patients. Infiltration is particularly in the portal areas and the sinusoids.[255] As in the spleen, hairy cells attach to the lining cells of sinusoids, destroying them and leading to the formation of pseudosinuses. These may be detected in hepatic biopsies in clusters which resemble angiomas. Massive dilation of sinuses may produce a lesion resembling peliosis hepatis.[256]

Lymph nodes

Lymphadenopathy is present in less than 10% of patients.[239] Infiltrated lymph nodes have hairy cells in the medulla and paracortical zone.[257] Plasma cells may also be increased in lymph nodes.

Other organs

Infiltration may be seen in the kidneys, lungs, pancreas, stomach, small intestine, adrenals, skin and pericardium. Plasma cells may be associated with infiltrating hairy cells. Rarely, meningeal infiltration occurs.[258] One case has been reported in which pulmonary infiltration caused pulmonary insufficiency and death.[259] Coexistence of hairy cell leukaemia and vasculitis (sometimes with the formation of microaneurysms) has been reported in six patients; in one case hairy cells were seen in the abnormal vessels.[260]

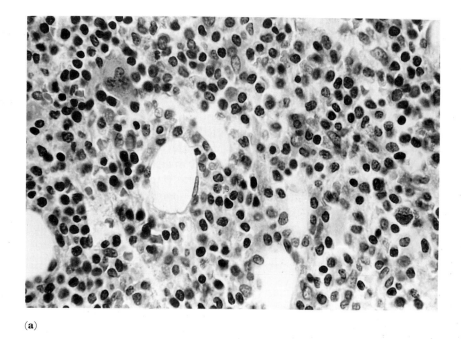

(a)

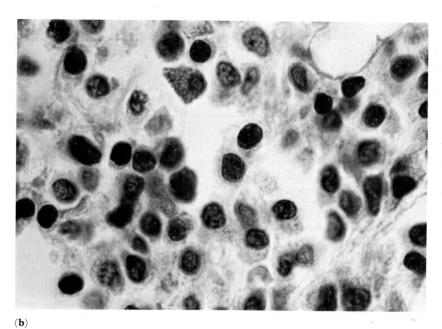

(b)

Fig. 6.33a,b Trephine biopsy of bone marrow from a patient with hairy cell leukaemia. The marrow is extensively infiltrated with leukaemic cells. The nuclei of hairy cells often appear to be more separated from one another when compared with the nuclei of the cells infiltrating the marrow in other lymphoproliferative diseases. At the higher magnification of (b), leukaemic cells showing ragged cytoplasm or hair-like surface projections can be recognized.

Haematoxylin–eosin   (a) × 375; (b) × 940

Infective complications

HCL patients show a marked susceptibility to infective complications: this is attributable to variable hypogammaglobulinaemia, neutropenia and monocytopenia. Bacterial infections are common; infections in which cell-mediated immunity is important are characteristic. The latter include tuberculosis and atypical mycobacterial infections (*Mycobacterium kansasi, M. intracellulare, M. fortuitum, M. gordonae, M. chelonei, M. scrofulaceum*), herpes simplex infection, legionnaires' disease, *Pneumocystis* infection, histoplasmosis, cryptococcosis, candidosis, coccidioidomycosis, blastomycosis and aspergillosis.[261, 262] In different series 10–25% of patients have had mycobacterial infection.[256] Granuloma formation may be defective.[261] Although the nature of the infections seen in HCL suggests poor cell-mediated immunity, T-cells have been reported to function normally *in vitro*.[263]

Treatment

The clinical course of HCL is very variable. Some patients survive for many years without treatment. If pancytopenia is present and the spleen is enlarged, splenectomy is often beneficial. Response to cytotoxic therapy is often poor. Interferon therapy is frequently of benefit.

ADULT T-CELL LEUKAEMIA-LYMPHOMA

Definition

Adult T-cell leukaemia–lymphoma (ATLL) is a lymphoproliferative disease resulting from malignant transformation of T-cells of mature phenotype and associated with a retrovirus infection.

Aetiology[264]

ATLL is strongly associated with the presence of a retrovirus (designated human T-cell leukaemia-lymphoma virus or human T-cell lymphocytopathic virus I, HTLV I) in the malignant lymphoid tissue. Retroviruses may be associated with leukaemia in animals by two possible mechanisms. In natural populations, retroviruses may cause malignant proliferation by activating cellular oncogenes (c-onc). In laboratory populations incomplete retroviruses, which need a helper virus for replication and which contain viral oncogenes (v-onc), may cause malignant proliferation. The mechanism in human ATLL (which has some similarity to a retrovirus-associated malignancy in cattle) is likely to be the former. Integration of provirus into cellular DNA may be at a random site and malignant transformation may occur only when integration is adjacent to a c-onc; this would explain the small proportion of virus-infected subjects who develop leukaemia. It is also possible that a second (unidentified) factor is required in addition to the retrovirus. Chromosomal abnormalities are common in the leukaemic cells.[265]

Prevalence

ATLL has its highest incidence in Japan (Kyushu district), in people of West Indian origin, and in blacks in the south-east of the USA. The areas with the highest incidence of ATLL are the areas with the greatest frequency of serological evidence of previous HTLV I infection. In Japan, ATLL is predominantly a disease of the elderly;[266] in the USA it is a disease predominantly of young Blacks.[267]

Pathogenesis

The pathological findings in ATLL are largely related directly to proliferation of the leukaemic cells, with lymphadenopathy, skin infiltration and to a lesser extent hepatomegaly and splenomegaly. Hypercalcaemia is a common[267] non-infiltrative complication. It is attributable to an osteoclast-stimulating factor secreted by the malignant T-cells; parathormone levels and parathyroid histology are normal.[268] The development of diabetes mellitus at the time of presentation or relapse has been observed in a number of cases.[267] A high incidence of opportunistic infections may be related to suppressor activities of the leukaemic lymphocytes.[266] Immunoglobulin levels may be reduced.[266]

Pathology

Peripheral blood

Malignant cells are usually but not invariably present in the peripheral blood. They are pleomorphic, 9–15 μm in diameter, and have a high nucleocytoplasmic ratio, clumped chromatin and inapparent nucleoli. Nuclei are deeply-lobulated (Figs 6.34 and 6.35), but not as complex and deeply-interwoven as in Sézary cells. The WBC may be very high. Anaemia is present in a minority and thrombocytopenia is unusual. The leukaemic cells form E-rosettes. The acid-phosphatase reaction is positive, with small scattered granules (rather than the focal pattern seen in some malignant T-cells).[269] The leukaemic cells may have Ia antigen. The TdT level may be high[270] or low.[269] Studies with monoclonal antibodies have revealed that the leukaemic cells usually have the phenotype of mature peripheral blood T-cells of helper phenotype (T3+, T4+, T8−). However, functionally they are of suppressor type.[266] They also give positive reactions with a monoclonal antibody, anti-Tac, which reacts with activated T-cells and may possibly be recognizing the receptor for T-cell growth factor.[271]

Bone marrow

At presentation bone marrow infiltration is detectable in about half of the patients. The infiltrate is sparse, with a focal and paratrabecular distribution.

Other organs

Various tissues may be infiltrated by pleomorphic leukaemic cells with lobulated nuclei. Skin lesions are usually disseminated and may take the form of erythroderma, papules, nodules and plaques. In addition to dermal infiltration, Pautrier epidermal microabscesses may occur.[267] Lymphadenopathy is generalized but the mediastinum is usually spared. Lymph nodes are usually diffusely replaced by leukaemic cells but the infiltrate may be predominantly in the T-zone;[189] repeated biopsy may show progression from

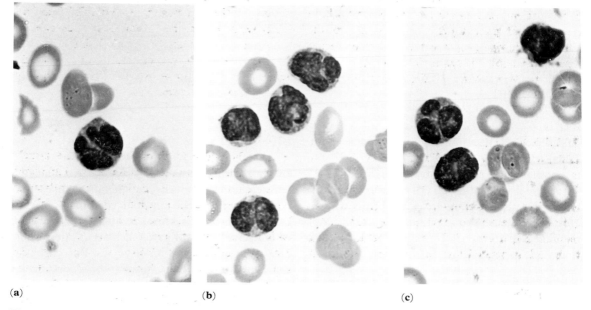

(a)   (b)   (c)

Fig. 6.34a,b,c Peripheral blood film of a patient with adult T-cell leukaemia-lymphoma (ATLL). The malignant cells show deeply-cleft (including clover-leaf-shaped) nuclei, as well as nuclei of highly irregular form.

May–Grünwald–Giemsa stain   × 940

The blood film was provided by Dr J.K. Wood and Dr D. Gill, Department of Haematology, Leicester Royal Infirmary, Leicester, UK

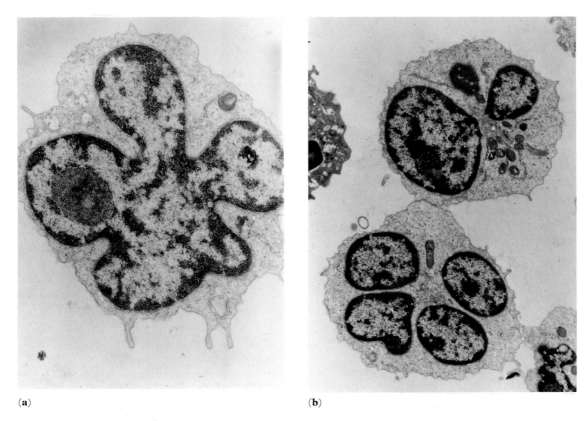

(a)   (b)

Fig. 6.35a,b Various ultrastructural appearances of the circulating lymphocytes from the patient with adult T-cell leukaemia-lymphoma whose blood film is illustrated in Figure 6.34. One of the cell profiles shows five deep nuclear clefts and the others show three or four separate nuclear masses which presumably result from tangential sectioning of deeply-cleft nuclei.

Courtesy of Dr J.K. Wood and Dr D. Gill, Department of Haematology, Leicester Royal Infirmary, Leicester, UK

paracortical infiltration to node effacement. Osteolytic lesions were rare in one series[268] but in another were found in five of 10 patients.[240] The bone lesions often do not contain detectable lymphoma cells but are areas of fibrosis and increased osteoclastic activity.[240] Leukaemic meningeal infiltration may occur.[240]

Disease progression

The condition is subacute or chronic but with a rapidly progressive terminal phase. The prognosis is poor despite initial responsiveness to chemotherapy. Opportunistic infections are common.

BIPHENOTYPIC LEUKAEMIA[272]

In blastic transformation of chronic granulocytic leukaemia the blast cells may be lymphoblasts, or blasts of any of the myeloid cell lines (myeloblasts, erythroblasts, megakaryoblasts) or mixtures of lymphoblasts and myeloid blasts. These cells of diverse phenotype all have the Ph[1] chromosome and are derived from a single precursor cell. Increasing evidence suggests that in acute leukaemia arising *de novo* a mixture of lymphoblasts and myeloblasts may also be present. Both types of blasts may be present at diagnosis, or only a single type may be initially detectable, the second type appearing as the first disappears in response to treatment. In biphenotypic leukaemia, it appears that the leukaemic change has occurred in a pluripotent stem cell capable of giving rise to lymphoid and myeloid progeny.

LEUKAEMOID REACTIONS

A leukaemoid reaction is a haematological response which simulates leukaemia, but which is secondary to a non-leukaemic pathological process. Necessarily, a leukaemoid reaction disappears when the primary pathological condition responsible for it is corrected. The distinction between leukaemia and a leukaemoid reaction may be difficult if the patient dies of the condition suspected of causing the leukaemoid reaction without haematological recovery. Diagnostic difficulties arise particularly in patients with tuberculosis as this disease may not only cause various types of leukaemoid reaction but also complicates the course of certain types of leukaemia which are associated with an impairment of immunological mechanisms. Many of the previously reported cases of 'leukaemoid reaction secondary to tuberculosis' were probably cases of leukaemia coexisting with tuberculosis as the case reports do not contain evidence of haematological recovery following effective anti-tuberculosis therapy.[273] Leukaemoid reactions are described as being myeloid or lymphoid depending on whether they mimic a myeloid or lymphoid leukaemia. Changes in white cells may be associated with anaemia or thrombocytopenia. Causes of leukaemoid reactions are shown in Table 6.13.

Conditions causing a marked neutrophil leucocytosis together with a left shift may simulate chronic granulocytic leukaemia. Distinction of such conditions from leukaemia may be aided by the following characteristics of this type of leukaemoid reaction: (1) lack of basophilia and eosinophilia; (2) the presence of toxic granulation or vacuolation of neutrophils or Döhle bodies; and (3) a normal or high neutrophil alkaline phosphatase score (which contrasts with the low score generally found in chronic granulocytic leukaemia). Some sarcomas and carcinomas causing a leukaemoid reaction contain malignant cells which secrete substances capable of stimulating the formation of granulocyte-macrophage colon-

Table 6.13 Conditions which may cause leukaemoid reactions

MYELOID LEUKAEMOID REACTIONS[274]
Simulating chronic granulocytic leukaemia
  Pneumococcal, meningococcal, staphylococcal, haemophilus and salmonella infections, diphtheria, tuberculosis, bubonic plague
  Following severe haemorrhage or rapid haemolysis
  Response to therapy in megaloblastic anaemia
  Recovery from agranulocytosis, particularly if accompanied by infection
  Eclampsia
  Burns
  Diabetic acidosis
  Carcinoma, with or without metastases
  Sarcoma
  Lymphoma—Hodgkin's disease or non-Hodgkin's lymphoma
  Mercury poisoning
Simulating juvenile myeloid leukaemia
  EB virus infection[275]

Simulating chronic myelomonocytic leukaemia
  Tuberculosis

Simulating acute myeloid leukaemia
  Bone marrow infiltration
  Tuberculosis
  Megaloblastic anaemia plus infection
  Infection complicating alcohol-induced marrow damage
  Infection complicating recovery from agranulocytosis
  Down's syndrome

LYMPHOID LEUKAEMOID REACTIONS
  Pertussis
  Infectious lymphocytosis
  Infectious mononucleosis (EB virus infection)
  Infectious hepatitis (hepatitis A infection)
  Cytomegalovirus infection
  Tuberculosis
  Congenital syphilis
  Carcinoma
  Sarcoma

ies *in vitro*.[276] It is therefore likely that in some patients with tumour-associated myeloid leukaemoid reactions, the haematological changes result from the secretion by the tumour cells of substances stimulating neutrophil granulocytopoiesis. In other patients, leucocytosis may be provoked by tumour necrosis or by bone marrow infiltration.

The peripheral blood picture of acute myeloid leukaemia, and particularly of aleukaemic or subleukaemic leukaemia, may be simulated by bone marrow infiltration or when bone marrow failure is accompanied by a strong stimulus to granulocytopoiesis (e.g. infection). In the latter situation, a bone marrow aspirate performed during an attempt at restoration of granulocytopoiesis may simulate acute myeloblastic leukaemia or acute promyelocytic leukaemia; the lack of Auer rods, the lack of abnormal granules in promyelocytes, and the presence of a normal karyotype help to exclude acute myeloid leukaemia.

Children with Down's syndrome suffer from an increased incidence of acute leukaemia and also show a tendency to develop self-limiting 'leukaemoid reactions' simulating acute myeloid leukaemia. However, some of these apparent leukaemoid reactions may be associated with abnormal chromosomes, in addition to trisomy 21,[277] and may therefore be more correctly regarded as transient leukaemias or spontaneously remitting leukaemias, rather than leukaemoid reactions.

Lymphoid leukaemoid reactions are mainly consequent on infections or non-haemopoietic malignancies. In pertussis and infectious lymphocytosis, the peripheral blood findings may simulate chronic lymphocytic leukaemia but the clinical setting and age allow ready distinction from leukaemia. Other infections characterized by the presence of immature lymphoid cells in the circulation may simulate acute lymphoblastic leukaemia; this type of leukaemoid reaction may occur in infectious mononucleosis, cytomegalovirus infection and infectious hepatitis. Bacterial infections, including congenital syphilis and tuberculosis, may also produce a similar reaction.

REFERENCES

1. Brunning RD. Hum Pathol 1970; 1: 99.
2. Skendzel LP, Hoffman GC. Am J Clin Pathol 1962; 37: 294.
3. Rebuck JW, Barth CL, Petz AJ. Fed Proc 1963; 22: 427.
4. Undritz VE. Schweiz Med Wochenschr 1964; 94: 1365.
5. Oski FA, Naiman JL, Allen DM, Diamond LK. Blood 1962; 20: 657.
6. Blume RS, Wolff SM. Medicine (Baltimore) 1972; 51: 247.
7. Virelizier J-L, Lagrue A, Durandy A, Arenzana F, Oury C, Griscelli C. N Engl J Med 1982; 306: 1055.
8. Argyle JC, Kjeldsberg CR, Marty J, Shigeoka AO, Hill HR. Blood 1982; 60: 672.
9. Oliver JM. Am J Pathol 1978; 93: 221.
10. Kitahara M, Eyre HJ, Simonian Y, Atkin CL, Hasstedt SJ. Blood 1981; 57: 888.
11. Larrocha C, Fernandez de Castro M, Fontana G, Viloria A, Fernandez-Chacon JL, Jimenez C. Scand J Haematol 1982; 29: 389.
12. Groover RV, Burke EC, Gordon H, et al. Semin Hematol 1972; 9: 371.
13. Good RA, Quie PG, Windhorst DR, Page AR, Rodey GE, White J, Wolfson JJ, Holmes BH. Semin Hematol 1968; 5: 215.
14. Johnston RB, Baehner RL. Pediatrics 1971; 48: 730.
15. Segal AW, Cross AR, Garcia RC, Borregaard N, Valerius NH, Soothill JH, Jones OTG. N Engl J Med 1983; 308: 245.
16. Cooper MR, de Chatelet LR, McCall CE, La Via MF, Spurr CL, Baehner RL. J Clin Invest 1972; 51: 769.
17. Matsuda I, Oka Y, Taniguchi N, Furuyama M, Kodama S, Arashima S, Mitsuyama T. J Pediatr 1976; 88: 581.
18. Fischer A, Trung PH, Descamps-Latscha B, et al. Lancet 1983; ii: 473.
19. Arnaout MA, Pitt J, Cohen HJ, Melamed J, Rosen FS, Colten HR. N Engl J Med 1982; 306: 693.
20. Rozenszajn L, Klajman A, Yaffe D, Efrati P. Blood 1966; 28: 258.
21. Boxer LA, Hedley-White ET, Stossel TP. N Engl J Med 1976; 291: 1093.
22. Donabedian H, Alling DW, Gallin JI. N Engl J Med 1983; 307: 290.
23. Burge PS, Johnson WS, Hayward AR. Br Med J 1976; 1: 742.
24. Shurin SB, Cohen HJ, Whitin JC, Newburger PE. Blood 1983; 62: 564.
25. Parmley RT, Tzeng DY, Baehner RL, Boxer LA. Blood 1983; 62: 538.
26. Boxer LA, Coates TD, Haak RA, Wolach JB, Hoffstein S, Baehner RL. N Engl J Med 1983; 307: 404.
27. Seger R, Wildfeuer A, Buchinger G, et al. Klin Wochenschr 1976; 54: 177.
28. Schofield KP, Stone PCW, Beddall AC, Stuart J. Br J Haematol 1983; 53: 15.
29. Itoga T, Laszlo J. Blood 1962; 20: 688.
30. Abernathy MR. Blood 1966; 27: 380.
31. Hernandez JA, Aldred SW, Bruce JR, Vanatta PR, Mattingly TL, Sheehan WW. Lancet 1980; ii: 642.
32. Boutilier MB, Hardy NM, Saffos RO. Lancet 1981; i: 53.
33. Faden H, Humbert J, Lee J, Sutyla P, Ogra PL. Blood 1981; 58: 221.
34. Tauber AI. Am J Med 1981; 70: 1237.
35. Gahmberg CG, Andersson LC, Ruutu P, et al. Blood 1979; 54: 4011.
36. Grange RW, Black MM, Carrington P, McKerron R. Lancet 1977; ii: 379.
37. Zielinski CC, Götz M, Ahmad R, Eibl MM. N Engl J Med 1982; 306: 486.
38. Palmblad J, Hallberg D, Engstedt L. Br J Haematol 1980; 44: 101.
39. Craddock PR, Yawata Y, Van Santen L, Gilberstadt S, Silvis S, Jacob HS. N Engl J Med 1974; 290: 1403.
40. Jayaswal U, Roper S, Roath S. J Clin Pathol 1983; 36: 449.
41. de Gruchy GC. Drug-induced blood disorders. Oxford: Blackwell Scientific Publications, 1975.
42. Arneborn P, Palmblad J. Acta Med Scand 1982; 212: 289.
43. Dameshek W, Colmes A. J Clin Invest 1936; 15: 85.

44. Hartl W. Semin Hematol 1965; 2: 313.
45. Pisciotta AV. Clin Pharmacol Ther 1971; 12: 1.
46. Pisciotta AV. Semin Hematol 1973; 10: 279.
47. Ritchie JC, Sloan TP, Idle JR, Smith RL. Ciba Foundation Symposium 76 on environmental chemicals, enzyme function and human disease. Amsterdam: Elsevier, 1980: 219.
48. Boxer LA, Greenberg MS, Boxer GJ, Stossel TP. N Engl J Med 1975; 293: 748.
49. Verheught FWA, von dem Borne AEG, van Noord-Bokhorst JC, Engelfriet CP. Br J Haematol 1978; 39: 339.
50. Verheught FWA, van Noord-Bokhorst JC, von dem Borne AEG, et al. Vox Sang 1979; 36: 1.
51. Halvorsen K. Acta Paediatr Scand 1965; 54: 86.
52. Bagby GC Jr, Lawrence J, Neerhout RC. N Engl J Med 1983; 309: 1073.
53. Agar JW, Hull JD, Kaplan M, Pletka PG. Ann Intern Med 1979; 90: 792.
54. Jacob HS, Craddock PR, Hammerschmidt DE, Moldow CF. N Engl J Med 1980; 302: 789.
55. Price TH, Lee MY, Dale DC, Finch CA. Blood 1979; 54: 581.
56. Kyle RA, N Engl J Med 1980; 302: 908.
57. Greenberg PL, Mara B, Steed S, Boxer L. Blood 1980; 55: 915.
58. Reimann HA, De Berardinis CT. Blood 1949; 4: 1109.
59. von Schulthess GK, Fehr J, Dehinden C. Blood 1983; 62: 320.
60. Krance RA, Spruce WE, Forman SJ, Rosen RB, Hecht T, Hammond WP, Blume KG. Blood 1982; 60: 1263.
61. Cutting HO, Lang JE. Ann Intern Med 1964; 61: 876.
62. Kostmann R. Acta Paediatr Scand 1956; 45: 105 (suppl).
63. Zucker-Franklin D, L'Esperance P, Good RA. Blood 1977; 49: 425.
64. De Vaal OM, Seynhaeve V. Lancet 1959; ii: 1123.
65. Shwachman H, Diamond LK, Oski FA, Khaw KT. J Pediatr 1964; 65: 645.
66. Aggett PJ, Harries JT, Harvey BAM, Soothill JF. J Pediatr 1979; 94: 391.
67. Lux SE, Johnston RB, August CS, Say B, Penchazadeh VB, Rosen FS, McKusick VA. N Engl J Med 1970; 282: 231.
68. Lonsdale D, Deodhar SD, Mercer RD. J Pediatr 1967; 71: 790.
69. Miller ME, Oski FA, Harris MB. Lancet 1971; i: 665.
70. Parmley RT, Crist WA, Ragab AH, et al. Blood 1980; 56: 465.
71. Beeson PB, Bass DA. The eosinophil. Philadelphia: Saunders, 1977.
72. Dvorak HF, Dvorak AM. Clin Haematol 1975; 4: 651.
73. Twomey JJ, Douglass CC, Sharkey O Jr. Blood 1973; 41: 187.
74. Rinehart JJ, Sagone AL, Balcerzak SP, Ackerman GA, Lo Buglio AF. N Engl J Med 1975; 292: 236.
75. Zacharski LR, Linman JW. Mayo Clin Proc 1971; 46: 168.
76. Kimura N, Niho Y, Yanase T. Scand J Haematol 1982; 28: 417.
77. Hocking W, Goodman J, Golde D. Blood 1983; 61: 600.
78. Slungaard A, Ascensao J, Zanjani E, Jacob HS. N Engl J Med 1983; 309: 778.
79. Bryant DH. Aust NZ J Med 1978; 8: 456.
80. Anonymous. Lancet 1983; i: 1417.
81. Spry CJF, Tai PC. Clin Exp Immunol 1976; 24: 423.
82. Brockington IF, Olsen EG. Am Heart J 1973; 85: 308.
83. Yakulis R, Bedetti CD. Arch Pathol Lab Med 1983; 107: 531.
84. Maldonado JE, Hanlon DG. Mayo Clin Proc 1965; 40: 248.
85. Krause JR, Kaplan SS. Scand J Haematol 1981; 28: 15.
86. Ahronheim G, Auger F, Joncas JH, Ghibu F, Rward G-E, Raab-Traub N. N Engl J Med 1983; 309: 313.
87. Purtilo DT. Lancet 1980; i: 300.
88. Hanto DW, Frizzira G, Gajl-Peczalska KJ, et al. N Engl J Med 1982; 306: 913.
89. Schubach WH, Hackman R, Neiman PE, Miller G, Thomas ED. Blood 1982; 60: 180.
90. Saemundsen AK, Berkel AI, Henle W, et al. Br Med J 1981; 282: 425.
91. Hochberg FH, Miller G, Schooley RT, Hirsch MS, Feorino P, Henle W. N Engl J Med 1983; 309: 745.
92. Amromin GD. Pathology of leukaemia. New York: Hoeber, 1968.
93. Kohler G, Milstein C. Nature 1975; 256: 495.
94. Foon KA, Schroff RW, Gale RP, et al. Blood 1982; 60: 1.
95. Schroff RW, Foon KA, Billing RJ, Fahey JL. Blood 1982; 59: 207.
96. Thurlow PJ, McKenzie IFC. Aust NZ J Med 1983; 13: 91.
97. Hsu S-M, Cossman J, Jaffe ES. Am J Clin Pathol 1983; 80: 21.
98. Shamoto M. J Clin Pathol 1983; 36: 307.
99. Stein H, Gerdes J, Mason DY. Clin Haematol 1983; 11: 531.
100. Knowles DM, Halper JP, Azzo W, Wang CY. Cancer 1983; 52: 1369.
101. Warnke RA, Gatter KC, Falini B, et al. N Engl J Med 1983; 309: 1275.
102. Breard J, Reinherz EL, Kung PC, Goldstein G, Schlossman SF. J Immunol 1980; 124: 1943.
103. Borne AEG Kr von dem. Vox Sang 1983; 45: 168.
104. Lund E, Lie SO. Scand J Haematol 1983; 31: 488.
105. Bennett JM, Catovsky D, Daniel MT, et al. Br J Haematol 1982; 51: 189.
106. Bennett JM, Catovsky D, Daniel MT, et al. Br J Haematol 1976; 33: 451.
107. Bennett JM, Catovsky D, Daniel MT, et al. Br J Haematol 1980; 44: 169.
108. Neel BG, Jhan War SC, Chaganti RSK, Hayward WS. Proc Natl Acad Sci USA 1982; 79: 7842.
109. Yunis JJ, Bloomfield CD, Ensrud K. N Engl J Med 1981; 305: 135.
110. Le Beau MM, Larson RA, Bitter MA, Vardiman JW, Golomb HM, Rowley JD. N Engl J Med 1983; 309: 630.
111. Kaneko Y, Rowley JD, Maurer HS, Variakojis D, Moohr JW. Blood 1982; 60: 389.
112. Golomb HM, Alimena G, Rowley JD, Vardiman JW, Testa JR, Sovik C. Blood 1982; 60: 404.
113. Burkhardt R, Frisch B, Bartl R. J Clin Pathol 1982; 35: 257.
114. Frei E, Fritz RD, Price E, Moore EW, Thomas LB. Cancer 1962; 16: 1089.
115. Burton JL. Br J Dermatol 1980; 102: 239.

116. Goodfellow A, Calvert H. Lancet 1979; ii: 478.
117. Burns CP, Armitage JO, Frey AL, Dick FR, Jordan JE, Woolson RF. Cancer 1981; 47: 2460.
118. Holt JM, Gordon Smith EC. Br J Ophthalmol 1969; 53: 145.
119. Neimann RS, Barcos M, Berard C, et al. Cancer 1981; 48: 1426.
120. Jetha N. Arch Pathol Lab Med 1981; 105: 683.
121. Bain BJ, Catovsky D, O'Brien M, et al. Blood 1981; 58: 206.
122. Lewis DS, Thompson M, Hudson E, Liberman MM, Samson D. Acta Haematol (Basel) 1983; 70: 236.
123. Chan WC, Brynes RK, Kim TH, et al. Blood 1983; 62: 92.
124. Lewis SM, Szur L. Br Med J 1963; ii: 472.
125. Ali NO, Janes WD. Cancer 1979; 43: 1211.
126. Weisenburgher DD. Am J Clin Pathol 1980; 73: 128.
127. Yeung K-Y, Trowbridge AA. Cancer 1977; 39: 359.
128. Bird T, Proctor SJ. Am J Clin Pathol 1977; 67: 512.
129. den Ottolander GJ, te Velde J, Bredervo P, et al. Br J Haematol 1979; 42: 9.
130. van Slyck EJ, Weiss L, Dully M. Blood 1970; 36: 729.
131. Clare N, Elson D, Manhoff L. Am J Clin Pathol 1982; 77: 762.
132. Peisson B, Benisch B. Radiology 1977; 125: 62.
133. Wintrobe MM, Lee GR, Boggs DR, et al. Clinical haematology. 8th ed. Philadelphia: 1981: 1457.
134. de Klein A, von Kessel AG, Grosveld G, et al. Nature 1982; 300: 765.
135. Spiers ASD, Bain BJ, Turner JE. Scand J Haematol 1977; 18: 25.
136. Burkhardt R. In: Catovsky D, ed. The leukaemic cell. Edinburgh: Churchill Livingstone, 1981: 49.
137. Burkhardt R, Frisch B, Bartl R. J Clin Pathol 1982; 35: 257.
138. Baccarani M, Zaccaria A, Santucci AM, et al. Ser Haematologica 1975; 8, No 4: 81.
139. Morse PH, McCready JL. Am J Ophthalmol 1971; 72: 975.
140. Jampol LM, Goldberg MF, Busse B. Am J Ophthalmol 1975; 80: 242.
141. Hine JE, Kingham JD. Ann Ophthalmol 1979; 11: 1867.
142. Green D, Dighe P, Ali NO, Katele GV. Cancer 1980; 46: 1763.
143. Bain BJ, Catovsky D, O'Brien M, Spiers ASD, Richards HGH. J Clin Pathol 1977; 30: 235.
144. Ondreyco SM, Kjedlsberg CR, Fineman RM, Vaninetti S, Kushner JP. Cancer 1981; 48: 957.
145. Srodes CH, Hyde EH, Boggs DR. J Clin Invest 1973; 52: 512.
146. Pedersen-Bjergaard J, Philip P, Mortensen BT, et al. Blood 1981; 57: 712.
147. Chessels JM, Sieff CA, Harvey BAM, Pickthall JT, Lawler SD. Br J Haematol 1981; 49: 129.
148. Greenberg PL. Blood 1983; 61: 1035.
149. Juneja SK, Imbert M, Joualt H, Scoazec J-Y, Sigaux F, Sultan C. J Clin Pathol 1983; 36: 1129.
150. Helmstädter V, Arnold H, Blume KG, et al. Acta Haematol (Basel) 1977; 57: 339.
151. Perona G, Guidi GC, Tummarello D, Mareni C, Battistuzzi G, Luzzatto L. Scand J Haematol 1983; 30: 407.
152. Kanatakis S, Chalevelakis G, Economopoulos Th, et al. Scand J Haematol 1983; 30: 89.
153. Breton-Gorius J, Houssay D, Vilde JL, Dreyfus B. Br J Haematol 1975; 30: 273.
154. Schmalzi F, Konwalinka G, Michlmayr G, Abbrederis K, Braunsteiner H. Acta Haematol (Basel) 1978; 59: 1.
155. Gralnick HR, Galton DAG, Catovsky D, Sultan C, Bennett JM. Ann Intern Med 1977; 87: 740.
156. Skinnider LF, Card RT, Padmanabh S. Am J Clin Pathol 1977; 67: 339.
157. Imbert M, Jarry MT, Tulliez M, Breton-Gorius J. J Clin Pathol 1983; 36: 1223.
158. Maldonado JE. Mayo Clin Proc 1976; 51: 452.
159. Seigneurin D, Audhuy B. Am J Clin Pathol 1983; 80: 359.
160. Faille A, Najean Y, Dresch C, et al. Scand J Haematol 1977; 19: 39.
161. Chui DHK, Clarke BJ. Blood 1982; 60: 362.
162. Coiffier B, Adeleine P, Viala JJ, et al. Cancer 1983; 52: 83.
163. Faille A, Dresch C, Poirier O, Balitrand N, Najean Y. Scand J Haematol 1978; 20: 280.
164. Lowenthal RM. Aust NZ J Med 1982; 12: 258.
165. Catovsky D, Pittman S, O'Brien M, et al. Am J Clin Pathol 1979; 72: 736.
166. Rowley JD. Nature 1983; 301: 290.
167. Roper M, Crist WM, Metzgar R, et al. Blood 1983; 61: 830.
168. Anonymous. Lancet 1975; i: 670.
169. Brouet JC, Valensi F, Daniel MT. Br J Haematol 1976; 33: 319.
170. Flandrin G, Brouet JC, Daniel MT, Preud'homme JL. Blood 1975; 45: 183.
171. Neftel KA, Stahel R, Müller OM, Morell A, Arrenbrecht S. Acta Haematol (Basel) 1983; 70: 213.
172. Stein P, Peiper S, Butler D, Melvin S, Williams D, Stass S. Am J Clin Pathol 1983; 79: 426.
173. Ho FCS, Chan GTC, Todd D. Br J Haematol 1983; 53: 171.
174. Sills RH, Stockman JA. Cancer 1981; 48: 110.
175. Breatnach F, Chessels JM, Greaves MF. Br J Haematol 1981; 49: 387.
176. Gafter U, Mandel EM, Weiss S, et al. Acta Haematol (Basel) 1976; 56: 355.
177. Kornberg A, Zimmerman J, Matzner Y, Polliack A. Arch Intern Med 1980; 140: 1236.
178. Goh TS, Le Quesne GW, Wong KY. Am J Dis Child 1978; 132: 1204.
179. Hann IM, Lees PD, Palmer MK, et al. Cancer 1981; 48: 207.
180. Mahoney DH, Fernbach DJ. N Engl J Med 1982; 306: 993.
181. Husta HO, Aur RJA. Clin Haematol 1978; 7: 313.
182. Fonken HA, Ellis PP. Arch Ophthalmol 1966; 57: 585.
183. Manoharan A, Catovsky D, Goldman JM, Lauria F, Lampert IA, Galton DAG. Br J Haematol 1980; 46: 330.
184. Begent R. Br J Hosp Med 1977; 18: 402.
185. Hughes IA. Clin Haematol 1976; 5: 329.
186. Vergani D, Locasciulli A, Masera G, et al. Lancet 1982; i: 361.
187. Chessels J. Br J Haematol 1983; 53: 369.
188. Shalet SM. J R Soc Med 1982; 75: 641.
189. Catovsky D, Linch DC, Beverley PCL. Clin Haematol 1982; 11: 661.
190. Sonner JA, Buchanan GR, Howard-Peebles PN, Rutledge J, Smith RD. N Engl J Med 1983; 309: 590.

191. Caligaris-Cappio F, Gobbi M, Bofill M, Janossy G. J Exp Med 1982; 155: 623.
192. McCann SR, Whelan CA, Willoughby R, Lawlor E, Greally J, Temperley IJ. Br J Haematol 1980; 46: 331.
193. Rai KR, Sawitsky A, Cronkite EP, Chanana AD, Levy RN, Pasternack BS. Blood 1975; 46: 219.
194. Chapman EH, Kurec AS, Davey FR. J Clin Pathol 1981; 34: 1083.
195. Binet JL, Vaugier G, Dighiero G, d'Athis P, Charron D. Am J Med 1977; 63: 683.
196. Pangalis GA, Nathwani BN, Rappaport H. Cancer 1977; 39: 999.
197. Sweet DL, Golomb HM, Ultmann JE. Clin Haematol 1977; 6: 141.
198. Prokocimer M, Polliack A. Am J Clin Pathol 1981; 17: 183.
199. Lipshutz MD, Mir R, Rai KR, Sawitsky A. Cancer 1980; 46: 1422.
200. Rozman C, Hernandez-Nieto L, Montserrat E, Brugues R. Br J Haematol 1981; 47: 529.
201. Bartl R, Frisch B, Burckhardt R, Hoffman-Fezer G, Demmler K. Br J Haematol 1982; 51: 1.
202. Charron D, Dighiero G, Raphael M, Binet JL. Lancet 1977; ii: 819.
203. Dick FR, Maca RD. Cancer 1978; 41: 283.
204. Schwartz JB, Shamsuddin AM. Hum Pathol 1981; 12: 432.
205. Dighiero G, Charron D, Debre P, et al. Br J Haematol 1979; 41: 169.
206. Lampert I, Catovsky D, Marsh GW, Cheld JA, Galton DAG. Histopathol 1980; 4: 3.
207. Martin B. Br J Ophthalmol 1968; 52: 781.
208. Glaser B, Smith JL. Br J Ophthalmol 1966; 50: 92.
209. Hansen MM. Scand J Haematol 1973; (suppl 18).
210. Dajani YF, Burke M. Cancer 1976; 38: 2442.
211. Applefeld MM, Milner SD, Vigorito RD, Shamsuddin AM. Cancer 1980; 46: 1479.
212. McMillan P, Mundy G, Mayer P. Br Med J 1980; 281: 1107.
213. Redmond J, Stites DP, Beckstead JH, George CB, Casavant CH, Gandara DR. Am J Clin Pathol 1983; 79: 616.
214. Liepman MK, Votaw ML. Cancer 1981; 47: 2482.
215. Davies GE. Cancer 1982; 50: 605.
216. Enno A, Catovsky D, O'Brien M, Cherchi M, Kumaran TO, Galton DAG. Br J Haematol 1975; 41: 9.
217. Kjeldsberg CR, Marty J. Cancer 1981; 48: 2447.
218. Long JC, Aisenberg AC. Am J Clin Pathol 1975; 63: 786.
219. Foucar K, Rydell RE. Cancer 1980, 46: 118.
220. Delsol G, Laurent G, Kuhlein E, Familiades J, Rigal F, Pris J. Am J Clin Pathol 1981; 76: 308.
221. Hocking WG, Singh R, Schroff R, Golde DW. Cancer 1983; 51: 631.
222. Catovsky D, Linch DC, Beverley PCL. Clin Haematol 1982; 11: 661.
223. Brouet J-C, Flandrin G, Sasportes M, Preud'homme J-L, Seligmann M. Lancet 1975; ii: 890.
224. Pandolfi F, Strong DM, Slease RB, Smith ML, Ortaldo JR, Herberman RB. Blood 1980; 56: 653.
225. Brisbane JU, Berman LD, Osband ME, Neiman RS. Am J Clin Pathol 1983; 80: 391.
226. Capron F, Perrot JY, Boucheix C, et al. J Clin Pathol 1982; 35: 167.
227. Nagasawa T, Abe T, Nakagawa T. Blood 1981; 57: 1025.
228. Aisenberg AC, Wilkes BM, Harris NL, Ault KA, Carey RW. Blood 1981; 58: 819.
229. Hoffman R, Kopel S, Hsu SD, Dainiak N, Zanjani ED. Blood 1978; 52: 255.
230. Costello C, Catovsky D, O'Brien M, Morilla R, Varadi S. Leuk Res 1980; 4: 463.
231. Catovsky D, Wechsler A, Matutes E, et al. Scand J Haematol 1982; 29: 398.
232. Costello C, Catovsky D, O'Brien M, Galton DAG. Br J Haematol 1980; 44: 389.
233. Martelli MF, Falini B, Tabilio A, Velardi A, Rossodivita M. Br J Haematol 1980; 46: 141.
234. Sadamori N, Han T, Minowada J, Bloom ML, Henderson ES, Sandberg AA. Blood 1983; 62: 729.
235. Bearman RM, Pangalis GA, Rappaport H. Cancer 1978; 42: 2360.
236. Golomb HM, Catovsky D, Golde DW. Ann Intern Med 1978; 89: 677.
237. Galton DAG, Maclennan ICM. Clin Haematol 1982; 11: 561.
238. Sebahoun G, Boufette P, Flandrin G. Leuk Res 1978; 2: 187.
239. Bartl R, Frisch B, Hill W, Burkhardt R, Sommerfeld W, Sund M. Am J Clin Pathol 1983; 79: 529.
240. Blayney DW, Jaffe ES, Blattner WA, et al. Blood 1983; 62: 401.
241. Tubbs RR, Savage RA. N Engl J Med 1983; 309: 616.
242. Rylwin AM. Histopathology of the bone marrow. Boston: Little, Brown and Company, 1976: 125.
243. Nenci GG, Gresele P, Agnelli G, Parise P. Thromb Haemost 1981; 46: 572.
244. Worman CP, Brooks DA, Hogg N, Zola H, Beverly PCL, Cawley JC. Scand J Haematol 1983; 30: 223.
245. Janckila AJ, Stelzer GT, Wallace JH, Yam LT. Am J Clin Pathol 1983; 79: 431.
246. Hernandez D, Cruz C, Carnot J, Dorticos E, Espinosa E. Br J Haematol 1978; 40: 504.
247. Semenzato G, Basso G, Cartei G, Pezzutto A, Cocito MG. Br J Haematol 1980; 46: 491.
248. Jansen J, Schuit HRE, Schreuder GMTH, et al. Blood 1979; 54: 459.
249. Burke JS. Am J Clin Pathol 1978; 70: 876.
250. Brearley RL, Chapman RM, Brozovic B. Ann Intern Med 1979; 91: 228.
251. Demanes DJ, Lane N, Beckstead JH. Cancer 1982; 49: 1697.
252. Pilon VA, Davey FR, Gordon GB. Arch Pathol Lab Med 1981; 105: 577.
253. Pilon V, Davey FR, Gordon GB, Jones DB. Cancer 1982; 49: 1617.
254. Lewis SM, Catovsky D, Hows JM, Ardalan B. Br J Haematol 1977; 35: 351.
255. Yam LT, Janchila AJ, Chan CH, Li C-Y. Cancer 1983; 51: 1497.
256. Case records of the Massachusetts General Hospital. N Engl J Med 1982; 307: 1693.
257. Janchila AJ, Wallace JH, Yam LT. Scand J Haematol 1982; 29: 153.
258. Cotelingam JD, Knop RH, Garvin DE, Mercado TC, Schumacher HR. N Engl J Med 1983; 308: 47.
259. Vardiman JW, Variakojis D, Golomb HM. Cancer 1979; 43: 1339.

260. Krol T, Robinson J, Bekeris L, Messmore H. Arch Pathol Lab Med 1983; 107: 583.
261. Rice L, Shenkenberg T, Lynch EC, Wheeler TM. Cancer 1982; 49: 1924.
262. Stewart DJ, Bodey GP. Cancer 1981; 47: 801.
263. Davey FR, Dock NL, Wolos JA. Br J Haematol 1980; 45: 29.
264. Gallo RC, Wong-Staal F. Blood 1982; 60: 545.
265. Ueshima Y, Fukuhara S, Hattori T, Uchiyama T, Takatsuki K, Uchino H. Blood 1981; 58: 420.
266. Yamada Y. Blood 1983; 61: 192.
267. Bunn PA, Schechter GP, Jaffe E, et al. N Engl J Med 1983; 309: 257.
268. Catovsky D, Greaves MF, Rose M, et al. Lancet 1982; i: 639.
269. Whitcomb CC, Olivella JE, Byrne GE. Cancer 1982; 52: 1202.
270. Nasu K, Tatsumi E, Takiuchi Y, et al. Am J Clin Pathol 1981; 76: 670.
271. Tsudo M, Uchiyama T, Uchino H, Yodoi J. Blood 1983; 61: 1014.
272. Anonymous. Lancet 1983; ii: 1179.
273. Coburn RJ, England JM, Samson DM, et al. Br J Haematol 1973; 25: 793.
274. Krumbhaar EB. Am J Med Sci 1926; 172: 519.
275. Herrod HG, Dow LW, Sullivan JL. Blood 1983; 61: 1098.
276. O'Brien HAW, Horton MA. J Clin Pathol 1984; 37: 665.
277. Denegri JF, Rogers PCJ, Chan KW, Sadoway J, Thomas JW. Blood 1981; 58: 675.

Abnormalities of the megakaryocytes and platelets

ASSESSMENT OF MEGAKARYOCYTOPOIESIS[1]

When the platelet count is in a steady state, the rate of production of new platelets by the marrow (i.e. the rate of effective thrombocytopoiesis) equals the rate of loss of platelets from the circulation. The latter can be calculated from the platelet life-span, which is determined using radioactively labelled autologous platelets and the total number of platelets in the vascular tree. The number of megakaryocytes in the marrow provides an index of total thrombocytopoietic activity. In practice, total thrombocytopoiesis is usually assessed qualitatively on an impression of the frequency of megakaryocytes in marrow smears or histological sections of trephine biopsies. For more precise studies the total megakaryocyte number, mean megakaryocyte volume and total megakaryocyte mass (i.e. the combined volume of all megakaryocytes in the body) have to be determined using a method involving detailed histological studies and the radioisotope dilution principle. The values obtained for these thrombokinetic indices in normal individuals are given in Table 7.1. In pathological states, thrombocytopoiesis is considered to be effective when any change in total thrombocytopoiesis is paralleled by a corresponding degree of change in effective thrombocytopoiesis. Thrombocytopoiesis is considered to be ineffective when an increase in total thrombocytopoiesis is not matched by a proportionate increase in effective thrombocytopoiesis or is associated with a decrease in the latter. The theoretical mechanisms underlying ineffective thrombocytopoiesis in-

273

Table 7.1 Thrombokinetic indices ($\pm$ s.d.) in normal adults[1]

Effective thrombocytopoiesis	Platelet count	$250 \pm 35 \times 10^9$/l of blood
	Platelet survival	9.9 ± 0.6 days
	Platelet recovery*	$64.6 \pm 4.1\%$
	Platelet turnover	$35 \pm 4.3 \times 10^9$/l of blood/day
Total thrombocytopoiesis	Total megakaryocyte number	6.1×10^6/kg
	Mean megakaryocyte volume	4700 ± 100 fl
	Total megakaryocyte mass	$2.8 \pm 0.3 \times 10^{10}$ fl/kg

*The proportion of ^{51}Cr-labelled platelets recoverable from the circulation immediately after the intravenous injection of labelled platelets

clude a disorder of megakaryocyte maturation leading to intramedullary death and a failure of platelet release.

ABNORMALITIES OF MEGAKARYOCYTE MORPHOLOGY AND PLOIDY[2,3,4]

In bone marrow smears, the cell outlines of normal megakaryocytes have areas which vary between 400 and 7 000 μm². A proportion of the megakaryocytes of patients with idiopathic thrombocytopenic purpura, polycythaemia rubra vera and essential thrombocythaemia are increased in size, sometimes with areas as large as 20 000 μm². By contrast, the size distributions of the megakaryocytes of patients with chronic granulocytic leukaemia show an increased proportion of small cells. Some patients with acute myeloid leukaemia, chronic granulocytic leukaemia and sideroblastic anaemia have a variable number of very small (70–300 μm²) megakaryocytes with pyknotic, irregular nuclei and scanty cytoplasm containing a few large platelet zones. The latter type of cell is quite distinct from the mononucleate and binucleate micromegakaryocytes (Fig. 7.1) which may be found in substantial numbers in myelodysplastic syndromes and acute myeloid leukaemia and in much smaller numbers in polycythaemia rubra vera and chronic granulocytic leukaemia. The individual nuclei of the mononucleate and binucleate micromegakaryocytes are oval or circular in outline, are similar in size to erythroblast or myelocyte

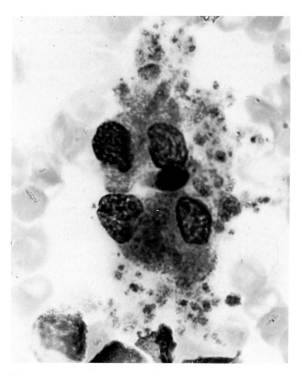

Fig. 7.1 Two binucleate micromegakaryocytes from the marrow smear of a patient with a myelodysplastic syndrome (from reference 4 by permission of the publishers).
May–Grünwald–Giemsa stain   × 940

nuclei, and usually have DNA contents between the 2 c and 4 c values (as in other diploid cells) (p. 57). These micromegakaryocytes therefore seem to suffer from a marked restriction of polyploidization.

ABNORMALITIES OF PLATELET NUMBER

A decrease in the number of platelets below the normal range is termed thrombocytopenia and an increase above the normal range is termed thrombocytosis. Platelets may also show abnormalities in function, either with or without accompanying abnormalities in number.

THROMBOCYTOPENIA

Thrombocytopenia may result from: (1) impaired production of platelets; (2) decreased platelet life-span; or (3) maldistribution of platelets due to splenic pooling.[1] In several conditions, the thrombocytopenia is caused by more than one of these mechanisms and in some conditions the pathophysiology has not yet been defined. The important clinical consequence of thrombocytopenia is haemorrhage. The bleeding may occur spontaneously or follow minor trauma. Thrombocytopenic patients may also bleed excessively after dental extraction and surgery. Small discrete haemorrhages commonly occur spontaneously into the skin (Fig. 7.2) and mucous membranes. This type of bleeding is described as purpura and is particularly prone to affect the lower limbs and areas of skin subjected to pressure. Pinpoint purpuric haemorrhages are known as petechiae and larger ones as ecchymoses. Bleeding from the gums and epistaxis are also common. Haemorrhagic bullae may occur in the buccal mucosa, particularly when the thrombocytopenia develops rapidly. Thrombocytopenic patients may also suffer from haematuria, menorrhagia, bleeding from the gastrointestinal tract, haemoptysis, and bleeding into internal organs. Cerebral haemorrhage is a common cause of death. Congenital thrombocytopenia is associated with the risk of intracranial haemorrhage following birth trauma.

The severity of the haemorrhagic tendency does not correlate very closely with the degree of reduction of the platelet count. However, in general, provided that platelet function is unimpaired, spontaneous bleeding is rare when the platelet count is above $80 \times 10^9/l$, occurs with in-

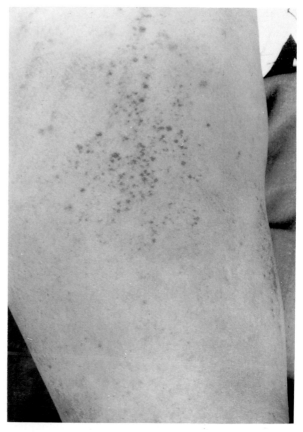

Fig. 7.2 Petechiae on the arm of a patient with idiopathic autoimmune thrombocytopenic purpura (platelet count $10 \times 10^9/l$). Some of the petechiae appeared spontaneously. Others followed a light scratch and these have a linear distribution.

creasing frequency as the count falls below $50 \times 10^9/l$ and is both usual and potentially dangerous with counts below $10-20 \times 10^9/l$.

Impaired production of platelets

The causes of impaired platelet production are listed in Table 7.2. The mechanisms underlying an impairment of platelet production are a reduction in the total number of megakaryocytes, ineffectiveness of thrombocytopoiesis, and disorders of the regulation of thrombocytopoiesis. Megakaryocytic hypoplasia occurs in Fanconi's syndrome, thrombocytopenia with absent radii, various trisomy syndromes, idiopathic aplastic anaemia and in some cases of marrow infiltration by malignant cells. It also occurs following some

Table 7.2 Causes of impaired platelet production

Congenital
  Fanconi's anaemia
  Thrombocytopenia with absent radii
  Trisomy syndromes
  Hereditary thrombocytopenias without associated
    congenital anomalies
  Tidal platelet dysgenesis and some cases of cyclic
    thrombocytopenia

Acquired
  Some chemicals and drugs
  Alcoholism
  Radiation
  Certain infections (e.g. live measles vaccine)
  Idiopathic aplastic anaemia
  Paroxysmal nocturnal haemoglobinuria
  Vitamin B$_{12}$ or folate deficiency
  Infiltration of the marrow by neoplastic cells
  Myelofibrosis
  Leukaemia and di Guglielmo's syndrome
  Myelodysplastic syndromes
  Iron deficiency anaemia

viral infections and after irradiation or the administration of certain drugs. Ineffective thrombocytopoiesis may be present in alcoholism, megaloblastic haemopoiesis due to vitamin B$_{12}$ or folate deficiency, di Guglielmo's syndrome, the myelodysplastic syndromes, paroxysmal nocturnal haemoglobinuria, and some hereditary thrombocytopenias. Rarely, iron deficiency anaemia may be associated with iron-responsive thrombocytopenia, particularly in young children; the thrombocytopenia seems to result from impaired platelet production but the mechanism underlying this impairment is not entirely clear.

Thrombocytopenia with absent radii (TAR syndrome, congenital megakaryocytic hypoplasia)[5,6]

This syndrome is characterized by neonatal thrombocytopenia, due to a marked reduction or absence of megakaryocytes, and bilateral absence of the radii. The white cells show a granulocytic leukaemoid picture in about half the cases. A variety of other congenital abnormalities may be present, including the absence of the ulna and the humerus and, less frequently, cardiac abnormalities, microcephaly and micrognathia. A high proportion of patients die within the first few months. The aetiology of this condition is uncer-

tain but the nature of the various congenital abnormalities suggests some form of intrauterine damage during the first eight weeks of gestation. In one case, the TAR syndrome was associated with treatment of the mother with thalidomide (W. St C. Symmers, personal communication).

Trisomy syndromes

Trisomy 18 has been associated with amegakaryocytic thrombocytopenia together with various other congenital abnormalities such as radial dysplasia, oesophageal atresia[7] and defects of the caecum and ascending colon.[8] Trisomy 13–15 has been associated with amegakaryocytic thrombocytopenia with multiple other congenital defects.[9]

Hereditary thrombocytopenias without associated congenital anomalies[10]

Most patients falling into this category have a normal platelet life-span and markedly ineffective thrombocytopoiesis. Inheritance is usually as an autosomal dominant character.

Tidal platelet dysgenesis[11] and cyclic thrombocytopenia

Tidal platelet dysgenesis is a rare condition in which there is a disturbance of the regulation of thrombocytopoiesis resulting in marked cyclical changes both in the number of megakaryocytes in the marrow and in the circulating platelet count. Thrombocytosis alternates with thrombocytopenia at intervals of about 40 days. This disorder may be related to the more common disorder known as cyclic thrombocytopenia,[12] which usually but not invariably affects females and in which thrombocytosis is usually not found. In both disorders, thrombocytopenia may be a manifestation of the potentially cyclical nature of haemopoiesis. However, it has been reported that cyclic changes in megakaryocyte number are not found in some cases of cyclic thrombocytopenia.

Infections

A mild thrombocytopenia associated with degenerating megakaryocytes in the marrow develops within a week of the administration of live measles vaccine, presumably as a result of the infection of megakaryocytes by the virus.[13] Between 40 and 80% of cases of the congenital rubella syndrome suffer from a thrombocytopenia, and marrow aspirates from a few such cases have been reported to show a reduced number or a total absence of megakaryocytes.[14] However, several other cases, including some in which detailed histological studies of the marrow were performed post mortem, have shown normal numbers of megakaryocytes;[15] in these cases the thrombocytopenia appears to be caused both by a shortening of platelet life-span and by a failure to increase megakaryocytopoiesis (see p. 279). Severe pancytopenia due to bone marrow hypoplasia develops in 0.1–0.2% of cases of viral hepatitis (non-A non-B).[16] This condition is associated with a high mortality; recovery, when it occurs, may take as long as 20 months.

Radiation, chemicals, drugs[17,18] and alcoholism

Ionizing radiation, certain chemicals and a long list of drugs may cause aplasia or hypoplasia of all haemopoietic lines including the megakaryocytes (see p. 188). A few drugs may cause a more or less selective thrombocytopenia by suppressing megakaryocytopoiesis (e.g. thiazide diuretics, mitomycin). Others cause thrombocytopenia by shortening platelet life-span; these are discussed on page 279.

Alcohol-related thrombocytopenia[19] is caused by ineffectiveness of thrombocytopoiesis resulting in a failure to adequately increase effective thrombocytopoiesis in response to an alcohol-induced reduction in platelet life-span. The megakaryocytes are increased in number but normal in size. The platelets of alcoholics also show functional abnormalities (see p. 285).

Decreased platelet life-span

Normal bone marrow can increase platelet production to four to eight times the basal rate. Therefore a moderate reduction in platelet life-span may not cause a thrombocytopenia provided that there is no associated impairment of megakaryocytopoiesis. Thrombocytopenia develops

Table 7.3 Mechanisms and causes of a shortening of platelet life-span

Immune platelet destruction
  Idiopathic autoimmune thrombocytopenic purpura
  Evans' syndrome
  Secondary autoimmune thrombocytopenic purpura (e.g. systemic lupus erythematosus, lymphoma, chronic lymphocytic leukaemia)
  Post-infective thrombocytopenia (e.g. after rubella)
  Drug-induced thrombocytopenia
  Feto-maternal incompatibility
  Post-transfusion purpura

Intravascular platelet consumption
  Infections
  Disseminated intravascular coagulation
  Haemolytic uraemic syndrome (Gasser's syndrome)
  Thrombotic thrombocytopenic pupura (Moschcowitz's disease)
  Giant haemangioma (Kasabach–Merritt syndrome)
  Congenital deficiency of a plasma factor
  Prosthetic valves and grafts

Intrinsic abnormalities of the platelet
  Bernard–Soulier syndrome (see p. 283)
  Wiskott–Aldrich syndrome (see p. 281 and Chapter 8)
  May–Hegglin anomaly (see p. 205)

Other mechanisms
  Massive haemorrhage
  Extracorporeal circulation

Uncertain mechanisms
  Alcoholism
  Graves' disease

when the bone marrow cannot adequately increase platelet production to compensate for a given degree of reduction of platelet life-span. The mechanisms and causes of a shortening of platelet life-span are given in Table 7.3.

Idiopathic autoimmune thrombocytopenic purpura (IATP, chronic idiopathic thrombocytopenic purpura)[20,21]

This disorder results from the production of an autoantibody against platelets. IATP should be distinguished from post-infective immune thrombocytopenia in which it is possible that platelet damage results from immune complexes rather than autoantibodies (see p. 278). Although IATP may occur both in children and in adults, in children thrombocytopenia often has a post-infective rather than an autoimmune basis. Adults show a genetic (high association with the antigen DRw2) and sex-linked predisposition (female:male ratio=2–4:1) to IATP. The anti-platelet autoantibody is usually IgG in type and sometimes IgM. In the majority of patients IgG can be detected on autologous platelets, and in some patients free antibody (which will coat normal platelets) is detectable in serum. The antibody shortens the survival of platelets from the normal 10 days to as little as 2 h or less; the antibody-coated platelets are mainly removed by the liver and spleen. Transfusion of plasma from a patient with IATP into a normal volunteer will cause thrombocytopenia. IATP of adults is usually characterized by an insidious onset, the absence of a history of a preceding infection, and a protracted course of months to years. Spleno-megaly is rare and its occurrence should cast doubts on the diagnosis.

The main changes in the blood are the thrombocytopenia and an abnormal degree of variation in the size and shape of platelets. Some platelets are very large, with a diameter of 3–4 μm or more. The larger platelets are haemostatically more effective than normal platelets so that the count may be as low as $10–20 \times 10^9/l$ before the bleeding time becomes prolonged and a bleeding tendency develops. Chronic blood loss may lead to the development of a hypochromic microcytic anaemia due to iron deficiency. An occasional patient with IATP also has autoimmune haemo-lytic anaemia (Evans's syndrome).[22]

The bone marrow usually shows megakaryo-cytic hyperplasia (increase of number and size) and there is a considerable increase in the rate of platelet production. However, some patients with chronic IATP are found to have subnormal platelet production despite a diminished platelet life-span; it has been postulated that this may result from damage to megakaryocytes by the antiplatelet antibody.[23]

Histological studies of the spleen show folli-cular hyperplasia, dilated sinusoids and lipid-containing macrophages; the lipid is derived from the destruction of platelets.

About 50% of patients with chronic IATP show a substantial rise in the platelet count within several days to a few weeks of commencing therapy with corticosteroids. However, relapse following cessation of therapy is common. If the response to corticosteroids is poor or the dose of corticosteroid required to prevent haemorrhage is unacceptably high, splenectomy may be useful; complete and sustained remissions follow splenectomy in 60–90% of cases. Some refractory patients respond to immunosuppressive therapy, Vinca alkaloids or danazol. Intravenous injections of high doses of immunoglobulin frequently cause a rise in the platelet count which usually lasts for only 1–3 weeks.

Babies born to mothers with chronic IATP often suffer from neonatal thrombocytopenia due to the passage of the mother's IgG platelet autoantibody across the placenta. This complication may even be seen in babies whose mothers have a normal platelet count following splenectomy.[24]

Secondary autoimmune thrombocytopenic purpura[25]

An autoimmune thrombocytopenia may precede other manifestations of SLE by several months or years or may complicate the course of SLE and other autoimmune diseases such as rheumatoid arthritis, mixed connective tissue disease, systemic sclerosis, pernicious anaemia, autoimmune thyroiditis and hyperthyroidism. An autoimmune thrombocytopenia also occurs in some patients with carcinoma, sarcoidosis,[26] lymphoproliferative disorders and plasma cell dyscrasias, in homosexual men with or without Kaposi's sarcoma[27] and in haemophiliacs treated with factor VIII concentrates (see p. 330).

There may be no essential difference between idiopathic and secondary autoimmune thrombocytopenic purpura; both may be a manifestation of some underlying defect of immunological mechanisms.[28]

Post-infective thrombocytopenic purpura[20,29]

Post-infective thrombocytopenia is most commonly seen in children aged less than 10 years. Both sexes are affected equally. It is characterized by the acute onset of thrombocytopenic bleeding and a history of an infection usually within 2–3 weeks preceding the development of the thrombocytopenia. The thrombocytopenia may be caused by the interaction of antigen-antibody complexes with platelets. Viral infections are the most frequent cause. Thrombocytopenia occurs not at the peak of the viraemia but 7–10 days later, at the time when specific antibody appears.[30] Platelet survival is shortened. Platelet production is normal or increased. Mild splenomegaly is seen in about 10% of affected children. Post-infective thrombocytopenia may follow specific viral infections (e.g. measles, rubella, mumps, influenza, infectious mononucleosis, chickenpox, viral epidemic haemorrhagic fevers) or may follow an upper respiratory tract infection of presumed viral origin. Immune-complex-induced thrombocytopenia may also follow bacterial and protozoal infections (e.g. scarlet fever, pertussis, toxoplasmosis[31] and tuberculosis). In post-infective thrombocytopenic purpura the platelet count is usually very low ($1-10 \times 10^9/l$) but in the great majority of cases the disease is self-limiting, remission occurring within 2–6 weeks. It is possible that some of the microorganisms mentioned above sometimes cause thrombocytopenia by precipitating disseminated intravascular coagulation (see pp. 280 and 335), damaging vascular endothelium and so increasing the rate of platelet utilization and/or by impairing platelet production rather than through the formation of antigen–antibody complexes.

Drug-induced immune thrombocytopenia[17,18,32]

An immunological mechanism has been implicated in the shortening of the platelet life-span in an occasional patient receiving quinine (Fig. 7.3), quinidine, apronal (allylisopropylacetylurea, Sedormid), stibophen, digitoxin, sodium aurothiomalate, frusemide,[33] cimetidine, novobiocin, co-trimoxazole, rifampicin,[34] sulphafurazole (sulfisoxazole), ampicillin, penicillin and heparin. In addition, an immunological mechanism is suspected but not experimentally proven in patients with thrombocytopenia induced by a wide variety of other drugs. Two mechanisms have been proposed to explain the thrombocytopenia. According to the first hypothesis, the drug or a metabolite binds to platelets, platelet destruction occurring as a result of the development of antibodies against the drug-platelet complex. The alternative possibility is that the drug or a meta-

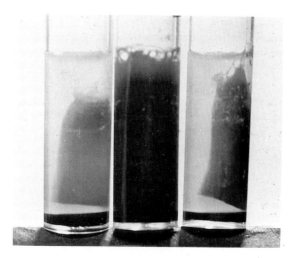

Fig. 7.3 Demonstration of inhibition of clot retraction by the addition of quinine to whole blood, in a patient with antiquinine antibodies who had recovered from an episode of quinine-induced thrombocytopenic purpura (central tube). The left- and right-hand tubes show that normal clot retraction has not been prevented by the addition of quinine to whole blood from a normal subject. The inhibition of clot retraction results from damage to platelets in the presence of the antiquinine antibody and quinine.

Courtesy of Dr Barbara J. Bain

bolite binds to a plasma protein and that antibodies develop against the drug-protein complex. In this case the thrombocytopenia would result from the interaction between platelets and immune complexes, the platelets being 'innocent bystanders'. The typical history is one of an acute onset of severe thrombocytopenic haemorrhage within 6–12 h of a single dose of drug in a patient previously exposed to that drug. Sometimes drug-induced immune thrombocytopenia may develop suddenly during the course of prolonged treatment with the drug. The thrombocytopenia may be associated with fever, joint pains and urticaria; it disappears spontaneously after withdrawal of the drug. The bone marrow shows an increased number of megakaryocytes.

Feto-maternal incompatibility[35,36]

Neonatal thrombocytopenia may occur in babies of healthy mothers due to feto-maternal incompatibility in platelet antigens. The mother forms IgG alloantibodies against a specific fetal platelet antigen (e.g. Pl^{A1}; see p. 38) or against HLA antigens which the fetus has inherited from the father and which are lacking in her. These antibodies cross the placenta and destroy fetal platelets. Immunization of the mother has usually occurred during previous pregnancies. About half the cases are in P1^A1-negative mothers bearing P1^A1-positive babies. As only about 3% of the population are P1^A1-negative, maternal immunization against the P1^A1 antigen is uncommon.

Post-transfusion purpura[37]

Very rarely, severe thrombocytopenia develops 5–8 days after the transfusion of donor blood, apparently as a result of the destruction of the recipient's platelets. Most patients have been P1^A1-negative with anti-P1^A1 in their serum. The anti-P1^A1 is thought to be an alloantibody formed as a result of pregnancy or previous transfusion which was boosted by the recent transfusion. However, the mechanism by which this alloantibody destroys the patient's P1^A1-negative platelets is uncertain (see p. 38). The thrombocytopenia may persist for up to 48 days. Plasmaphaeresis has been reported to effect a rapid remission.[38]

Disseminated intravascular coagulation (DIC) (see also p. 335)

Widespread activation of the haemostatic mechanisms leads to intravascular deposition of fibrin and thrombocytopenia due to the consumption of platelets. DIC may develop either acutely or more chronically and at all ages, from birth onwards. Septicaemia may precipitate DIC in the newborn as at any age. Other factors that predispose to DIC in the newborn are birth asphyxia, hypoxia, prematurity, hypothermia, shock, Rhesus isoimmunization and obstetric complications in the mother (pre-eclampsia and abruptio placentae). Thrombocytopenia occurs frequently in neonates with the congenital rubella syndrome or with congenital cytomegalovirus infection, and occasionally in those with congenital toxoplasmosis, congenital syphilis and generalized herpes simplex infection. In all these conditions the thrombocytopenia disappears after the first few weeks and (except in some cases of the congenital rubella syndrome—see p. 277) seems to be due to disseminated intravascular coagulation. Causes of DIC in adults include obstetric complications (abruptio placentae, amniotic fluid embolism, eclampsia, pre-eclampsia and retention of a dead fetus), malignant disease (carcinoma, lymphoma and leukaemia, especially promyelocytic leukaemia), shock and acute intravascular haemolysis.

Thrombotic thrombocytopenic purpura (Moschcowitz's disease)[39]

This serious illness usually affects young adults but may affect individuals of all ages. The disease is characterized by fever, haemolytic anaemia, thrombocytopenia, fluctuating or stable neurological symptoms and disturbed renal function. Fragmented red cells may be seen in the blood. About half of the cases show a neutrophil leucocytosis. Platelet life-span is markedly shortened due to an extracorpuscular defect. The bone marrow shows normal or increased numbers of megakaryocytes and erythroid hyperplasia. The characteristic histological finding at necropsy or in biopsy specimens is the occlusion of some capillaries and arterioles of virtually all tissues by granular platelet thrombi which become hyalinized: the affected vessels may show endothelial proliferation; microaneurysmal dilatation is a characteristic feature. These lesions occur particularly in the heart, brain, kidneys, pancreas and adrenal glands. In contrast to immune vasculitis, a perivascular cellular infiltrate is lacking. Electron microscope studies show that the hyaline substance is composed of platelet aggregates with some fibrin and a few red cells and leucocytes. The thrombocytopenia appears to be caused by the incorporation of platelets into the microthrombi that form throughout the body. The red cell fragmentation is attributed to damage whilst circulating past the microthrombi. Despite the presence of some fibrin in the microthrombi and occasional elevation of the levels of fibrin degradation products in the serum, the fibrinogen level and prothrombin time are usually normal. If untreated, the clinical course is rapidly fatal. The aetiology of thrombotic thrombocytopenic purpura is uncertain, but recent work indicates that affected patients lack a plasma factor which is normally involved in stimulating prostacyclin synthesis by endothelial cells. It has been proposed that this reduced vascular prostacyclin synthesis permits platelet deposition and the formation of platelet thrombi in the microcirculation. A number of patients have responded to infusions of fresh-frozen plasma or to plasmaphaeresis and replacement with fresh-frozen plasma.

Haemolytic uraemic syndrome (HUS, Gasser's syndrome[40,41,42])

This syndrome is seen most frequently during the first year of life and is rare over the age of 6 years. It is characterized by the sudden onset of fever, intravascular haemolysis, renal failure and, commonly, thrombocytopenia. Hypertension develops in more than half the cases. The blood film shows many fragmented red cells and some microspherocytes. Serum levels of fibrin degradation products are raised. In comparison with thrombotic thrombocytopenic purpura (described above), neurological symptoms are less frequent, renal impairment is more severe and vascular lesions are usually limited to the afferent arterioles and glomerular capillaries of the kidneys. The aetiology of the haemolytic uraemic syndrome is uncertain. The disorder frequently occurs in an epidemic form following an episode of diarrhoea and vomiting or a non-specific febrile illness in infants. Furthermore, a recent study has shown that the stools of some sporadic cases of HUS contain a faecal cytotoxin and cytotoxin-producing *Escherichia coli*,[43] raising the possibility that bacterial toxins may play a role in the pathogenesis of this condition. HUS may also follow vaccination against poliomyelitis, smallpox or measles, suggesting that the disorder may sometimes be caused by virus-induced or immune-complex-induced damage to renal glomeruli. In addition, there are recent data suggesting that in some (but not all) affected children, HUS may be caused by a decreased ability of endothelial cells to synthesize prostacyclin due to the deficiency of a stimulatory factor normally present in the plasma.[44,45] Prostacyclin inhibits platelet deposition on the vessel wall and seems to be the substance which normally protects against the formation of thrombi. It is possible that in some unknown way certain infections cause a deficiency of the plasma factor involved in prostacyclin synthesis. With modern management of the renal failure, children in whom 50% or less of the glomeruli are affected frequently make a complete clinical recovery. Treatment with fresh-frozen plasma may be efficacious.[46]

HUS may develop in pregnancy or postpartum.[47] It has developed after therapy with certain drugs[48,49] (e.g. oral contraceptives, fluorouracil plus mitomycin) and after solvent abuse[50] (e.g. glue sniffing).

Giant haemangioma (Kasabach–Merritt syndrome)[51]

Thrombocytopenia and microangiopathic haemolytic anaemia may occur due to thrombosis within a massive subcutaneous haemangioma or a haemangioendothelioma of the liver. Levels of fibrinogen, factor V and factor VIII are also frequently reduced.

Congenital deficiency of a plasma factor[52]

In two children, recurrent attacks of thrombocytopenia and microangiopathic haemolytic anaemia (p. 150), sometimes associated with infections, seemed to have resulted from a congenital deficiency of a factor present in normal plasma which protects against shortened platelet and red cell survival under certain abnormal circumstances. Transfusion of normal plasma repeatedly resulted in the rapid elevation of the platelet count.

Wiskott–Aldrich syndrome[5, 10, 53, 54]

This syndrome consists of moderate to severe thrombocytopenia, eczema and recurrent life-threatening infections due to defects in both cellular and humoral immunity. Infecting organisms include the pneumococcus, herpes viruses and *Pneumocystis carinii*. The disorder is inherited as an X-linked recessive character. The bone marrow contains normal numbers of megakaryocytes and the circulating platelets are abnormally

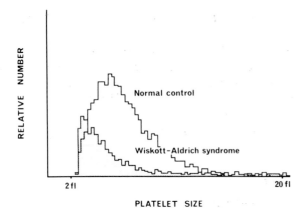

Fig. 7.4 Platelet volume distribution curves obtained on a Coulter counter, model S plus IV, with blood from a patient with the Wiskott–Aldrich syndrome (stippled area) and from a normal subject. It is evident that the modal platelet volume is substantially reduced in the patient.

small (Fig. 7.4) with a markedly reduced life-span. Affected individuals usually die in childhood from an overwhelming infection, massive haemorrhage or malignant disease arising in lymphoid cells.

Other disorders

The transfusion of large volumes of platelet-poor, stored blood to a bleeding patient results in a moderate degree of thrombocytopenia as does exchange transfusion with stored blood.

Patients subjected to extracorporeal circulation usually show a 50% reduction of the platelet count because of damage to platelets in the perfusion apparatus; occasionally a more severe degree of thrombocytopenia develops.

There is a reduction of platelet life-span in ethanol-related thrombocytopenia.[19] The same is true in Graves' disease which may be associated with mild thrombocytopenia.[55] Impaired megakaryocytopoiesis contributes to the thrombocytopenia in both these conditions.

Increased splenic pooling[1,56,57]

Patients with splenomegaly from any cause may develop thrombocytopenia. This is mainly the result of increased pooling of platelets within the spleen; large spleens may contain 50–90% or more of the total platelet mass. Expansion of the plasma volume, which occurs in proportion to the size of the spleen, contributes to the thrombocytopenia. Platelet life-span is normal or only modestly reduced. The rate of platelet production is increased but the marrow response is sub-optimal for the degree of thrombocytopenia, perhaps as a result of some effect of the intrasplenic platelets on the regulation of thrombocytopoiesis. There is no evidence of ineffective thrombocytopoiesis.

Undefined pathophysiology

Epstein's syndrome[58,59]

This syndrome consists of hereditary thrombocytopenia, macrothrombocytes and the two features of Alport's syndrome, namely nerve deafness and nephritis. It is inherited as an autosomal dominant character.

THROMBOCYTOSIS[60]

The causes of thrombocytosis are listed in Table 7.4. A transient physiological thrombocytosis develops rapidly after the administration of adrenaline or after vigorous exercise and appears to

Table 7.4 Causes of thrombocytosis

Exercise, adrenaline
Haemorrhage, haemolysis
Postpartum
Following surgery and trauma
Rebound (recovery from thrombocytopenia)
Tidal platelet dysgenesis
Chronic myeloproliferative disorders (including essential thrombocythaemia)
Splenectomy, splenic agenesis or atrophy
Acute and chronic infections
Chronic inflammatory disease (e.g. ulcerative colitis, regional enteritis, rheumatoid arthritis, sarcoidosis)
Malignant disease (e.g. Hodgkin's disease, carcinoma of breast and lung, other neoplasms)
Iron deficiency anaemia

be caused by the mobilization of platelets pooled in organs such as the spleen and lungs. In the other conditions listed in Table 7.4, the thrombocytosis is caused by an increased rate of production of platelets and is associated with increased numbers of megakaryocytes in the marrow.

Essential (idiopathic, primary or haemorrhagic) thrombocythaemia[61,62]

A raised platelet count due to increased platelet production may occur in any of the chronic myeloproliferative disorders, which include polycythaemia rubra vera (p. 196), primary idiopathic myelofibrosis (p. 184), chronic granulocytic leukaemia (p. 235) and essential thrombocythaemia. Essential thrombocythaemia is a disorder which affects middle-aged or elderly individuals. It is characterized by a very high platelet count (usually $1-4 \times 10^{12}/l$), abnormal platelet morphology and function, a hypercellular bone marrow with a gross increase in megakaryocytes, and both haemorrhagic and microvascular occlusive episodes. Splenomegaly is present at diagnosis in about 60% of cases but splenic atrophy may eventually result from repeated splenic infarction. There may be spontaneous haemorrhages into the subcutaneous tissue or gastrointestinal tract and thrombosis involving both veins and smaller arteries. Arterial thrombosis may result in peripheral gangrene or transient cerebral ischaemic attacks. Platelets show bizarre morphology with many irregularly-shaped and giant forms. There may be a moderate neutrophil leucocytosis (e.g. up to $30 \times 10^9/l$) with some neutrophil metamyelocytes and myelocytes. Basophilia may be present. The neutrophil alkaline phosphatase score is often raised. The marked increase in the number of megakaryocytes can be clearly seen in histological sections of trephine biopsies which also show an increase in reticulin. The marrow cells do not contain the Ph[1] chromosome. The disease runs a chronic course and occasionally transforms into myelofibrosis. Treatment is aimed at reducing the platelet count, using busulphan, melphalan or ^{32}P and, if necessary, inhibiting platelet aggregation with drugs such as aspirin and dipyridamole.

DISORDERS OF PLATELET FUNCTION

The role of platelets in normal haemostasis is discussed on page 21. There are a number of congenital and acquired defects of platelet function which cause impairment of haemostasis. The congenital disorders are very much rarer but better understood than the acquired ones.

Congenital disorders[63]

Bernard–Soulier syndrome

This is characterized by giant platelets (Fig. 7.5), some of which are as large as 8 μm in diameter,

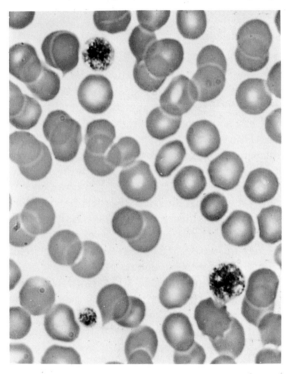

Fig. 7.5 Blood film from a patient with the Bernard–Soulier syndrome showing giant platelets.

a normal or slightly low platelet count, a prolongation of the bleeding time and an autosomal recessive inheritance. Platelet life-span may be reduced.[64] In those cases with a low platelet count, both the prolongation of the bleeding time and the severity of the haemorrhagic tendency are quite disproportionate to the extent of the thrombocytopenia. The disease appears to be caused by a deficiency in the platelet cell membrane of glycoprotein Ib which is required for the adhesion of platelets to exposed vascular subendothelium. This glycoprotein which is rich in sialic acid also carries the binding sites for the von Willebrand factor. The function of the adhesion of platelets to subendothelial fibrils is reflected in the ability of ristocetin to induce platelet aggregation *in vitro*. The defect of adhesion in the Bernard–Soulier syndrome can be detected by a failure of ristocetin-induced aggregation. The affected platelets aggregate normally in response to collagen or ADP. This pattern of response to platelet aggregating agents is similar to that seen in von Willebrand's disease (Fig. 7.6).

Storage pool deficiency[63,64,65]

In a small number of patients, the platelets are congenitally deficient in the dense bodies (see p. 20) which contain the storage pool of ADP concerned with secondary platelet aggregation. Such platelets show defective release of ADP after stimulation with aggregating agents such as collagen and thrombin. Storage pool deficiency has been reported in a few patients in the absence of abnormalities affecting other cell types and in some of these patients the disorder has been inherited as an autosomal dominant trait. In the Hermansky–Pudlak syndrome, a storage pool deficiency is associated with a normal platelet count, a mild to moderate haemorrhagic tendency, tyrosinase-positive oculocutaneous albinism, the presence of ceroid-like pigment in bone marrow macrophages, and an autosomal recessive inheritance. Storage granules may also be deficient in patients with the Chédiak–Higashi syndrome (see p. 205), Wiskott–Aldrich syndrome (see p. 281) and thrombocytopenia with absent radii (see p. 276).

Thrombasthenia (Glanzmann's disease)

The features of this disease are a moderately severe bleeding tendency, a normal platelet count, normal platelet morphology, a prolonged bleeding time, abnormal clot retraction and an autosomal recessive inheritance. The platelets

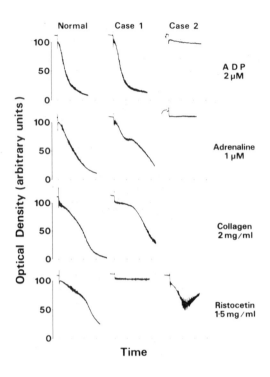

Fig. 7.6 Platelet aggregometer tracings showing the aggregation of platelets following the addition of adenosine diphosphate (ADP), adrenaline (epinephrine), collagen or ristocetin to platelet-rich plasma. Aggregation of platelets causes a decrease of optical density. One division on the time axis is equivalent to one minute. Case 1 is a patient with von Willebrand's disease in whom aggregation was normal with ADP, adrenaline and collagen, but absent with ristocetin. The biphasic adrenaline-induced aggregation shown by this case may also be seen in normal individuals; the second phase results from the release of ADP from platelets during the platelet release reaction. Case 2 is a patient with Glanzmann's thrombasthenia in whom there was no aggregation following the addition of ADP or adrenaline. The platelets aggregated after the addition of ristocetin but subsequently disaggregated spontaneously. In some patients with thrombasthenia, the platelets do not show any ristocetin-induced aggregation.

show no abnormality of adhesion and undergo normal shape-changes in response to various stimuli. They display a normal release reaction in response to collagen and thrombin but not ADP. They bind ADP and thrombin normally but completely fail to aggregate in the presence of these substances or collagen (Fig. 7.6). There is a deficiency in the platelet membrane of glycoproteins IIb and IIIa, which come together to form a complex during platelet activation. The IIb/IIIa complex carries the fibrinogen binding site and the failure of thrombasthenic platelets to aggregate appears to be a consequence of their failure to bind fibrinogen. Platelet fibrinogen and α-actinin are reduced. The platelet antigen P1^{A1} is absent or reduced suggesting that it is conveyed by the IIb/IIIa complex.[66]

Acquired disorders[63]

Disturbances of platelet composition and function are seen in many diseases and in individuals taking ethanol or a wide variety of drugs. These acquired disturbances include reductions of

Table 7.5 Some conditions associated with 'vascular purpura'

Condition	Main features
Congenital disorders	
Hereditary haemorrhagic telangiectasia (Rendu–Osler–Weber disease)	Multiple vascular malformations up to 3 mm in diameter affect the skin and mucous membranes; recurrent internal and external haemorrhage may occur from such lesions. Autosomal dominant inheritance.
Ehlers–Danlos syndrome, osteogenesis imperfecta, Marfan's syndrome and pseudoxanthoma elasticum	Abnormalities of the connective tissue of blood vessels and perivascular tissue result in ecchymoses, haematomas and other haemorrhagic manifestations.
Acquired disorders	
Henoch–Schönlein purpura (allergic purpura)	Probably caused by an allergic vasculitis resulting from a reaction to streptococcal infection or other antigenic stimulus. Results in purpura, severe abdominal colic, vomiting, gastrointestinal bleeding, arthritis and, occasionally, focal proliferative glomerulonephritis. Rarely runs a fulminant course with death from acute renal failure.
Scurvy (vitamin C deficiency)	Abnormality of endothelium and vascular connective tissue causes perifollicular haemorrhages and ecchymoses (often in a 'saddle distribution'), sometimes with gingivitis and bleeding gums. Infants may have subperiosteal haemorrhages.
Drug-induced vascular purpura	Occasionally follows treatment with frusemide, indomethacin, phenobarbitone, phenytoin, quinine, sodium aurothiomalate. Commonly follows prolonged treatment with moderate or high doses of corticosteroids.
Septicaemias due to meningococcal and other bacterial infections	Vascular purpura is occasionally accompanied by severe shock due to bilateral adrenal haemorrhage (*Waterhouse–Friderichsen syndrome*).
Polyarteritis nodosa and other collagen diseases	Widespread purpura due to a generalized vasculitis may develop, usually as a terminal feature.
Senile purpura	Develops in old age secondary to fragility of the vessels of the skin as a result of a decrease of the connective tissue of the skin and a loss of subcutaneous fat. A similar clinicopathological picture develops in cachectic patients at any age (purpura cachectica).

glycoprotein I, α-adrenergic receptors, or thrombin-binding sites in the platelet membrane, reduced synthesis of thromboxane A_2, and a storage pool or α-granule deficiency. Conditions associated with one or more acquired defects of platelet function include thrombocythaemia, chronic granulocytic leukaemia, polycythaemia rubra vera, myelofibrosis, acute leukaemia, myelodysplastic syndromes, uraemia, liver failure, disseminated intravascular coagulation and fibrinolytic therapy, cyanotic heart disease, chronic hypoglycaemia, paraproteinaemias, immune thrombocytopenia (including SLE), pernicious anaemia, scurvy, severe burns, giant haemangioma, and following cardiopulmonary bypass. Drugs which impair platelet function include aspirin, phenylbutazone, indomethacin, sulphinpyrazone, dipyridamole, clofibrate, chloroquine, phenothiazines (e.g. chlorpromazine), tricyclic antidepressants (e.g. amitriptyline), dihydroergotamine and high doses of penicillins and cephalosporins. Aspirin and other non-steroidal anti-inflammatory drugs inhibit platelet cyclooxgenase (p. 21) and thus impair the platelet release reaction and secondary platelet aggregation. Ethanol inhibits both primary and secondary ADP-induced aggregation. Dietary constituents (e.g. ginger and garlic) may decrease platelet function.

DIFFERENTIAL DIAGNOSIS OF PLATELET-RELATED PURPURA

In the present chapter, a variety of conditions have been described in which purpuric bleeding into the skin and mucous membranes (see p. 275) is associated with a reduction in the number or an impairment of the function of platelets. In von Willebrand's disease, there is a haemorrhagic tendency which is associated both with an impairment of the adhesion of platelets to subendothelium and a reduction of factor VIII coagulation activity (see p. 330); the former may give rise to purpuric bleeding and the latter to deep haemorrhages (e.g. into muscles and joints). Purpura as well as other forms of haemorrhage may also occur in various disorders of blood vessels. Some of these disorders, which are sometimes grouped under the heading 'vascular purpura', are listed in Table 7.5.

REFERENCES

1. Harker LA, Finch CA. J Clin Invest 1969; 48: 963.
2. Albrecht M, Fülle H-H. Blut 1974; 28: 109.
3. Queisser U, Olischläger A, Queisser W, Heimpel H. Acta Haematol (Basel) 1972; 47: 21.
4. Wickramasinghe SN. Human bone marrow. Oxford: Blackwell Scientific Publications, 1975.
5. Lusher JM, Barnhart MI. Semin Thromb Hemost 1977; 4: 123.
6. Hall JG, Levin J, Kuhn JP, Ottenheimer EJ, van Berkum KAP, McKusick V. Medicine 1969; 48: 411.
7. Rabinowitz JG, Moseley JE, Mitty HA, Hirschhorn K. Radiology 1967; 89: 488.
8. Christodoulou C, Werner B. Acta Genet Med Gemellol (Roma) 1967; 17: 77.
9. Mehes K, Bata G. Lancet 1965; i: 1279.
10. Murphy S. Clin Haematol 1972; 1: 359.
11. Engström K, Lundquist A, Söderström N. Scand J Haematol 1966; 3: 290.
12. Cohen T, Cooney DP. Scand J Haematol 1974; 12: 9.
13. Oski FA, Naiman JL. N Engl J Med 1966; 275: 352.
14. Berge T, Brunnhage F, Nilsson LR. Acta Paediatr Scand 1963; 52: 349.
15. Zinkham WH, Medearis DN, Osborn JE. J Pediatr 1967; 71: 512.
16. Camitta BM, Storb R, Thomas ED. N Engl J Med 1982; 306: 645 and 712.
17. de Gruchy GC. Drug-induced blood disorders. Oxford: Blackwell Scientific Publications, 1975.
18. Miescher PA, Graf J. Clin Haematol 1980; 9: 505.
19. Cowan DH. Semin Hematol 1980; 17: 137.
20. Doan CA, Bouroncle BA, Wiseman BK. Ann Intern Med 1960; 53: 861.
21. Karpatkin S. Blood 1980; 56: 329.
22. Evans RS, Takahashi K, Duane RT, Payne R, Liu CK. Arch Intern Med 1951; 87: 48.
23. Grossi A, Vannucchi AM, Casprini P, et al. Scand J Haematol 1983; 31: 206.
24. Cines DB, Dusak B, Tomaski A, Mennuti M, Schreiber AD. N Engl J Med 1982; 306: 826.
25. Helmerhost FM, van Leeuwen EF, Pegels JG, van der Plas-van Dalen C, Eengelfriet CP, von dem Borne AEG Kr. Scand J Haematol 1982; 28: 319.
26. Thomas LLM, Alberts C, Pegels JG, Balk AG, von dem Borne AEG Kr. Scand J Haematol 1982; 28: 357.
27. Morris L, Distenfeld A, Amorosi E, Karpatkin S. Ann Intern Med 1982; 96: 714.
28. Stuart MJ, Tomar RH, Miller ML, Davey FR. JAMA 1978; 239: 939.
29. Cohn J. Scand J Haematol 1976; 16: 226.
30. Myllylä G, Vaheri A, Vesikari T, Penttinen K. Clin Exp Immunol 1969; 4: 323.
31. Kucera JC, Davis RB. Am J Clin Pathol 1983; 79: 644.
32. Kelton JG, Meltzer D, Moore J, et al. Blood 1981; 58: 524.
33. Duncan A, Moore SB, Barker P. Lancet 1981; i: 1210.
34. Hadfield JW. Postgrad Med J 1980; 56: 59.
35. Pochedly C. Obstet Gynecol Surv 1971; 26: 63.

36. von dem Borne AEG Kr, van Leeuwen EF, von Riesz LE, van Boxtel CJ, Engelfriet CP. Blood 1981; 57: 649.
37. Mueller-Eckhardt C, Lechner K, Heinrich D, et al. Blut 1980; 40: 249.
38. Abramson N, Eisenberg PD, Aster RH. N Engl J Med 1974; 291: 1163.
39. Machin SJ. Br J Haematol 1984; 56: 191.
40. Brain MC. Semin Hematol 1969; 6: 162.
41. Hammond D, Lieberman E. Arch Intern Med 1970; 126: 816.
42. Anonymous. Lancet 1978; i: 26.
43. Karmali MA, Steele BT, Petric M, Lim C. Lancet 1983; i: 619.
44. Remuzzi G, Mecca G, Livio M, et al. Lancet 1980; i: 656.
45. Webster J, Rees AJ, Lewis PJ, Hensley CN. Br Med J 1980; 281: 271.
46. Remuzzi G, Misiani R, Marchesi D, et al. Clin Nephrol 1979; 12: 279.
47. Strauss RG, Alexander RW. Obstet Gynecol 1976; 47: 169.
48. Jones BG, Fielding JW, Newman CE, Howell A, Brookes VS. Lancet 1980; i: 1275.
49. Morel-Maroger L. Kidney Int 1980; 18: 125.
50. Locatelli F, Pozzi C. Lancet 1983; ii: 220.
51. Rodriguez-Erdmann F, Button L, Murray JE, Moloney WC. Am J Med Sci 1971; 261: 9.
52. Upshaw JD. N Engl J Med 1978; 298: 1350.
53. Baldini MG. Ann NY Acad Sci 1972; 201: 437.
54. Stiehm ER, McIntosh RM. Clin Exp Immunol 1967; 2: 179.
55. Kurata Y, Nishioeda Y, Tsubakio T, Kitani T. Acta Haematol (Basel) 1980; 63: 185.
56. Cooney DP, Smith BA. Arch Intern Med 1968; 121: 332.
57. Aster RJ. J Clin Invest 1966; 45: 645.
58. Eckstein JD, Filip DJ, Watts JC. Ann Intern Med 1975; 82: 639.
59. Bernheim J, Dechavanne M, Bryon PA, et al. Am J Med 1976; 61: 145.
60. Addiego JE, Mentzer WC, Dallman PR. J Pediatr 1974; 85: 805.
61. Frick PG. Helv Med Acta 1969; 35: 20.
62. Silverstein MN. Arch Intern Med 1968; 122: 18.
63. Hardisty RM. Br Med Bull 1977; 33: 207.
64. Gröttum KA, Solum NO. Br J Haematol 1969; 16: 277.
65. Weiss HJ, Witte LD, Kaplan KL, et al. Blood 1979; 54: 1296.
66. Clemetson KJ, Capitanio A, Pareti FI, McGregor JL, Luscher EF. Thromb Res 1980; 18: 797.

Abnormalities of immunoglobulin synthesizing cells and immune deficiency syndromes

PLASMA CELL DYSCRASIAS

The plasma cell dyscrasias are malignancies of cells which correspond to the terminal stages of differentiation of the B-lymphocyte lineage, the antibody secreting cells: the malignant cells may have the morphology of plasma cells or of lymphocytes with plasmacytoid features. The malignant population is derived from a single cell and is, therefore, a clone and the protein secreted is therefore designated a monoclonal protein; it has a single light chain type (κ or λ) and a single heavy chain type ($\gamma, \alpha, \mu, \delta, \varepsilon$). Furthermore, all molecules have the same structure and in particular have the same structure in the variable regions of the light and heavy chains, i.e. they are of the same idiotype. Because all molecules of a monoclonal protein have an identical structure, they form a discrete narrow band on electrophoresis. Such discrete bands have been designated M-bands (because of their occurrence in *m*ultiple *m*yeloma and *m*acroglobulinaemia). They have also been designated paraproteins, suggesting that they differ in structure from normal immunoglobulins, and the corresponding diseases have been called paraproteinaemias. However, only a proportion of paraproteins have major structural abnormalities. Some paraproteins have demonstrable antibody activity which, since paraproteins are monoclonal, is directed against a single antigen. The term monoclonal gammopathy has also been used to refer to diseases in which a monoclonal immunoglobulin is produced. The plasma cell dyscrasias fall within the broader group of malignant lympho-proliferative disorders.

MULTIPLE MYELOMA[1]

Definition

Multiple myeloma (myelomatosis) is a malignant disease resulting from a monoclonal proliferation of cells of the B-lymphocyte lineage in which the malignant cells (myeloma cells) are functionally similar to plasma cells and are morphologically similar to either plasma cells or plasmacytoid lymphocytes. The great majority of patients with multiple myeloma have cells which secrete a monoclonal immunoglobulin or a monoclonal light chain or both immunoglobulin and light chain (derived from the same clone). A small minority have cells which are morphologically similar but do not secrete a paraprotein.

Incidence

Multiple myeloma is predominantly a disease of the middle-aged and elderly. In two Caucasian populations studied, the incidence and the mortality rate were approximately 3 cases/100 000 of population/year[2,3] while in another the annual mortality in Caucasians was of the order of 10 per 100 000 of population aged above 65 years.[4] The incidence and mortality rate are appreciably higher in Blacks than in Caucasians.[3,4]

Aetiology

The aetiology is unknown. Results of studies with murine plasma cell tumours indicate that both genetic factors and antigenic stimuli may play a role. The finding of an increased incidence of paraproteins in the relatives of patients with multiple myeloma suggests that genetic factors may also operate in man. An increased incidence of myeloma was found following exposure to atomic explosions.[5] Cytogenetic changes may be present in myeloma cells and may be relevant to aetiology. Thus, translocations involving chromosome 14 and the breakpoint q 32 (14q+), which are characteristic of Burkitt's lymphoma and certain other B-cell malignancies, are seen

also in multiple myeloma, and an equivalent abnormality is seen in mouse plasmacytoma. The donor chromosome differs between individuals and between different lymphoproliferative disorders. The translocation t(11,14) (q 13, q 32) may be seen in multiple myeloma.[6] As the genes coding for the constant region of the immunoglobulin heavy chain are adjacent to the band q 32 it seems possible that the translocation may be a factor in tumorigenesis. The presence of idiotypic markers on peripheral blood B-cells indicates that the target cell in the malignant transformation is usually a B-cell, and sometimes a pre-B-cell.[7,8]

Pathogenesis

The malignant clone appears to have a rapid rate of growth at the subclinical stage but shows a marked decrease of doubling time at the symptomatic stage. The manifestations of multiple myeloma result directly from the malignant proliferation of myeloma cells and indirectly from the effects of the paraprotein. Proliferating plasma cells may cause tumours in soft tissue and in bone. Bones may also show multiple lytic lesions, most characteristically in the skull (Fig. 8.1), or there may be diffuse osteoporosis. Crush fractures of vertebrae (Figs 8.2 and 8.3a) and other pathological fractures (Fig. 8.3b) may occur. Dissolution of bone is contributed to not only by proliferation of myeloma cells but also by activation of osteoclasts by humoral factors secreted by the myeloma cells.[9] Bone lesions may lead to hypercalcaemia. Bone repair is poor so that osteosclerotic lesions are much less common than osteolytic lesions, and alkaline phosphatase is seldom elevated—usually only in relation to a healing fracture. Proliferation of myeloma cells in the bone marrow may lead to anaemia and less often neutropenia, thrombocytopenia or a leuco-erythroblastic blood film. Increased turnover of myeloma cells commonly leads to hyperuricaemia, which may contribute to renal failure. The paraprotein produced may be either IgG (κ or λ) or IgA (κ or λ) immunoglobulin, IgG or IgA plus the corresponding free light chain, or light chain only (κ or λ). Rarely, myeloma cells secrete IgD or IgE. IgG and IgA paraproteins may cause

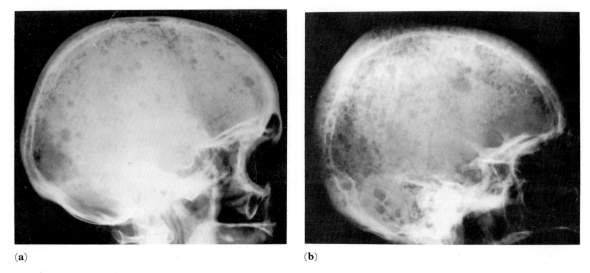

(a)   (b)

Fig. 8.1a,b Radiological abnormalities in the skulls of two patients with multiple myeloma. (a) Radiograph showing multiple radiolucent lesions which are, characteristically, not associated with a sclerotic reaction around them. At the apex of the vault, a radiolucent lesion is seen in profile. (b) Skull X-ray of a patient with both Paget's disease of bone and multiple myeloma. The characteristic radiolucent lesions of multiple myeloma are seen, in addition to thickening of the skull and sclerosis due to Paget's disease.

Courtesy of Departments of Radiology, St Mary's Hospital, London and St Charles's Hospital, London, UK.

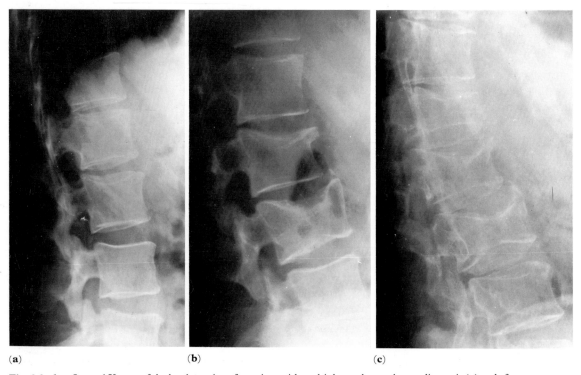

(a)   (b)   (c)

Fig. 8.2a,b,c Lateral X-rays of the lumbar spine of a patient with multiple myeloma taken at diagnosis (a) and after one year (b) and two years (c). Progressive vertebral destruction and collapse has occurred.

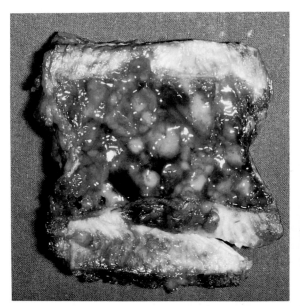

(a)

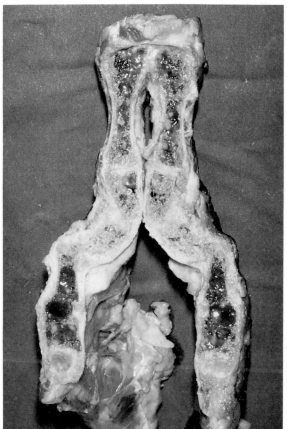

(b)

Fig. 8.3a,b Post-mortem findings in the patient with multiple myeloma whose X-rays are shown in Figure 8.2. (a) Longitudinal section of a lumbar vertebra; the pale nodules are myelomatous deposits. (b) Longitudinal section of the sternum showing pale nodular myelomatous deposits in the red bone marrow. The deformity of the sternum is a consequence of previous pathological fractures.

hyperviscosity of the blood (with neurological manifestations, cardiac failure, overexpanded blood volume, and characteristic retinal changes); hyperviscosity is much more likely with IgA paraproteins than with IgG, because of the greater propensity of the former to polymerize. Paraproteins may also be cryoglobulins and may cause tissue damage by precipitating in the cold (see cryoglobulinaemia, p. 307). Rarely, paraproteins may exhibit antibody activity which leads to clinical manifestations; bleeding may be consequent on anti-factor VIII activity, and xanthomatosis may be consequent on a paraprotein complexing with lipid.[1] In one patient a recurrent bullous eruption appeared to be due to a paraprotein with antibody activity against the basal cell layer of epidermis.[10]

Light chains of immunoglobulins were first detected by their ability to precipitate on heating to 50–60°C and to redissolve on heating to 90–100°C. They have been designated Bence Jones proteins (BJP) after Bence Jones who first described this property in 1847. More sensitive means of detecting free light chains are now available (see below). BJP, because of their low molecular weight (approximately 22 000), are filtered by the glomerulus and appear in the urine. Considerable reabsorption and metabolism by renal tubular cells occurs. BJP are nephrotoxic. BJP which are more cationic (high isoelectric point) appear to be more nephrotoxic[11] and lowering the urinary pH below the pI may increase nephrotoxicity. If the pH equals the pI, precipitation as casts may be more likely. Rarely BJP may damage renal tubules in such a manner as to cause an adult Fanconi syndrome.[12]

An immune paresis accompanies multiple myeloma. Both humoral and cellular immunity are impaired but humoral immunity more severely. Levels of normal immunoglobulins are reduced due both to decreased synthesis and increased catabolism. The reduction in the levels of normal immunoglubulins is not due solely to the presence of a high level of total immunoglobulin since it is seen also in Bence Jones myeloma. The number of normal B-cells in the peripheral blood is reduced.[13] An imbalance between helper and suppressor T-cells[8] may contribute to impaired humoral immunity. In advanced disease, total T-lymphocytes are decreased. The immune paresis is associated with an increased incidence of infections. Among infective complications are pneumonia, with pneumococcal infections being particularly common, and herpes zoster.

Laboratory studies of paraproteins

A paraprotein, being the product of a single clone of cells, is composed of identical molecules which are uniform in their characteristics. A paraprotein thus forms a discrete band on electrophoresis (Figs 8.4 and 8.5). Serum paraprotein bands are

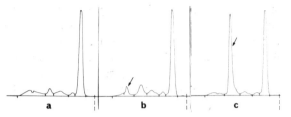

Fig. 8.5a,b,c Densitometric tracings of electrophoretic patterns shown in Figure 8.4. (**a**) Normal serum showing, from right to left, the albumin band and the α_1-, α_2-, β- and γ-globulin bands. (**b**) Serum from a patient with multiple myeloma showing a narrow paraprotein band (arrowed) in the γ region; normal γ globulin is reduced and β globulin is increased. (**c**) Serum from a patient with multiple myeloma showing a heavy paraprotein band (arrowed) in the β region; normal γ globulin is reduced.

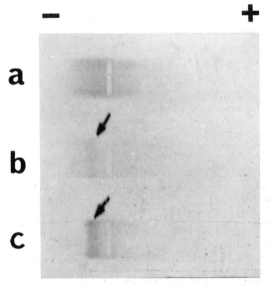

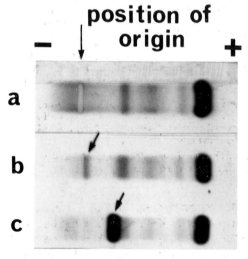

Fig. 8.4a,b,c Electrophoretic patterns obtained by electrophoresis of serum on 1% agarose gel using barbital buffer at a pH of 8.6. (**a**) Normal serum showing, from right to left, the albumin band and the α_1-, α_2-, β- and γ-globulin bands. (**b**) Serum from a patient with multiple myeloma showing a narrow paraprotein band (arrowed) in the γ region; normal γ globulin is reduced and β globulin is increased. (**c**) Serum from a patient with multiple myeloma showing a heavy paraprotein band (arrowed) in the β region; normal γ globulin is reduced.

Courtesy of Miss Carol Hughes, Department of Chemical Pathology, St Mary's Hospital, London, UK.

Fig. 8.6a,b,c Demonstration of an IgMκ paraprotein in a patient with a plasma cell dyscrasia by the technique of immunofixation. After serum proteins were separated by electrophoresis on agarose gel, a strip of cellulose acetate soaked with the antibody was placed on the agarose. Once the immunoprecipitate was formed, the unprecipitated protein was eluted off and the precipitate stained with amido black. The clear areas indicate the sites of application of the patient's serum for electrophoresis.
(**a**) Immunofixation using anti-λ-chain antibodies; the diffuse staining is caused by the reaction of the antibody with λ light chains in the normal, polyclonal immunoglobulins present in the patient's serum.
(**b**) Immunofixation using anti-κ-chain antibody demonstrating a κ-chain-containing paraprotein (arrowed).
(**c**) Immunofixation using anti-μ-chain antibody showing a μ-chain-containing paraprotein (arrowed).

Courtesy of Miss Carol Hughes, Department of Chemical Pathology, St Mary's Hospital, London, UK.

most often in the γ-globulin region but may also be in the β- or even the α-globulin zone. The immunoglobulin class and the light chain type of the paraprotein may be demonstrated by immunofixation (Figs 8.6 and 8.7), or by immunoelectrophoresis which shows an alteration of the

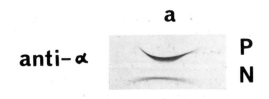

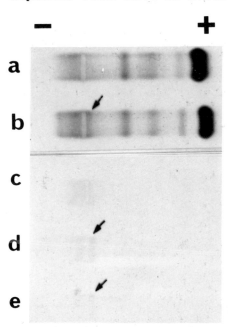

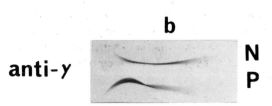

Fig. 8.8a,b Immunoelectrophoresis (IEP) of serum from two patients with paraproteins. Agar gel was poured on to a glass plate and allowed to set. A longitudinal central trough was cut and two wells were punched out, one on either side of the centre of the trough. The patient's serum (P) was placed in one of the wells and normal serum (N) in the other. The sera were subjected to electrophoresis, and the separated proteins were then reacted against specific antibody which was placed in the longitudinal trough. The occurrence of a reaction between the antibody and the corresponding antigen is indicated by the formation of a precipitation arc. (**a**) IEP with anti-α-chain antibody showing the formation of an abnormal, bowed precipitation arc with the patient's serum. A smooth arc has formed with normal serum. IEP of the patient's serum with anti-κ-chain antibody also resulted in the formation of a bowed arc. The patient had IgAκ multiple myeloma. (**b**) IEP with anti-γ-chain antibody showing bowing of the precipitation arc formed with the patient's serum. IEP with anti-κ-chain antibody showed a similar abnormality. The patient had IgGκ multiple myeloma.

Courtesy of Miss Carol Hughes, Department of Chemical Pathology, St Mary's Hospital, London, UK.

Fig. 8.7a–e Electrophoresis of serum followed by immunofixation to demonstrate clearly the presence of an IgMλ paraprotein band. The technique of immunofixation is outlined in the legend describing Figure 8.6. (**a**) Electrophoresis of normal serum. (**b**) Electrophoresis of patient's serum; a paraprotein band in the γ region (arrowed) is barely apparent. (**c**) Immunofixation showing diffuse staining with anti-κ-chain antibody, consequent on the presence of polyclonal immunoglobulins. (**d,e**) Immunofixation with anti-λ-chain and anti-μ-chain antibodies, respectively. The presence of a discrete paraprotein band is now readily seen.

Courtesy of Miss Carol Hughes, Department of Chemical Pathology, St Mary's Hospital, London, UK.

shape of the normally smooth arc of heterogeneous immunoglobulins (Figs 8.8 and 8.9). Immunoelectrophoresis is a more sensitive technique than electrophoresis and may occasionally detect small amounts of paraprotein which have not been detected by the latter technique. If a cryoglobulin is suspected, the blood sample must be kept warm until the serum has been separated from the red cells. Rarely, two or more discrete bands may be seen on serum electrophoresis; this

may be due to the presence of light chain as well as immunoglobin in the serum in a patient with renal failure, the presence of both monomers and polymers of IgA, or the presence of more than one paraprotein. The presence of two different paraproteins does not necessarily indicate biclonality; the two paraproteins may have the same light chain, be of the same idiotype and be secreted by the same cells.[14] Rarely, the same cells may secrete two paraproteins of the same idiotype but of different light chain type.[15] This indicates an aberration of the rearrangement of light chain genes (see p. 25). Serum electropho-

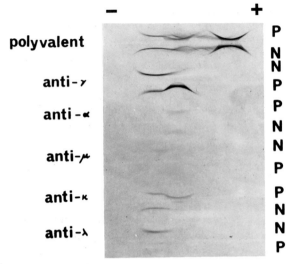

Fig. 8.9 Immunoelectrophoresis of serum from a patient with an IgG paraprotein. The technique of immunoelectrophoresis is outlined in the legend describing Figure 8.8. The antisera used are shown on the left of the figure. P indicates the side containing the electrophoresed proteins from the patient's serum and N the side containing a normal serum. With anti-α-chain, anti-μ-chain, anti-λ-chain antibodies, the patient's serum has formed smooth arcs similar to those formed by the normal serum; however, the patient's serum has formed much fainter arcs with anti-μ-chain and anti-λ-chain antibodies than the normal serum because of the lowered concentration of normal immunoglobulins (immune paresis) in the patient. With anti-γ-chain and anti-κ-chain antibodies, the patient's serum has formed abnormal bowed arcs due to the presence of an IgGκ paraprotein, in addition to normal polyclonal γ-chain-containing and κ-chain-containing immunoglobulins. Comparison of the patterns of precipitation arcs given by the patient's serum when reacted with specific antisera with the pattern given when reacted with the polyvalent antiserum (anti-human-serum proteins) allows the identification in the IEP with polyvalent antibody of abnormal arcs similar to and in the same position as those given by anti-γ-chain and anti-κ-chain antibodies.

Courtesy of Miss Carol Hughes, Department of Chemical Pathology, St Mary's Hospital, London, UK.

resis usually demonstrates not only a paraprotein band, but also a depletion of normal immunoglobulins (a reflection of immune paresis). In a patient who is secreting only a Bence Jones protein, a depletion of normal immunoglobulins is usually the only abnormality detected on serum protein electrophoresis. Quantitation of immunoglobulin using the radial immunodiffusion (RID) technique may be inaccurate when part of the immunoglobulin is a paraprotein, since the paraprotein may not diffuse normally. Inaccuracy

may also occur when immunoglobulins are quantitated by the RID technique and other immunochemical methods because of the use of antibodies directed against normal polyclonal immunoglobulins rather than the monoclonal immunoglobulin in question.[16]

Urinary Bence Jones protein may be detected by the heat test, if present in large amounts, but for reliable detection electrophoresis of urine concentrated 200-fold or more is needed (Fig. 8.10). Urine should be filtered and passed

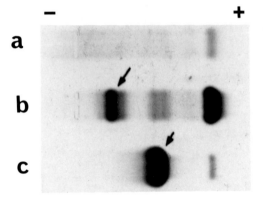

Fig. 8.10a,b,c Electrophoretic patterns obtained by electrophoresis of urine which had been concentrated 200-fold. Electrophoresis was performed on 1% agarose gel (barbital buffer, pH 8.6). (**a**) Urine lacking a paraprotein but containing albumin and traces of normal serum globulins (this pattern is shown when there is renal tubular damage). (**b**) Urine containing normal serum proteins and also a Bence Jones protein (arrowed) moving between β and γ globulins. (**c**) Urine containing a small amount of albumin, and also a Bence Jones protein moving in the α2 region.

Courtesy of Miss Carol Hughes, Department of Chemical Pathology, St Mary's Hospital, London, UK.

through ultrafilters prior to electrophoresis, as bacteria may destroy BJP in a matter of hours.[17] To facilitate interpretation, the patient's serum and concentrated urine should be electrophoresed in parallel (Fig. 8.11). As for serum, immunofixation and immunoelectrophoresis can be used to demonstrate that a discrete band is either κ or λ light chain. It should be noted that tests such as 'Albustix' which depend on the 'protein error of indicators' for the detection of urinary protein are unsatisfactory for the detection of BJP, since they give negative results with about 50% of BJP. Sulphosalicylic acid precipitation or

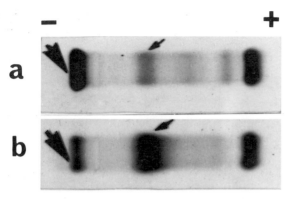

Fig. 8.11a,b Electrophoresis of serum and urine of a patient with multiple myeloma whose myeloma cells produced both an IgGλ paraprotein and a λ Bence Jones protein. Electrophoresis was performed on 1% agarose gel (barbital buffer, pH 8.6). (**a**) Electrophoresis of serum. The major abnormal band present is the IgGλ paraprotein (large arrow) but, because of a degree of renal insufficiency, the λ Bence Jones protein is also being retained in the serum and is seen superimposed on the normal β-globulin band (small arrow). (**b**) Electrophoresis of urine concentrated 200-fold. The major abnormal band is the λ Bence Jones protein (small arrow) but because of renal damage, albumin is appearing in the urine (band at far right) as is the larger molecular weight IgGλ paraprotein (large arrow).

Courtesy of Miss Carol Hughes, Department of Chemical Pathology, St Mary's Hospital, London, UK.

Bradshaw's ring test (in which urine is layered on to concentrated hydrochloric acid) are more satisfactory since approximately 97% and 95% of BJP are detected by the respective tests. As a small percentage of Bence Jones proteins are not detected by screening tests for urinary protein it may be necessary to carry out electrophoresis of concentrated urine despite negative screening tests in patients in whom there is a strong clinical suspicion of multiple myeloma or a related disorder.

The paraprotein produced is IgG ($\pm$ BJP) in 50–60% of cases of myeloma, IgA ($\pm$ BJP) in 20–25%, BJP alone in approximately 25% and IgD or IgE ($\pm$ BJP) in approximately 1%.[1,18] Rare patients who have the clinical features of multiple myeloma rather than Waldenström's macroglobulinaemia produce an IgM paraprotein. The distribution of light chain types in patients with multiple myeloma is κ in approximately two-thirds of cases and λ in the other third. BJP may appear in the urine for the first time during the course of myeloma; this may represent intra-

clonal evolution. A small percentage of patients have no demonstrable paraprotein in serum or concentrated urine. They are designated as having non-secretory multiple myeloma. A paraprotein may be demonstrable within the plasma cells of some of these cases[19,20] but not in all of them.[21] A distinction could thus be drawn between non-secretors and non-producers.

Pathology

Peripheral blood

Anaemia is usual, and neutropenia and thrombocytopenia are quite common. Anaemia is due not only to bone marrow infiltration but also to increased plasma volume, 'the anaemia of chronic disorders' (see Chapter 5) and, sometimes, renal failure. The blood film is often leucoerythroblastic. Myeloma cells may be seen in the peripheral blood, usually in small numbers. If large numbers of plasma cells are present, the condition is designated *plasma cell leukaemia*. The presence of a paraprotein in the blood leads to a

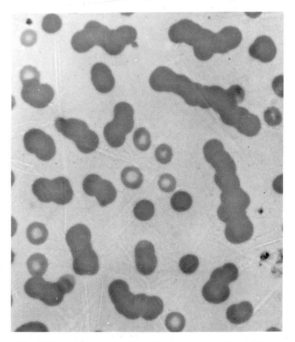

Fig. 8.12 Peripheral blood film from a patient with multiple myeloma showing increased background staining and rouleaux formation.

May–Grünwald–Giemsa stain   × 375

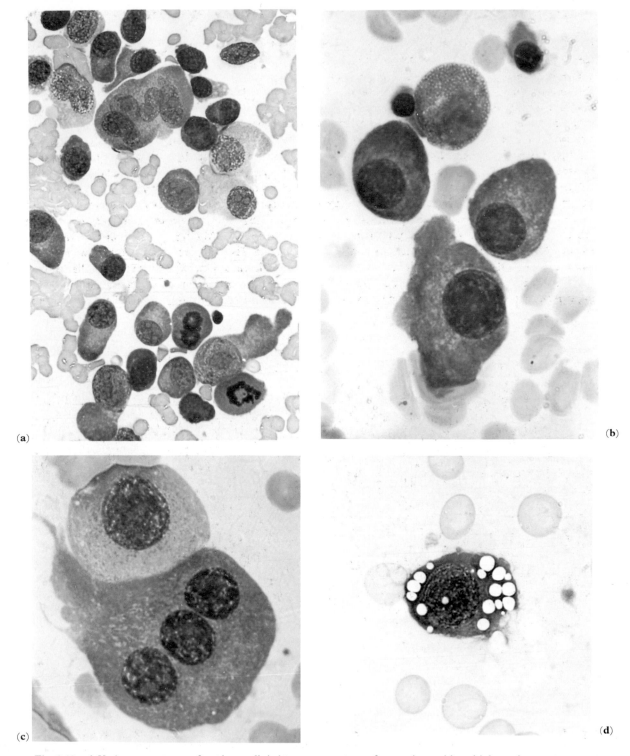

(a)

(b)

(c)

(d)

Fig. 8.13a–d Various appearances of myeloma cells in bone marrow smears from patients with multiple myeloma.
(a) Myeloma cells showing nucleo-cytoplasmic dissociation; the nucleus is immature (presence of a nucleolus, lack of chromatin clumping) in relation to the degree of cytoplasmic maturation. One binucleate and one multinucleate plasma cell and two plasma cells in mitosis are present. (b) Myeloma cells showing a milder degree of nucleo-cytoplasmic dissociation than the cells in (a). (c) Two myeloma cells showing nuclear immaturity and a marked increase in cell size; one cell is trinucleate.
(d) Myeloma cell showing extensive cytoplasmic vacuolation.   May–Grünwald–Giemsa stain   (a) × 375; (b,c,d) × 940

coating of erythrocytes with protein and a lessening of the electrical charges which normally repel the cells from one another; this leads to rouleaux formation (Fig. 8.12) and an increase in the erythrocyte sedimentation rate (ESR), often to greater than 100 mm/h. Large amounts of paraprotein cause an increased basophilic background-staining in blood smears which is apparent both microscopically and macroscopically. A paradoxically very low ESR may be seen in patients with marked hyperviscosity. Changes in the ESR and increased background-staining are not seen in patients who are producing only Bence Jones protein, or in the minority of patients with non-secretory myeloma.

It has been demonstrated that morphologically-normal lymphocytes in the peripheral blood may belong to the same clone as the myeloma cells.[13]

Bone marrow and bone

The bone marrow is infiltrated by abnormal cells whose appearances range from those of mature lymphocytes with slightly plasmacytoid features (cytoplasmic basophilia, Golgi zone) to dysmorphic plasma cells (Figs 8.13 and 8.14). Plasmacytoid lymphocytes are seen in a minority of patients and cells resembling plasma cells in the majority. Myeloma cells vary from those showing few atypical features to large, pleomorphic cells with very immature nuclei (diffuse chromatin pattern and nucleoli). Nucleo-cytoplasmic dissociation is common, with the nucleus

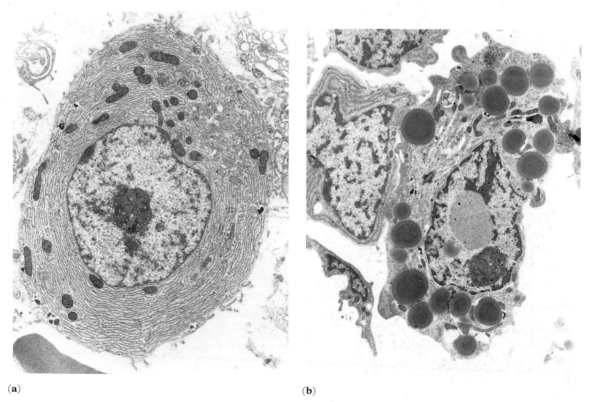

(a)

(b)

Fig. 8.14 Ultrastructure of two myeloma cells from the bone marrows of two different patients with multiple myeloma. (**a**) Myeloma cell displaying considerable asynchrony between nuclear and cytoplasmic differentiation (compare with normal plasma cells in Fig. 3.23, p. 65). The nucleus is immature-looking with relatively little condensed chromatin and a prominent nucleolus. The cytoplasm contains many parallel strands of rough endoplasmic reticulum. (**b**) Myeloma cell containing several unusual rounded inclusions. The majority of the myeloma cells of this patient contained such inclusions. In Romanowsky-stained smears the malignant cells appeared vacuolated, as illustrated in Figure 8.13d.

Uranyl acetate and lead citrate   (**a**) × 6000; (**b**) × 11 650

being immature but the cytoplasm showing a Golgi zone and basophilia. Mitotic figures may be common and bi-, tri- and multinucleate forms may be increased; when there is more than one nucleus per cell, the nuclei may differ considerably from one another in size and morphology. Myeloma cells may show scanty or numerous cytoplasmic vacuoles and cytoplasmic or intranuclear inclusions. 'Flaming' pink cytoplasm may be seen but, contrary to early reports, is not confined to IgA myeloma. Asynchronous development of nucleus and cytoplasm and pronounced multinuclearity ($\geqslant$ four nuclei per cell) are helpful in distinguishing multiple myeloma from reactive conditions but Mott cells and Russell bodies are of little help (see p. 83).[22] Intranuclear inclusions (Dutcher bodies) may be a more significant indicator of myeloma; however, they may be seen in other plasma cell dyscrasias and to a lesser extent in reactive conditions (e.g. bacterial and viral infections, cirrhosis, collagen disorders and carcinoma). Rarely, myeloma cells are haemophagocytic.[23] Because bone marrow infiltration in multiple myeloma is characteristically patchy, the bone marrow aspirate does not always show an increased proportion of plasma cells. Although the plasma cells (myeloma cells) are usually present in large numbers, in a minority of patients an aspirate may contain as little as 5 or 10% of plasma cells. If, in addition, the cellular atypia is only moderate, diagnosis may be difficult. In some patients, it may be necessary to aspirate bone marrow from more than one site, or to aspirate from an area of bony tenderness or radiological abnormality in order to obtain a diagnostic aspirate. Focal accumulations of large numbers of plasma cells may be more readily detected in 'squash' preparations of bone marrow-fragments, or in histological sections of bone marrow fragments or of a trephine biopsy. A trephine biopsy of bone marrow may also facilitate diagnosis by sampling a larger amount of tissue. Histological sections show both solid collections of plasma cells with an associated increase in reticulin fibres and also interstitial infiltration.[24] Focal aggregates have an endosteal and perivascular distribution[22] (Fig. 8.15); when the infiltrate is heavy, the predilection for an endosteal and perivascular distribution is lost. The detec-

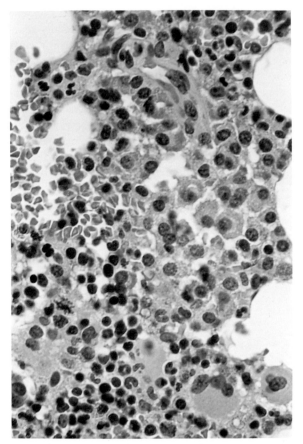

Fig. 8.15 Histological section of an aspirated bone marrow particle from a patient with multiple myeloma. The myeloma cells have a predominantly perivascular distribution.

Haematoxylin–eosin   × 375

tion of plasma cells in histological sections may be facilitated by a PAS stain for cytoplasmic carbohydrate or by a methyl-green-pyronine stain which identifies cells with large amounts of ribosomal RNA. The monoclonal nature of a plasma cell infiltrate may be demonstrated by the immunoperoxidase technique using antisera against specific heavy chains and light chains. A rare finding in myeloma is a sarcoid-like granulomatous reaction in infiltrated bone marrow.[25] Remodelling of bone by osteoclastic and osteoblastic activity is seen in association with myelomatous deposits; osteoclasts lie against the scalloped surface of rarefied trabeculae.[22] Osteoclasts may be particularly increased in areas where plasma cell infiltration is heavy.[9] Osteolytic lesions are most characteristic of multiple myeloma. Uncommonly, mixed lytic and sclerotic lesions occur, and rarely localized or diffuse osteosclerosis may be seen.[26] Because lesions are usually osteolytic, ^{99m}Tc radioisotopic bone scanning is generally an insensitive method for detecting myelomatous deposits; radiology is much more sensitive (Figs 8.1 and 8.2).

The bones most commonly affected by lytic lesions in multiple myeloma are the vertebral column, the ribs, the pelvis and the skull.

Other tissues

Approximately 70% of patients with multiple myeloma have extraosseous lesions.[27,28] These may be extensions of bony lesions, or disseminated lesions of blood-borne origin. Extraosseus lesions which have risen by direct spread from intramedullary lesions are most commonly paracostal, paravertebral or epidural within the spinal canal.[29] Spinal epidural lesions commonly result in paraplegia from cord compression and extensions from skull lesions may involve the orbit or may cause cranial nerve lesions. Disseminated lesions consequent on blood-borne spread are most common in the spleen, liver and lymph nodes, but virtually any tissue may be involved.[27,28,29]

The spleen is infiltrated in 45–70% of patients. The infiltrate is usually diffuse and is found in the red pulp and within sinuses; less often, it is nodular. Follicles are usually hypoplastic.[27,28,29] The liver is infiltrated in 27–56% of patients. The infiltration may be diffuse or nodular. Diffuse infiltration has a predilection for the sinusoids and the periportal region.[27–31] Liver infiltration may be severe enough to cause jaundice and ascites[31] though this is relatively uncommon. Ascitic fluid has the characteristics of an exudate, and sometimes contains plasma cells.[31] In the case of both the liver and the spleen, there is a poor correlation between organomegaly and the likelihood of infiltration.[29]

Lymph nodes are infiltrated in 22–64% of patients, with infiltration being least commonly detected in the more recent series.[27, 28, 29] Lymph nodes may be completely replaced by myeloma cells, or may contain nodules of these cells. When infiltration is diffuse there is a predilection for the medullary cords and the interfollicular area.[28, 29] Germinal centres are reduced in size and number.[28]

Other organs are infiltrated less often. The kidneys, lungs and heart are next most commonly involved, but virtually any organ may be. Renal infiltration may be diffuse interstitial, nodular, or within capillaries. Pleural infiltration may result in pleural effusions. Meningeal myelomatosis is rare; when it occurs, myeloma cells and the paraprotein may both be detected in the cerebrospinal fluid.[32]

Non-infiltrative lesions

Non-infiltrative lesions may also occur in multiple myeloma. They include amyloidosis, infective complications and the effects of paraproteins. Amyloidosis occurs in 7–10% of patients with myeloma. The distribution of amyloid is very similar to that in other types of immunocyte-derived or primary amyloidosis (see p. 301).

Infective lesions are common. Bacterial infections (bronchopneumonia, urinary tract infections and septicaemia) predominate.[29] Progressive multifocal leucoencephalopathy has occurred. This lesion is now known to be of viral aetiology, and its occurrence may be related to the immune paresis of multiple myeloma.

Renal lesions are very common. In one autopsy series, the kidneys were normal in only 12% of patients.[29] In addition to infiltrative lesions, amyloidosis and acute and chronic pyelonephritis, the kidneys may show tubular atrophy and interstitial fibrosis, casts (often laminated or fractured and sometimes containing protein crystals), giant cell reactions, nephrocalcinosis (tubular and interstitial) and glomerular lesions (fusion of foot-processes, basement membrane thickening, and an increase of mesangial cells and matrix).[1,29,33] A rare lesion is an acquired Fanconi syndrome consequent on tubular damage by Bence Jones protein. This may precede any other evidence of multiple myeloma.[12]

Neurological lesions are common. In addition to those due to infiltration or pressure, and those due to amyloidosis, neural damage may be due to a direct effect of paraprotein. Axonal degeneration in the absence of plasma cell infiltration or amyloidosis is the commonest lesion underlying peripheral neuropathy.[34] An unusual syndrome with dermatoendocrine alterations in addition to polyneuropathy has been described in patients with monoclonal gammopathies, some of whom can be categorised as having a plasmacytoma or multiple myeloma.[35]

Treatment

Chemotherapy with an alkylating agent (melphalan or cyclophosphamide) with or without corticosteroids causes a modest improvement in prognosis. Combination chemotherapy with larger numbers of drugs is also used. Radiotherapy provides effective palliative therapy for localized lesions. Current forms of treatment reduce the number of myeloma cells to a plateau but do not eliminate them. In the plateau phase the proliferative activity of the tumour cells is relatively low.[36]

Disease progression

The median survival of multiple myeloma is two to three years. Death may be due to infection, haemorrhage or renal failure, to refractoriness of the myeloma to therapy, or to a secondary acute leukaemia or dysmyelopoietic state (see Chapter 6). The most characteristic dysmyelopoietic state is refractory pancytopenia with sideroblastic changes in the bone marrow. The latter progresses to acute myeloid leukaemia if death does not occur in the preleukaemic phase. Multiple myeloma may also transform to an immunoblastic sarcoma of B-cell type with the immunoblasts bearing the same monoclonal markers as the myeloma cells.[37] This transformation may occur within or outside the marrow and is associated with a poor prognosis. It is likely that some patients described as having reticulum cell sarcoma following multiple myeloma actually had immunoblastic sarcoma.

PLASMA CELL LEUKAEMIA[1]

Plasma cell leukaemia is not a distinct disease but part of the spectrum of multiple myeloma; it occurs in 1–2% of patients with myeloma. The term plasma cell leukaemia is applied to those patients who have a large number of myeloma cells in the peripheral blood: a relative plasma cell count of more than 20% of the peripheral blood leucocytes and an absolute plasma cell count of greater than $2 \times 10^9/l$ have been suggested as criteria for this diagnosis.[38] Plasma cell leukaemia may occur as the terminal event in multiple myeloma which has become refractory to treatment. Patients who have plasma cell leukaemia at presentation tend to be younger than other patients with multiple myeloma, and have a higher incidence of hepatomegaly and splenomegaly and a worse prognosis. IgD myeloma is especially likely to manifest itself as plasma cell leukaemia; nevertheless, only a small proportion of patients with IgD myeloma present in this way. Of 11 patients reported with IgE myeloma, three have had plasma cell leukaemia.[39]

SOLITARY PLASMACYTOMA[40, 41]

A solitary plasmacytoma is a single localized tumour (in soft tissue or bone) which is due to local proliferation of a clone of malignant plasma cells. Those in bone marrow may be termed solitary myeloma and those in soft tissues extramedullary plasmacytoma. Extramedullary plasmacytomas have a predilection for the upper respiratory tract and the oral cavity; the underlying bone may be involved. The malignant cell is morphologically and functionally the same as the malignant cell in multiple myeloma. Paraproteins may be secreted and may appear in serum and urine. In some patients who appear to have a solitary plasmacytoma, careful study of the bone marrow may disclose evidence of multiple myeloma. In others no such evidence is found, and the occasional apparent cure of solitary plasmacytoma suggests that such tumours are indeed localized in a proportion of patients. Solitary plasmacytomas may recur locally, may metastasize (e.g. to regional lymph nodes) or may evolve into multiple myeloma. Prognosis is better than in multiple myeloma. Radical local treatment (surgery plus radiotherapy) is indicated.

IMMUNOCYTE-DERIVED AMYLOIDOSIS (INCLUDING PRIMARY AMYLOIDOSIS)[42, 43]

Definition

Amyloid fibrils, although structurally similar, show great chemical diversity. Immunocyte-derived amyloidosis is that type of amyloidosis in which the amyloid fibrils are derived from the light chains of immunoglobulin molecules.

Pathogenesis

Amyloidosis may be associated with overt plasma cell dyscrasias, such as multiple myeloma, Waldenström's macroglobulinaemia and heavy chain disease and less often with other malignancies of B-lymphocyte lineage. In such patients, deposition of amyloid in various tissues can be demonstrated in addition to the pathological lesions of the basic disease. In other cases, designated primary amyloidosis, there is no overt plasma cell dyscrasia but features suggestive of such a condition may be found. These features include a monoclonal immunoglobulin or Bence Jones protein, a reduction of levels of normal immunoglobulins, and a monoclonal proliferation of plasma cells in the bone marrow. There is no sharp demarcation between patients with an overt plasma cell dyscrasia and those with an occult one. Not all light chains are equally amyloidogenic, λ light chains being more likely than κ to be associated with amyloidosis. One subclass of λ light chains (VλI) was found to be particularly likely to form amyloid-like fibrils after digestion with pepsin in vitro.[44] Studies of a culture of bone marrow cells from a patient with multiple myeloma have shown that macrophages may process light chains to form amyloid.[45] In tissue sections, for example of the bone marrow, amyloid deposits may occur in conjunction with plasma cell infiltrates. Amyloidosis may be complicated by a haemorrhagic tendency due to the binding of factor X, and to a lesser extent other coagulation factors, to the amyloid.[46]

Pathology

A modest increase of bone marrow plasma cells (5–15% of nucleated marrow cells) is common in primary amyloidosis. A bone marrow biopsy shows the presence of amyloid in about a quarter of patients and is therefore a useful initial diagnostic procedure (see p. 102). The tissue distribution of amyloid in immunocyte-derived amyloidosis tends to differ from that in secondary, or reactive systemic amyloidosis. Common sites of amyloid distribution in immunocyte-derived amyloidosis are peripheral nerves, autonomic nerves, tongue, heart, pulmonary parenchyma, skin, joints, kidneys, liver, spleen, gastrointestinal tract and adrenals.[1, 42] In reactive systemic amyloidosis, kidneys, spleen and liver are characteristically involved, with deposition in other tissues being less common. In immunocyte-derived amyloidosis the usual histochemical features of amyloid (positive reaction with Congo red with green birefringence in polarized-light, yellow-green fluorescence with thioflavine -T) are seen and electron microscopy shows characteristic non-branching hollow fibrils. Amyloid deposits sometimes give positive results on immunofluorescence using antisera against the light chain type from which they are derived. Amyloid confined to a single organ (localized amyloidosis) may also be derived from immunoglobulin light chains[43] even though localized amyloidosis is unassociated with a circulating monoclonal protein.

Therapy

The demonstration that an occult or overt plasma cell dyscrasia underlies primary amyloidosis has led to trials of cytotoxic drugs and corticosteroids in patients in whom amyloidosis is the only clinical manifestation of the plasma cell dyscrasia. Although randomised controlled trials have not shown any improvement in survival,[47] individual patients appear to have benefited, with improvement in the nephrotic syndrome[47] and improvement in hepatic and renal function.[48, 49]

Disease progression

Prognosis is poor with a reported median survival in primary amyloidosis of 13 months.[50] Secondary acute myeloid leukaemia has been reported in two patients with primary amyloidosis who received prolonged melphalan therapy.[51]

WALDENSTRÖM'S MACROGLOBULINAEMIA[52]

Definition

Waldenström's macroglobulinaemia (WM) is a disorder characterised by a malignant monoclonal proliferation of B-lymphocytes which often have plasmacytoid features (plasmacytoid lymphocytes) and which secrete an IgM paraprotein. WM is part of the spectrum of lymphoplasmacytoid lymphomas, being distinguished by a clinical presentation consequent on the presence of the paraprotein.

Incidence

In one Australian survey, there were 0.5 new cases per 100 000 population per year.[3]

Pathogenesis

Manifestations of the disease result directly from lymphoproliferation, and indirectly from effects of the paraprotein. A few manifestations result from antibody activity of the paraprotein. Lymphoproliferation leads to lymphadenopathy, hepatomegaly and splenomegaly. Lymphoid infiltration of pleura, lungs and kidneys may occur. Osteolytic lesions are uncommon. The paraprotein generally causes hyperviscosity[53] and may also act as a cryoglobulin (Raynaud's phenomenon, vascular occlusion after cold exposure) or cause bleeding by coating platelets and impairing their function. BJP may also be present and amyloidosis occurs in about 10% of patients. The paraprotein may be deposited in the glomeruli. Serum levels of normal immunoglobulins are less reduced than in multiple myeloma. T-cell function is impaired and the incidence of fungal infections and tuberculosis is increased.

Laboratory studies of the paraprotein[1]

As the IgM paraprotein may be a cryoglobulin, the specimen should be kept at 37°C until serum is separated from red cells. In order to detect a cryoglobulin, serum should be left at 4°C and inspected daily for the presence of a precipitate for at least 48 hours and preferably for one week. The Sia test is a crude screening test for high levels of macroglobulins; as both false negative results and false positive results may occur, it is not recommended.

The IgM paraprotein is readily detected on serum electrophoresis. On immunoelectrophoresis the abnormal heavy chain arc is easily detected but the light chain arc may be difficult to detect unless the sample is pretreated with a reducing agent such as a mercaptoethanol. Immunochemical methods of assaying IgM are often inaccurate when an IgM paraprotein is present. With the technique of radial immunodiffusion (RID), the zone of precipitation is sometimes faint because of antigen excess, and may remain unrecognised until the sample is diluted. A significant part of the IgM may be present as a monomer (with a sedimentation coefficient of 7S) which diffuses more rapidly than 19S (pentameric) IgM and leads to overestimation of total IgM both with the RID technique and with electroimmunoassay (Laurell rocket technique). Immunochemical methods based on the measurement of turbidity and light scattering may also be inaccurate and it may be necessary to quantitate the paraprotein by densitometric measurements of the electrophoretic strip.

As in multiple myeloma, BJP may be present in the urine.

Pathology

Peripheral blood

Normocytic normochromic anaemia is usual; it is consequent on diminished erythropoiesis, shortened red cell life-span, increased plasma volume and splenomegaly. Rouleaux formation and the ESR are usually strikingly increased. A lymphocytosis may be present. In some patients, peripheral blood lymphocytes may be pleomorphic

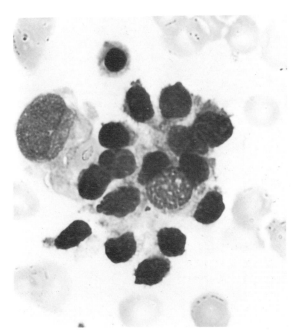

Fig. 8.16 Marrow smear of a patient with Waldenström's macroglobulinaemia (WM) showing a group of lymphocytes surrounding a macrophage. We have observed this close association between tumour cells and macrophages in two cases of WM; other cases have not shown this feature.

May–Grünwald–Giemsa stain   × 940

but in others they may be indistinguishable from CLL cells, even though the lymphocytes infiltrating tissues show plasmacytoid features.[54] The peripheral blood lymphocytes are often of the same clone as those in tissue infiltrates, even in patients without a lymphocytosis[55] and if sensitive techniques are used, a monoclonal blood lymphocyte population may be found in all patients.[56]

Bone marrow

The bone marrow is generally infiltrated by plasmacytoid lymphocytes but the morphology of the infiltrating cells may range from mature small lymphocytes to well-developed plasma cells[1] (Figs 8.16 and 8.17). Large PAS-positive intranuclear inclusions (Dutcher bodies) may be seen within the lymphoid cells. Cytoplasmic vacuoles or inclusions may also occur.[52, 57] On electron microscopy, variable amounts of rough endoplasmic reticulum are evident; ribosomal-lamellar complexes may be seen in some of the lymphoid cells of occasional cases of Waldenström's macroglobulinaemia, but this abnormality is more characteristic of hairy cell leukaemia (see

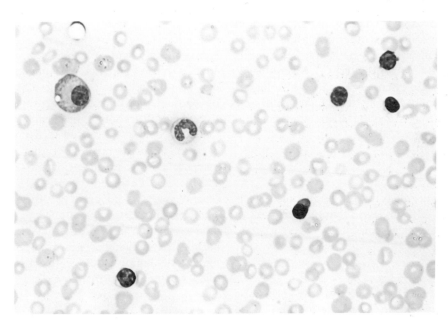

Fig. 8.17 Photomicrograph of a bone marrow smear from a patient with Waldenström's macroglobulinaemia. One plasma cell, one plasmacytoid lymphocyte and four lymphocytes are present.

May–Grünwald–Giemsa stain   × 350

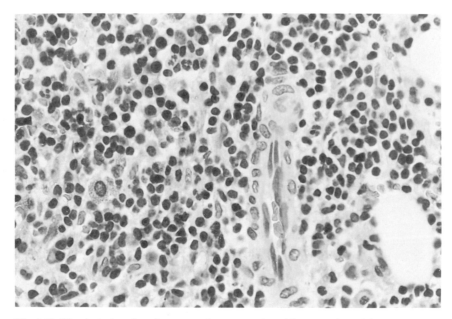

Fig. 8.18 Histological section of a marrow fragment aspirated from a patient with Waldenström's macroglobulinaemia. The marrow is diffusely infiltrated by many lymphocytes and some plasma cells.

Haematoxylin–eosin   × 350

p. 260 and Fig. 6.32). Immunofluorescence (IF) techniques demonstrate μ and either κ or λ light chains within the cytoplasm. IF can also be used to demonstrate the J chain which is found in more mature cells resembling plasma cells.[58] PAS-positive material may be seen in vessel walls and intra- and extravascularly.[59] Macrophages and mast cells are often increased. In histological sections, the infiltrate may be nodular or diffuse[60] (Fig. 8.18). Sinuses may be dilated and reticulin deposition increased.[60]

Lymph nodes

Lymph node histology is that of a diffuse, well-differentiated, lymphocytic lymphoma with a variable degree of plasmacytoid differentiation.

Kidneys

Renal failure is common and the nephrotic syndrome may occur. Renal lesions[33] include amyloidosis, infiltration by lymphoid cells (which may cause massive renal enlargement),[61] deposition of IgM on the endothelial aspect of the base-ment membrane, proliferative glomerulonephritis and the formation of casts.

Other tissues

Hepatomegaly and splenomegaly are found in about a third of patients. The lung and the pleura may also be infiltrated. Lytic lesions of bones are uncommon. Peripheral neuropathy may be due to cellular infiltration of the perineurium or endoneurium or may be related to deposition of the paraprotein in the myelin sheath.[34] Paraproteins may have anti-myelin or anti-Schwann-cell specificity.[62] Peripheral neuropathy may occur several years in advance of other evidence of Waldenström's macroglobulinaemia. An uncommon association of Waldenström's macroglobulinaemia is lymphangiectasia of the intestine and mesenteric lymph nodes;[63] this may be consequent on hyperviscosity of lymph.

Treatment

Alkylating agents such as chlorambucil may be of benefit. In patients whose symptoms are due mainly to hyperviscosity or the presence of a cryo-globulin, plasmaphaeresis may be of use, either for acute complications or occasionally for maintenance therapy; the predominantly intravascular distribution of IgM (Table 2.1, p. 26) makes this form of therapy feasible. The disease may terminate as immunoblastic sarcoma.[64]

IDIOPATHIC COLD HAEMAGGLUTININ DISEASE (CHAD)

Definition

Chronic idiopathic cold haemagglutinin disease (CHAD) is characterized by the occurrence of a cold-related haemolytic anaemia or cold-related vascular disturbance consequent on the presence of antibody which agglutinates autologous red cells at low temperatures.

Pathogenesis

The cold agglutinin of idiopathic CHAD is of monoclonal origin and CHAD is thus a clinical syndrome resulting from a plasma cell dyscrasia. The abnormal clone expands slowly and for many years the clinical manifestations may be confined to those due to the antibody activity of the paraprotein. The antibody is complement-binding IgM. Specificity is usually anti-I but may be anti-i or occasionally anti-Sp. Clinical features may be predominantly either those of haemolytic anaemia or of peripheral vascular disturbances. Haemolysis is chronic with exacerbations following exposure to the cold; haemolysis occurs on rewarming as complement is not fixed at low temperatures. Haemolysis is intravascular with haemoglobinuria. The vascular disturbance takes the form of reversible acrocyanosis on exposure to the cold due to obstruction of the capillaries in the cooler extremities by red cell agglutinates; some chronic tissue damage may occur. The underlying lymphoproliferative disorder is usually initially occult but in a minority of patients is clinically manifest.[65, 66]

Pathology

Peripheral blood

Anaemia is normocytic and normochromic in type. Agglutinates are present on blood films spread in cool conditions (see Fig. 5.34a) but not on those spread in warm conditions. A factitious elevation of the MCV and MCH and reduction of the RBC is usual in blood counts from automated counters, consequent on agglutinates rather than single cells passing through counting orifices. The reticulocyte count is increased. The direct antiglobulin test is positive with anticomplement reagents; commonly, only an inactive complement component (C3d) is present on red cells. Serum complement levels may be reduced. The titre of cold-agglutinin in serum is markedly elevated. In the usual case with anti-I specificity, the titre against adult red cells is much higher than the titre against normal red cells obtained from the umbilical cord, the latter having many fewer I antigen sites. In patients with a strong haemolytic element, the antibody may show increased thermal amplitude, e.g. may be active at temperatures above 30°C. The usual features of intravascular haemolysis are present (see p. 114). The IgM level may be increased and the amount of paraprotein present may be sufficient to cause a discrete band on serum protein electrophoresis and to be identified as monoclonal on immuno-electrophoresis. Light chain type is usually κ, but may be λ. Blood taken for immunological studies should be kept at 37°C both whilst clotting and during the separation of the serum.

Bone marrow and other tissues

In some patients, the marrow is infiltrated by cells resembling those seen in Waldenström's macroglobulinaemia or lymphoplasmacytoid lymphoma; in others, no such infiltrate is detectable.

Treatment

Avoidance of exposure to the cold may ameliorate haemolysis. Cytotoxic drugs may reduce the synthesis of the cold haemagglutinin.

Table 8.1 Classification of cryoglobulinaemia

Classification	Nature of cryoglobulin	Dominant clinical features	Clinical setting
Type I	Monoclonal paraprotein (usually IgM or IgG; rarely IgA or Bence Jones protein)	Cold-induced symptoms; hyperviscosity symptoms	(i) Primary (essential monoclonal cryoglobulinaemia) (ii) Secondary to lymphoproliferative disorder (e.g. multiple myeloma, Waldenström's macroglobulinaemia, lymphoma, chronic lymphocytic leukaemia and heavy chain disease)
Type II	Immune complex containing monoclonal paraprotein (usually IgM, may be IgG or IgA) with antibody activity against polyclonal IgG	Symptoms and signs due to immune-complex vasculitis affecting the skin (purpura), joints, kidneys and nervous system; hepatomegaly and splenomegaly are also common	(i) Primary (essential mixed cryoglobulinaemia) (ii) Secondary to lymphoproliferative disorder (iii) Associated with autoimmune disease, hepatitis or acute or chronic infections
Type III	Immune complex containing polyclonal immunoglobulin with antibody activity against IgG	As in type II cryoglobulinaemia	(i) Primary (essential mixed cryoglobulinaemia) (ii) Associated with autoimmune disease (e.g. rheumatoid arthritis, systemic lupus erythematosus, Sjögren's syndrome, progressive systemic sclerosis, allergic vasculitis, immune-complex nephritis) (iii) Associated with acute and chronic infections (e.g. hepatitis B infection, cytomegalovirus infection, subacute bacterial endocarditis, infectious mononucleosis, lepromatous leprosy)

Disease progression

In patients whose lymphoproliferative disorder is initially overt, the prognosis is related mainly to the primary disorder and not to cold-related phenomena. In patients without an overt lymphoproliferative disorder, the disease progresses very slowly. Spontaneous regression may occur.[54] A monoclonal band and clinical features of lymphoma may develop during the course of the disease. About 15% of such patients die of malignant lymphoma.[54]

CRYOGLOBULINAEMIA[67,68,69]

Definition

Cryoglobulinaemia is the presence in the serum of a globulin which precipitates on cooling and redissolves on rewarming (Fig. 8.19). Small amounts of cryoglobulin (less than 80 μg/ml) are found in the serum of normal people and are of no pathological significance.

Pathogenesis

The majority of cryoglobulins of clinical importance are composed of, or contain, immunoglobulins (Table 8.1); C-reactive protein may occasionally act as a cryoglobulin and cryofibrinogen may precipitate on cooling plasma.[70] A paraprotein may itself be a cryoglobulin (type I). Alternatively it may have antibody activity against polyclonal IgG (i.e. rheumatoid factor activity) and the immune complex formed may be a cryoglobulin (type II). Occasionally, immune complexes formed by polyclonal antibodies with rheumatoid factor activity may act as cryoglobulins (type III). Cryoglobulins may cause purpura and cold intolerance with acrocyanosis and cutaneous ulceration; these manifestations dominate in type I cryoglobulinaemia. In types II and III cryoglobulinaemia, signs and symptoms due to immune-complex vasculitis

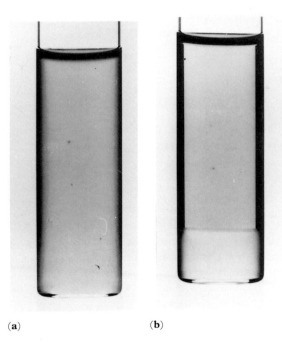

(a)   (b)

Fig. 8.19a,b Demonstration of a paraprotein which has the properties of a cryoglobulin in a patient with multiple myeloma. (**a**) The patient's serum at 37°C. (**b**) The patient's serum after chilling to 4°C followed by centrifugation; the cryoglobulin is now apparent at the bottom of the test tube.

Courtesy of Dr Helen Dodsworth

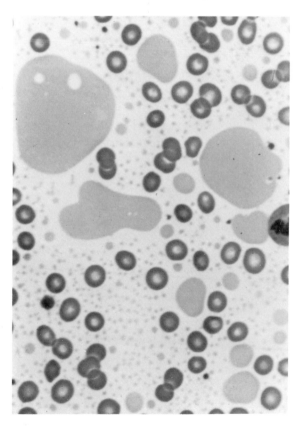

Fig. 8.20 Peripheral blood film spread at room temperature showing precipitated cryoglobulin.

May-Grünwald-Giemsa stain.

tend to dominate over cold-related symptoms. Serum complement is low and vasculitic lesions contain IgG, IgM and complement. Vasculitic lesions are common in skin, joints, kidney and nervous system. Proliferative glomerulonephritis may occur. Rarely, a cryoglobulin may also be a cold agglutinin so that the patient also has features of cold haemagglutinin disease[67] (see p. 305.

Peripheral blood and bone marrow

There are no specific abnormalities in the peripheral blood. Rarely, a cryoglobulin may precipitate in a blood film (Fig. 8.20). In essential monoclonal cryoglobulinaemia, the bone marrow may show an increase of lymphocytes or plasma cells, or intermediate forms. In patients in whom the bone marrow is initially normal, non-Hodgkin's lymphoma or other lymphoproliferative disorder may subsequently appear.[67]

HEAVY CHAIN DISEASES

Definition

The heavy chain diseases (HCD) are plasma cell dyscrasias in which the malignant cells secrete a heavy chain, or part of a heavy chain, rather than a complete immunoglobulin molecule. The heavy chain secreted may be γ, α or μ.

Aetiology

αHCD can be related both to host factors (HLA linkage, familial incidence) and to environmental factors (geographic distribution—possibly intestinal infections).[71]

Clinical features

Epidemiological and clinical features vary between γ heavy chain disease (γHCD), α heavy chain disease (αHCD) and μ heavy chain disease (μHCD) (Table 8.2). μHCD usually occurs as a feature of chronic lymphocytic leukaemia, often of long standing. αHCD is a form of 'Mediterranean lymphoma'. It is preceded by a prelym-phomatous polyclonal infiltration of the small intestine which is associated with malabsorption and is responsive to antibiotics.

Studies of immunoglobulins

On serum electrophoresis the heavy chains are usually found as a broad band in the γ or β regions or extending from the γ to the α_2 region. In some cases, the abnormal protein may be undetectable or may simulate a polyclonal increase. On immunoelectrophoresis (IEP), the protein is seen to react with a heavy chain antiserum but not with any light chain antiserum. On IEP, the free heavy chains migrate more rapidly than complete Ig with the same heavy chain. Because of their relatively low molecular weight, γ, α and μ heavy chains may all be found in urine. In αHCD, free α chains may be found in jejunal secretions or in the plasma cell infiltrate even when they are not found in serum or in urine. In μHCD, free light chains (BJP) may be found in the urine; although both light chains and heavy chains are synthesized, the defective heavy chain is not joined to the light chain.

Pathology

Peripheral blood and bone marrow

The features of the peripheral blood and bone marrow vary between the three types of HCD (see Table 8.2).

Other pathological features

Amyloidosis has been reported in γ- and μHCD (suggesting that some light chain secretion may occur in the former as has been demonstrated in the latter).

Disease progression

γ heavy chain disease is often rapidly progressive with bacterial infections being common. αHCD may respond to chemotherapy and radiotherapy; it may terminate in an immunoblastic sarcoma derived from the original clone of cells.

Table 8.2 Clinical and pathological features of the heavy chain diseases

	gamma (γ)	alpha (α)	mu (μ)
Age	Usually elderly	Usually young	Usually elderly
Epidemiology		Prevalent around the Mediterranean	
Hepatomegaly	+	−	+
Splenomegaly	+	−	+
Peripheral lymphadenopathy	+	−	−
Abdominal lymphadenopathy		Spread initially to mesenteric then retroperitoneal nodes	+
Particular features	May have uvular and palatal oedema	Small intestine infiltration with lymphocytes and plasmacytoid cells; supervenes on a prelymphomatous polyclonal infiltration Rarely may involve respiratory rather than gastrointestinal tract	
Peripheral blood	Atypical lympho-plasmacytoid cells and plasma cells in some; may have overt plasma cell leukaemia; may have pancytopenia and eosinophilia	Usually no specific features	Usually chronic lymphocytic leukaemia
Bone marrow	Lymphocytic or plasmacytoid infiltration, may have eosinophilia	Usually normal	Resembles chronic lymphocytic leukaemia but may also have plasma cells
Immunoglobulins			
Serum	Broad band in β region, normal Igs reduced	Broad band or apparently diffuse increase extending from α_2 to γ; monoclonal on IEP; normal Igs reduced	Broad band, or electrophoresis may show only hypogammaglobulinaemia with immunoelectrophoresis being required for diagnosis; normal Igs reduced
Urine	Broad band in β region in about half	Broad band	May have Bence Jones protein (free light chain)

MONOCLONAL GAMMOPATHY OF UNDETERMINED SIGNIFICANCE (MGUS)[72,73]

Definition

This phrase is used to describe the presence in the serum of a monoclonal immunoglobulin, in the absence of definite evidence of multiple myeloma or other plasma cell dyscrasia or lympho-proliferative disorder. The term MGUS is preferable to benign monoclonal gammopathy or benign monoclonal paraproteinaemia since prediction of a continuing benign course in all cases is not possible. Idiopathic Bence Jones proteinuria[74] is the presence in the urine of a monoclonal light chain, in the absence of any evidence of a plasma cell dyscrasia or lymphoproliferative disorder.

In MGUS the paraprotein is usually present in a relatively low concentration and Bence Jones protein (BJP) if present is usually excreted in relatively low amounts (e.g. 100–500 mg/day).[72, 75] Larger amounts of BJP (1–6 g/day) may be excreted in patients with idiopathic Bence Jones proteinuria.[74]

Pathogenesis

MGUS is due to proliferation and consequent expansion of a clone of antibody-secreting plasma cells but the extent of the expansion is less than in multiple myeloma. The abnormal plasma cells are found in the marrow together with lymphocytes of the same clone. Occasionally monoclonal plasma cells and lymphocytes are detectable in the peripheral blood. Although it has been suggested that there is an increased incidence of MGUS in patients with non-haemopoietic malignancy, this association has been disputed.[72, 73]

Pathology

Plasma cells usually make up less than 5% of the cells in bone marrow but may be up to 10%. Atypical plasma cells may be present; however the occurrence of asynchronous development of nucleus and cytoplasm suggests multiple myeloma rather than MGUS.[22] The presence of a large proportion of plasma cells containing cytoplasmic J chains supports a diagnosis of malignant rather than benign monoclonal gammopathy.[76]

Disease progression

Prolonged follow-up has shown that more than a quarter of patients who have not died of unrelated causes develop multiple myeloma, Waldenström's macroglobulinaemia, primary amyloidosis, or other lymphoproliferative disorder, sometimes as long as 15–20 years after the initial diagnosis. Others show progression of the disorder (rise of serum paraprotein or appearance of BJP) but do not develop overt plasma cell dyscrasia. Even on prolonged follow-up, more than half the cases do not show progression; in occasional patients the paraprotein disappears. The likelihood of progression cannot be predicted on the basis of paraprotein level, presence of BJP, diminution of normal immunoglobulins, or percentage of bone marrow plasma cells.[72] Idiopathic Bence Jones proteinuria is usually a precursor of multiple myeloma but some patients show no progression on prolonged follow-up.[74]

IMMUNE DEFICIENCY[77, 78]

INHERITED DEFECTS OF IMMUNE FUNCTION[79]

Congenital abnormalities of immune function may involve humoral immunity (B-cell defects), cellular immunity (T-cell defects) or both. The various inherited defects of immunity are listed in Table 8.3.

Inherited defects of humoral immunity

Defects of humoral immunity are characterised by hypo- or agammaglobulinaemia, or a lack of a specific class of gammaglobulin.

Sex-linked agammaglobulinaemia is the most severe defect of this type. B-lymphocytes and plasma cells are lacking from the blood and tissues, though in some cases pre-B-cells may be present in the bone marrow.[81] Germinal centres are absent from lymphoid tissue. Immunoglobulins are absent and the γ-globulin band is absent on serum protein electrophoresis. On blood grouping, anti-A and anti-B are absent. Patients with agammaglobulinaemia are particularly prone to bacterial infection but also have decreased ability to deal with certain other infections (infectious hepatitis, *Pneumocystis carinii* infection). There is an increased incidence of leukaemia, lymphoproliferative disorders, amyloidosis, and disorders which appear to be autoimmune in nature.

In *selective deficiency of IgG and IgA with elevated IgM*, B-cells are present but there is a failure of lymphocytes to switch isotype secretions from IgM to IgG, A and E.[82] Some individuals with *selective IgA deficiency* are healthy; others have sinopulmonary disease, allergy and auto-

Table 8.3 Inherited defects of immunity (AR = autosomal recessive; AD = autosomal dominant)

	Condition	Inheritance
Defective humoral immunity (B-cell defect)	Sex-linked agammaglobulinaemia	X-linked
	IgA deficiency	AR or AD
	IgM deficiency	Uncertain
	Lesch-Nyhan syndrome (see p. 181) (IgG↓)	X-linked
	Transcobalamin II deficiency (see p. 178)	AR
	IgG and IgA deficiency with elevated IgM	X-linked or AR
	Dystrophia myotonica (IgG↓)	AD
	Partial albinism with immunodeficiency (Ig↓)	AR
Defective cellular immunity (T-cell defect)	Thymic hypoplasia (di George syndrome)	May be AR (but usually not familial)
	Chronic mucocutaneous candidosis (± endocrinopathy) (defective T-cell response to *Candida*)	AR(?)
	Purine nucleoside phosphorylase deficiency	AR
	Hereditary orotic-aciduria[80] (see p. 181)	AR
	Duncan's syndrome (defective T-cell response to EB virus) (see p. 223)	X-linked recessive
Combined defect of cellular and humoral immunity (B- + T-cell defect)	Severe combined immunodeficiency (SCID)	AR or X-linked
	SCID with short-limbed dwarfism with or without cartilage-hair hypoplasia (T-cell deficiency may dominate)	AR
	SCID with aleucocytosis (reticular dysgenesis) (see p. 215)	AR
	Ataxia-telangiectasia	AR
	Wiskott-Aldrich syndrome (see p. 314)	X-linked
	Adenosine deaminase deficiency (T-cell deficiency may dominate)	AR
	Bare lymphocyte syndrome	AR
	Multiple biotin-dependent carboxylase deficiency	AR

immune disease. Those who are totally lacking in IgA may develop antibodies to IgA which can cause anaphylactic reactions following blood transfusion. Low IgG levels in *dystrophia myotonica* are consequent on hypercatabolism of IgG.

Inherited defects of cellular immunity

Di George syndrome

This syndrome is characterized by severe thymic hypoplasia associated with defective development of the third and fourth pharyngeal pouches. Inheritance is autosomal recessive. The thymus is absent or rudimentary. T-cells are lacking in the peripheral blood and in the T-dependent areas of lymphoid organs. There is usually lymphopenia.

Delayed hypersensitivity, graft rejection, and the development of antibodies to thymus-dependent antigens is defective. There is increased susceptibility to viral, fungal and protozoan infections and also to certain bacteria (mycobacteria, listeriae). Subjects with the di George syndrome also have abnormal facies, hypoparathyroidism and congenital heart disease. Permanent reconstitution of T-cell function occurs with fetal thymus transplantation.

Chronic mucocutaneous candidosis[83]

This disorder results from a specific inability of T-cells to respond to *Candida*. At least some cases appear to be inherited, probably as an autosomal recessive character, but others may have an autoimmune basis.

Table 8.4 Conditions associated with acquired defects of immunity*

Condition	Nature of defect
Prolonged physiological hypogammaglobulinaemia of infancy	Slow maturation of B-cell function; common in premature infants[81]
Common variable hypogammaglobulinaemia ($\pm$ thymoma, $\pm$ nodular lymphoid hyperplasia of intestine)	B-cell $\pm$ T-cell defect[81]
Sporadic acquired IgA deficiency	B-cell defect
IgA deficiency associated with phenytoin, gold or penicillamine therapy	B-cell defect
Phenytoin immunoblastosis	B-cell defect (general, or specific lack of IgA)
Nephrotic syndrome	Loss of immunoglobulin
Exudative skin disease	Loss of immunoglobulin
Protein-losing enteropathy and purgative abuse	Loss of immunoglobulin $\pm$ T-cell defect
Intestinal lymphangiectasia	Loss of immunoglobulin; loss of lymphocytes, particularly T-cells
Burns	Loss of immunoglobulin; destruction of T- and B-cells
Intensive plasma exchange with albumin solutions	Loss of immunoglobulins
Splenectomy and hyposplenism	Some antibody responses decreased
Sickle cell disease	Some antibody responses decreased
Infections[84]	
Cytomegalovirus and EB virus	T-cell defect; reduced T4/T8 ratio
Measles (natural disease or immunisation), chickenpox, infectious hepatitis, influenza	T-cell defect
Congenital rubella	T- and B-cell defects
Mycoplasma	T-cell defect
Leprosy, particularly lepromatous leprosy	T-cell defect
Tuberculosis	T-cell defect
Trypanosomiasis	T- and B-cell defects[85]
Sarcoidosis	Mild T-cell defect
Lymphoproliferative disorders	
Multiple myeloma	Decreased synthesis and increased catabolism of immunoglobulin; alteration of T-cell subsets (Tμ/Tγ ratio reduced[8,13])
Waldenström's macroglobulinaemia	B-cell defect in many patients
Chronic lymphocytic leukaemia	T- and B-cell defects; B-cell defect predominant; alteration of T-cell subsets (Tμ/Tγ ratio reduced); reduced NK and ADCC[86]
Follicular lymphoma	B-cell defect— hypogammaglobulinaemia in 20 per cent[54]

Condition	Nature of defect
Hodgkin's disease	T-cell defect predominant[87,88]
Hairy cell leukaemia	T-cell and monocyte/macrophage defects; lack of NK cells;[89] altered subsets in some studies but not others[90,91]
Angioimmunoblastic lymphadenopathy	T-cell defect
Advanced carcinoma	T-cell defect
Liver disease	T-cell defect
Uraemia	T-cell defect
Malnutrition	T-cell defect
Zinc deficiency	T-cell defect
Surgery and trauma	T-cell defect[92]
Anaesthesia	T-cell defect
Corticosteroid therapy	B-cell, T-cell and macrophage defects
Cytotoxic chemotherapy	B- and T-cell defects
Following bone marrow transplantation	B- and T-cell defects due to slow reconstitution; B-cell functional defect which may be due to earlier reconstitution of T8 subset than of T4 subset[81,93]
Graft-versus-host disease	T-cell defect; alteration of T-cell subsets; T4/T8 ratio reduced due to absolute or relative increase of T8 subset;[93] thymic involution; hyposplenism;[94] some degree of B-cell defect
Antilymphocyte globulin	T-cell defect
Cyclosporin A	T-cell defect, reduced T-helper and possibly T-cytotoxic-effector subsets[95]
Radiotherapy	Reduced T-cells due to selective reduction of T4 subset[88]
Acquired immunodeficiency syndrome (AIDS) of homosexuals and others, due to HTLV III infection	T-cell defect predominant, particularly reduction of T4 subset
Normal ageing	Decline of T-cell number and function; increased incidence of autoantibodies

*ADCC = cells mediating antibody-dependent cellular cytotoxicity; B-cell = B-lymphocyte; NK = natural killer cells; T-cell = T-lymphocyte; $T\mu$ and $T\gamma$ = T-cells with receptors for the $Fc\mu$ and $Fc\gamma$ fragments of immunoglobulin molecules, respectively; T4 = T-cells identified by monoclonal antibodies as being of helper phenotype; T8 = T-cells identified by monoclonal antibodies as being of suppressor phenotype.

Combined defects of humoral and cellular immunity

Severe combined immunodeficiency

The syndrome of severe combined immunodeficiency (SCID), which is inherited as an autosomal recessive characteristic, results from gross defects of both T- and B-cells.

Severe hypogammaglobulinaemia coexists with lymphopenia and defective cell-mediated immunity. T-cells are absent or very low but, in the majority, B-cells are present despite the failure to produce antibody.[78] There is susceptibility to bacterial, fungal, viral and protozoan infections. Death has followed the administration of live attenuated virus vaccines. Graft rejection is delayed. An inability to reject donor lymphocytes may allow graft-versus-host disease to occur after blood transfusion. The condition is uniformly fatal in childhood (in the absence of a successful bone marrow transplantation). SCID with sex-linked recessive inheritance is similar but somewhat less severe.

Ataxia-telangiectasia

This is a condition with autosomal recessive inheritance in which the thymus resembles the embryonic thymus and a major defect in T-cell function is associated with a variable defect of immunoglobulin synthesis. The latter is due to both an intrinsic B-cell defect and a deficiency of helper T-cells. IgM-secreting B-cells are normal but there is a failure to switch to IgA and IgE synthesis, and IgG synthesis is sometimes also defective. The pathogenetic mechanism may be a defect of lymphoid tissue maturation secondary to failure of DNA synthesis, repair, or both.[84]

Wiskott–Aldrich syndrome

The Wiskott–Aldrich syndrome (see also p. 281) is an X-linked defect in which there is eczema, recurrent pyogenic infections and thrombocytopenia. The thrombocytopenia (platelet count 5–$100 \times 10^9/l$) is present at birth. Platelets are decreased in size. Platelet life-span is reduced due to an intrinsic defect. Megakaryocytes are normal or increased. T-cell numbers are reduced, as are IgM levels and the antibody response to polysaccharide antigens.

Immunodeficiency consequent on enzyme deficiency

Certain enzyme deficiencies, particularly those involved in purine synthesis, may cause immunodeficiency (Table 8.3), probably as a consequence of accumulation of intermediates of purine metabolism. In adenosine deaminase deficiency, the transfusion of red cells, which supply the missing enzyme, is sometimes but not always of benefit. When successful, deoxyadenosine disappears from urine and plasma, and T-lymphocyte numbers rise.

ACQUIRED DEFECTS OF IMMUNE FUNCTION[77,78,81]

A large number of conditions are associated with acquired defects of immune function and these are summarized in Table 8.4. The defects of immune function commonly involve both humoral and cellular immunity and often have a multifactorial basis. Impaired humoral immunity may be due to defective synthesis of immunoglobulins (transient hypogammaglobulinaemia of infancy, chronic lymphocytic leukaemia), to increased catabolism or loss of immunoglobulins (nephrotic syndrome, burns), or to both (multiple myeloma). Lymphocytes as well as immunoglobulin may be destroyed or lost from the body (burns, intestinal lymphangiectasia). Defects of antibody synthesis may be due to a lack or defect of B-cells, an excess or increased activity of suppressor T-cells, or a lack of helper T-cells. For example, *common variable immunodeficiency* (CVID) is a heterogeneous group of conditions in which there may be a marked deficiency of B-cells (particularly if a thymoma is present); more commonly, there are normal numbers of B-cells which, however, are functionally immature, being capable of producing IgM but little IgG or IgA.[81] In a minority of patients with CVID, B-cells are mature but are reduced in number, and suppressor T-cells are increased.[81] *Transient hypogammaglobulinaemia of infancy* may be related to a lack of helper T-cells.[81]

REFERENCES

1. Kyle RA, Bayrd ED. The monoclonal gammopathies: multiple myeloma and related plasma cell disorders. Springfield: Thomas, 1976.
2. Wintrobe MM, Lee GR, Boggs DR, et al. Clinical haematology. 8th ed. Lea & Febiger, Philadelphia, 1981: 1457.
3. Lowenthal R. Aust NZ J Med 1982; 12: 258.
4. Blattner WA, Blair A, Mason TJ. Cancer 1981; 48: 2547.
5. Ishimaru T, Finch SC. N Engl J Med 1979; 301: 439.
6. Fukuhara S, Uchino H. N Engl J Med 1983; 308: 1603.
7. Greaves M, Janossy G. Biochim Biophys Acta 1978; 516: 193.
8. Mellstedt H, Holm G, Pettersson D, Peest D. Clin Haematol 1982; 11: 65.
9. Mundy GR, Raisz LG, Cooper RA, Schechter GP, Salmon SE. N Engl J Med 1974; 291: 1041.
10. Vincendeau P, Claudy A, Thivolet J, Tessier R, Texier L. Arch Dermatol 1980; 116: 681.
11. Clyne DH, Pesce AJ, Thompson RE. Kidney Int 1979; 16: 345.
12. Maldonado JE, Velosa JA, Kyle RA, et al. Am J Med 1975; 58: 354.
13. Abdou NI, Abdou NL. Ann Intern Med 1975; 83: 42.
14. Rudders RA, Yakulis V, Heller P. Am J Med 1973; 55: 215.
15. Bouvet JP, Buffe D, Oriol R, Liacopoulos P. Immunology 1974; 27: 1095.
16. Whicher JT, Warren C, Chambers RE. Ann Clin Biochem 1984; 21: 78.
17. Hobbs JR. Adv Clin Chem 1971; 41: 219.
18. Hobbs JR. Br J Haematol 1969; 16: 599.
19. Mancilla R, Davis GL. Am J Med 1977; 63: 1015.
20. van Camp B, de Bock B, Peetermans M. Br J Haematol 1977; 35: 670.
21. River GL, Tewksbury DA, Fudenberg HH. Blood 1972; 40: 204.
22. Bartl R, Frisch B, Burkhardt R, et al. Br J Haematol 1982; 51: 361.
23. Wirt DP, Grogan TM, Payne CM, et al. Am J Clin Pathol 1983; 80: 75.
24. Rywlin AM. Histopathology of the bone marrow. Boston: Little, Brown and Company, 1976: 83.
25. Falini B, Tabilio A, Velardi A, Cernetti C, Aversa F, Martelli MF. Scand J Haematol 1982; 29: 211.
26. Raman S, Frame B, Saeed SM, Tolia K, Raju U, Kottamasu S. Am J Clin Pathol 1983; 80: 84.
27. Hayes DW, Bennett WA, Heck FJ. Arch Pathol 1952; 53: 262.
28. Churg J, Gordon AJ. Am J Clin Pathol 1950; 20: 934.
29. Kapadia SB. Medicine (Baltimore) 1980; 59: 380.
30. Young GP, Bhathal PS, Wall AJ, Sullivan JR, Hurley TH. Aust NZ J Med 1978; 8: 14.
31. Thomas FB, Clausen KP, Greenberger NJ. Arch Intern Med 1973; 132: 195.
32. Spiers ASD, Halpern R, Ross SC, Neiman RS, Harawi S, Zipoli TE. Arch Intern Med 1980; 140: 256.
33. Porter K. In: Symmers W St C, ed. Systemic pathology. 2nd ed. London: Churchill Livingstone, 1978: vol. 4, 1375.
34. Vital C, Vallat JM, Deminiere C, Loubet A, Leboutet MJ. Cancer 1982; 50: 1491.
35. Moya-Mir MS, Martin-Martin F, Barbadillo R, Cuervas-Mono V, Martin-Jiminez T, Sanchez-Miro I. Postgrad Med J 1980; 56: 427.
36. Durie BGM, Russell DH, Salmon SE. Lancet 1980; ii: 65.
37. Falini B, de Solas I, Levine AM, Parker JW, Lukes RJ, Taylor CR. Blood 1982; 59: 923.
38. Kyle RA, Maldonado JE, Bayrd ED. Arch Intern Med 1974; 133: 813.
39. Endo T, Okumura H, Kikuchi K, et al. Am J Med 1981; 70: 1127.
40. Bataille R, Sany J. Cancer 1981; 48: 845.
41. Bataille R. Clin Haematol 1982; 11: 113.
42. Glenner GG. N Engl J Med 1980; 302: 1333.
43. Kyle RA. Clin Haematol 1982; 11: 151.
44. Linke RP, Tischendorf FW, Zucker-Franklin D, Franklin EC. J Immunol 1973; 111: 24.
45. Durie BGM, Persky B, Soehnlen BJ, Grogan TM, Salmon SE. N Engl J Med 1982; 307: 1689.
46. McPherson R, Onstad J. Am J Clin Pathol 1977; 67: 205.
47. Kyle RA, Greipp PR. Blood 1978; 52: 818.
48. Horne McDK. Ann Intern Med 1975; 83: 281.
49. Bradstock K, Clancy R, Uther J, Basten A, Richards J. Aust NZ J Med 1978; 8: 176.
50. Barth WF, Willerson JT, Waldmann TA, Decker JL. Am J Med 1969; 47: 259.
51. Kyle RA, Pierre RV, Bayrd ED. Blood 1974; 44: 333.
52. McCallister BD, Bayrd ED, Harrison EG, McGuckin WF. Am J Med 1967; 43: 394.
53. MacKenzie MR, Lee TK. Blood 1977; 49: 507.
54. Galton DAG, MacLennan ICM. Clin Haematol 1982; 11: 561.
55. van Camp B, Reynaert P, Broodtaerts L. Clin Exp Immunol 1981; 44: 82.
56. Smith BR, Robert NJ, Ault KA. Blood 1983; 61: 911.
57. Ricci A, Monahan RA, Paradise C, Robinson S, Dvorak AM. Arch Pathol Lab Med 1982; 106: 452.
58. Bast BJEG, Boom SE, Ballieux RE. Blood 1982; 60: 608.
59. Rywlin AM, Civantos F, Ortega RS, Dominguez CJ. Am J Clin Pathol 1975; 63: 769.
60. Chalazzi G, Bettini R, Pinotti G. Lancet 1979; ii: 965.
61. Grossman ME, Bia MJ, Goldwein MT, Hill G, Goldberg M. Arch Intern Med 1977; 137: 1613.
62. Dellagi K, Dupouey P, Brouet JC, et al. Blood 1983; 62: 280.
63. Harris M, Burton IE, Scarffe JH. J Clin Pathol 1983; 36: 30.
64. Abe M, Takahashi K, Mori N, Kojima M. Cancer 1982; 49: 2580.
65. Isbister JP, Cooper DA, Blake HM, Biggs JC, Dixon RA, Penny R. Am J Med 1978; 64: 434.
66. Lee CH, Cherian R, Hughes WG, Nurbhai M. Aust NZ J Med 1979; 9: 602.
67. Invernizzi F, Galli M, Serino G, et al. Acta Haematol (Basel) 1983; 70: 73.
68. Brouet J-C. Clauvel J-P, Danon F, Klein M, Seligman M. Am J Med 1974; 57: 775.
69. Barnett EV, Bluestone R, Cracchiolo A, Goldberg LS, Kantor GL, McIntosh RM. Ann Intern Med 1970; 73: 95.
70. Clinicopathological Conference. Am J Med 1980; 68: 757.
71. Khojasteh A, Haghshenass M, Haghighi P. N Engl J Med 1983; 308: 1401.

72. Kyle RA. Clin Haematol 1982; 11: 123.

73. Anonymous (Editorial). Br Med J 1980; 208: 273.

74. Kyle RA, Greipp PR. N Engl J Med 1982; 306: 564.

75. Pick A1, Shoenfield Y, Frohlichmann R, Weiss H, Vana D, Schreibman S. JAMA 1979; 241: 2275.

76. Bast JEG, van Camp B, Boom SE, Jaspers FCA, Ballieux RE. Clin Exp Immunol 1981; 44: 375.

77. Ammann AJ, Fudenberg H. In: Fudenberg HH, Stites DP, Caldwell JL, Wells JV, eds. Basic and clinical immunology. 3rd ed. Los Altos: Lange, 1980: 409.

78. Siegal FP, Good RA. Clin Haematol 1977; 6: 355.

79. Hirschhorn R. N Engl J Med 1983; 308: 714.

80. Girot R, Hamet M, Perignon J-L, et al. N Engl J Med 1983; 308: 700.

81. Pereira RS, Platts-Mills TAE. Clin Haematol 1982; 11: 589.

82. Levitt D, Haber P, Rich K, Cooper MD. J Clin Invest 1983; 72: 1650.

83. Hermans PE, Ulrich JA, Markowitz H. Am J Med 1969; 47: 503.

84. Waldmann TA, Misiti J, Nelson DL, Kraemer KH. Ann Intern Med 1983; 99: 367.

85. Askonas BA, Lehner T. J R Soc Med 1981; 74: 382.

86. Platsoucas CD, Fernandes G, Gupta SL, et al. J Immunol 1980; 125: 1216.

87. Posner MR, Reinherz E, Lane H, Mauch P, Hellman S, Schlossman SF. Blood 1983; 61 705.

88. Lauria F, Foa R, Gobbi M, et al. Cancer 1983; 52: 1385.

89. Ruco LP, Procopio A, Maccallini V, et al. Blood 1983; 61: 1132.

90. Worman CP, Cawley JC. Scand J Haematol 1982; 29: 338.

91. Catovsky D, Linch DC, Beverley PCL. Clin Haematol 1982; 11: 661.

92. Munster AM. Lancet 1976; i: 1329.

93. Janossy G, Prentice HG. Clin Haematol 1982; 11: 631.

94. Prentice HG. J Clin Pathol 1983; 36: 1207.

95. Kahan BD. Clin Haematol 1982; 11: 743.

9

Blood coagulation, fibrinolysis and the disorders

Normal haemostasis involves vasoconstriction of small vessels, formation of a platelet plug and blood coagulation. Platelet plug formation and blood coagulation both require an interaction between coagulation factors, platelets and subendothelial or extravascular tissues. In addition to the coagulation factors, blood plasma contains inhibitors of coagulation, and proteins of other systems which interact with the coagulation factors. Specifically, these are proteins of the fibrinolytic, complement, and kinin systems.

THE COAGULATION FACTORS AND NORMAL HAEMOSTASIS

The coagulation factors are primarily contained in the blood plasma, although fibrinogen, factors XI, V and XIII and factor-VIII-related antigen (VIIIR:Ag) are also found in or on the platelet. With the exception of the factor VIII molecule, the coagulation factors are probably all synthesized in the parenchymal cells of the liver. The interactions of the coagulation factors during blood coagulation are shown in Figure 9.1. Coagulation may be initiated by two pathways. The intrinsic pathway is initiated when factor XII (Hageman factor) is activated by exposure to a foreign surface, with a cascade of catalytic reactions then continuing through factors XI, IX, X and II. Each of these factors is present as a procoagulant which when cleaved becomes an active serine protease, and then cleaves its own substrate. In this cascade high molecular weight kininogen (HMWK), factors VIII and V and

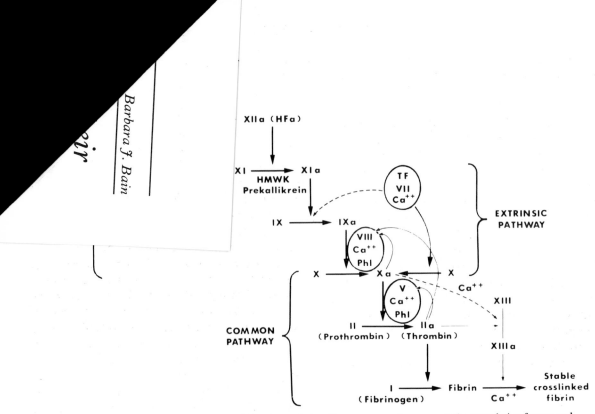

Fig. 9.1 The intrinsic and extrinsic pathways of blood coagulation. Roman numerals represent the coagulation factors and 'a' indicates the activated form. HF = Hageman factor; HMWK = high molecular weight kininogen; Phl = phospholipid; TF = tissue factor. (The slow activation of XIII by Xa may not be of physiological significance.)[1]

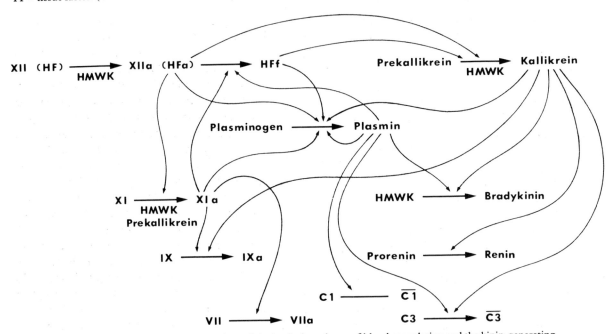

Fig. 9.2 The interaction between the contact phase of the intrinsic pathway of blood coagulation and the kinin-generating, complement and fibrinolytic systems. HF = Hageman factor; HFa = activated Hageman factor; HFf = Hageman factor fragment; Cl, C3 = complement components; $\overline{C1}$, $\overline{C3}$ = activated complement components; HMWK = high molecular weight kininogen.

calcium and phospholipid are cofactors. Coagulation may also be initiated through the extrinsic pathway when the exposure of factor VII to tissue factor in the presence of calcium leads to the formation of a complex which activates factor X and thus II. Activation of the extrinsic pathway also leads to activation of factor IX,[2] thus bypassing factors XII and XI (Fig. 9.1). Whether this activation of factor IX is of any physiological significance is uncertain,[3] though it does provide a possible explanation for the relatively mild haemorrhagic disorder in factor XI deficiency and the lack of any haemorrhagic disorder in deficiency of factor XII or the other contact factors. Factor XI may also be bypassed by a pathway involving kallikrein[4] (Fig. 9.2). Factor Xa greatly enhances the cofactor activity of factor VIII[5] and IIa greatly enhances the cofactor activity of both factor VIII and factor V (Fig. 9.1); thus activated factors which may be the product of either the extrinsic or the intrinsic system have an enhancing effect on the intrinsic system.

The vitamin-K-dependent factors[6]

These are closely related to one another in structure and function and include not only the four procoagulant factors, factors II, VII, IX and X, but also protein C which, when activated, has an anticoagulant action. They are designated serine proteases since after cleavage they have a serine residue at their enzymatically active centre. They all undergo a post-translational vitamin-K-dependent carboxylation reaction in which γ-carboxyl groups are added to glutamic acid residues at the amino-terminal end of the molecule. The γ-carboxyglutamic acid residues make possible the binding of calcium ions by the activated molecule, and thus allow complexing of factors IXa, VIII, X and platelet phospholipid, and similarly of factors Xa, V, II and platelet phospholipid (PF3). Acarboxy- or partly carboxylated coagulation factors have a reduced ability to bind calcium and thus a reduced coagulation activity; such defective factors are formed when there is vitamin K deficiency or when vitamin K antagonists (coumarins and indanediones) are administered. Prior to an understanding of the bio-

chemical defect they were designated PIVKAs—proteins induced by vitamin K absence or antagonist.

Factor VIII

The factor VIII molecule has functions beyond the coagulation cascade, being necessary for some of the functions of normal platelets. Factor VIII appears to be a complex of a large polymer, the synthesis of which is controlled by an autosomal gene, and a smaller component, the synthesis of which is controlled by an X-chromosome gene. The smaller component has a molecular weight of approximately 150 000–255 000 and has factor VIII coagulation activity (factor VIII:C) and its own antigenic determinants recognized by antibodies developed in haemophiliacs or uncommonly in non-haemophiliacs (VIII:C Ag). The large polymer is composed of four, six or more identical subunits each with a mol. wt. of 200 000–250 000 so that the mol. wts of the polymers vary between 850 000 and $12–20 \times 10^6$; it is recognized by a precipitating antibody raised in rabbits injected with factor VIII and is therefore called the factor-VIII-related antigen (VIIIR:Ag). The larger polymers ($>1 \times 10^6$ daltons) have ristocetin cofactor activity (factor VIII:RiCoF) (see p. 284) and other von Willebrand factor (factor VIII:VWF) activities such as involvement in the adhesion of platelets to subendothelium and collagen fibrils and to glass beads, and shortening of the bleeding time. The existence of polymers of different molecular weight causes the formation of an arc on crossed immunoelectrophoresis; if polymers of different size are not present in the normal ratio then the precipitation arc will be abnormal in position (variant von Willebrand's disease).

Specific antibodies can be raised against low molecular weight factor VIII (with VIII:C activity) and high molecular weight factor VIII (with VWF activity) respectively[7] suggesting that VIII:C does not merely consist of one of the subunits making up VIII/VWF. The synthesis of factor VIII:C appears to be dependent on the prior synthesis of VIIIR:Ag (VIII:VWF), since transfusion of normal serum or haemophiliac plasma into a patient with von Willebrand's disease (VWD) leads to the synthesis of VIII:C.

Factor VIIIR:Ag has been detected in endothelial cells, platelets, and megakaryocytes. It is generally considered that factor VIIIR:Ag is synthesized by endothelial cells[8, 9] though others have suggested that it is not synthesized by these cells but taken up from plasma.[10] Within the platelet, factor VIIIR:Ag is found in the cytosol and in granules (see Table 1.8); exogenous VIIIR:Ag does not enter the granules, suggesting that synthesis occurs in the megakaryocyte.[11]

The initiation of the extrinsic pathway[12]

Factor VII interacts with and is altered by tissue factor, a phospholipid-apoprotein complex released from damaged cell membranes. Altered factor VII, in the presence of tissue factor, cleaves factor X to Xa, and Xa in turn cleaves VII to VIIa—a two-chain form with a greatly enhanced proteolytic effect on factor X. The tissue-factor—factor-VII complex may activate factor IX, and factor Xa may also activate factor IX thus enhancing the conversion of factor X to Xa. Factor VII may also be activated by factor XIIa.

The action of thrombin: conversion of fibrinogen to fibrin; fibrin stabilization

The fibrinogen molecule is composed of three pairs of peptide chains designated the Aα, Bβ and γ chains. Thrombin cleaves fibrinopeptide A from the Aα chain and, at a slower rate, fibrinopeptide B from the Bβ chain and thus converts fibrinogen to fibrin monomer.

Fibrin monomer undergoes spontaneous polymerization, by means of hydrogen bonds, to form fibrin polymer. Thrombin also activates factor XIII to XIIIa which acts as a transamidase and stabilizes fibrin polymer by forming covalent bonds between pairs of α and pairs of γ chains (Fig. 9.1). Thrombin also enhances the activity of factors VIII and V, with more prolonged exposure leading to their degradation. A stable fibrin clot is important in allowing fibroblast proliferation and normal wound healing.

Contact factors and contact activation[13]

Contact activation of factor XII involves conformational change rather than cleavage of the molecule. Factor XIIa is able to activate XI but is itself cleaved by XIa, plasmin and kallikrein (Fig. 9.2). The smaller of the cleavage products designated HFf activates prekallikrein to kallikrein, which in turn activates the complement cascade and activates high molecular weight kininogen (HMWK) to bradykinin, factor IX to IXa and prorenin to renin. Prekallikrein is a cofactor in the activation of factor XI, and HMWK is a cofactor in the activation of prekallikrein and factors XII and XI. Consequently, deficiency of prekallikrein or HMWK produces an *in vitro* abnormality of coagulation tests such as the activated partial thromboplastin time (aPTT) which are based on contact activation of the intrinsic pathway. Prekallikrein has also been designated Fletcher factor and HMWK has been designated Fitzgerald factor. Patients described as having deficiency of Flaujeac factor or Williams factor have had deficiencies of both high and low molecular weight kininogen. Platelets may also be involved in contact activation since ADP-aggregated platelets activate factor XII and platelets exposed to collagen activate factor XI. The latter pathway may explain why the *in vitro* defect of factor XII deficiency is not associated with a haemorrhagic disorder. The close interrelationships of the contact factors with the fibrinolytic, complement and kinin systems are shown in Figure 9.2. Furthermore, Fletcher factor (prekallikrein) appears to be essential for the release of plasminogen activator after venous occlusion.[14] The effects of these close interrelationships are seen in disseminated intravascular coagulation (DIC) (see p. 335) in which coagulation factors, complement, plasminogen, prekallikrein and high molecular weight kininogen are all consumed. The four systems also share an inhibitor—C1 esterase inhibitor—which inhibits activated C1, plasmin, kallikrein and factor XII. Utilization of the inhibitor by one activated factor may allow uncontrolled activity of other factors. During the symptomatic phase of hereditary angioneurotic oedema, kallikrein and HMWK are reduced in addition to complement components.[15]

THE FIBRINOLYTIC SYSTEM AND OTHER MECHANISMS FOR PREVENTING UNCONTROLLED COAGULATION

The aggregation of platelets and the coagulation cascade, both of which are initiated by vascular injury, allow rapid clot formation with cessation of haemorrhage. Mechanisms are needed to prevent platelet aggregation and coagulation in undamaged vessels, to prevent uncontrolled coagulation following vascular damage and to lyse clots which are formed. Protective mechanisms, which are multiple, are shown in Table 9.1.

THE FIBRINOLYTIC SYSTEM

Activation of the contact factors of the coagula-

tion cascade leads to conversion of the inactive precursor, plasminogen, to the active serine protease, plasmin, by two routes. Factor XIIa activates blood proactivator to plasminogen activator which converts plasminogen to plasmin; factor XIIa also activates prekallikrein to kallikrein which in turn converts plasminogen to plasmin (Fig. 9.2). Plasminogen is also activated by vascular activator, secreted by endothelial cells, and by tissue activators. Fibrin has considerable affinity for both plasminogen and plasminogen activator and enhances the action of plasminogen activator so that conversion to plasmin occurs preferentially at sites of fibrin deposition with consequent clot lysis. Plasmin also has the capacity to destroy fibrinogen and factor VIII but circulating plasmin is bound to its major inhibitor, α_2 antiplasmin, so that lysis of circulating fibrinogen and factor VIII is generally prevented.

Table 9.1 Factors preventing uncontrolled coagulation

Action	Mechanism	Defect
Inhibition of platelet aggregation	Prostacyclin secreted by endothelial cells	May be defective in thrombotic thrombocytopenic purpura, and haemolytic uraemic syndrome
Inactivation of factor V and VIII	(1) Thrombin initially activates V and VIII but subsequently inactivates them	Deficiency of protein C may be associated with venous thrombosis
	(2) Protein C, a vitamin-K-dependent serine protease, is activated by thrombin and in turn inactivates V and VIII	
Inhibition or inactivation of thrombin	(1) Thrombin is autoregulatory since it cleaves the calcium-binding amino-terminal end of the prothrombin molecule	Congenital or acquired deficiency of ATIII is associated with a thrombotic tendency
	(2) Thrombin is adsorbed on to fibrin	
	(3) Thrombin is inhibited by ATIII (as are IXa, Xa, and XIa)	
	(4) Thrombin (like other proteolytic enzymes) is inhibited by α_2 macroglobulin	
Removal of coagulation-pathway-activators (collagen, bacteria), activated coagulation factors and small fibrin strands	Reticuloendothelial system with fibronectin as a major opsonin[16]	
Lysis of clots	The fibrinolytic system is activated whenever coagulation is activated	Plasminogen deficiency, dysplasminogenaemia and familial defective release of vascular plasminogen activator are associated with a thrombotic tendency

ATIII = antithrombin III

THE LABORATORY DIAGNOSIS OF COAGULATION DEFECTS

An overall assessment of coagulation is best obtained by performing a prothrombin time (PT), activated partial thromboplastin time (aPTT), thrombin time, and bleeding time. In many clinical situations estimation of fibrinogen and of fibrin/fibrinogen degradation products (FDP) is also useful. The principles underlying these and other coagulation tests, and possible causes of abnormal results, are shown in Table 9.2. With the exception of the whole blood clotting time (WBCT) and FDP determination,

which are performed on native blood and serum respectively, coagulation tests are usually performed on platelet-poor-plasma prepared from blood to which citrate has been added to prevent clotting. During performance of the test, sufficient Ca^{++} is added to neutralize the citrate and allow clotting to occur. If the aPTT or PT are found to be prolonged, further information may be obtained by mixing the patient's plasma with normal plasma (the defect corrects unless an inhibitor is present), with aluminium hydroxide-adsorbed plasma (correction occurs if there is a lack of factor XII, XI, VIII or V) and with aged serum (correction occurs if there is a lack

Table 9.2 Principles underlying coagulation tests and causes of abnormal results

Test	Principle	Causes of abnormality
Whole blood clotting time (WBCT)	Contact activation by glass test tube activates the intrinsic pathway	Severe deficiencies of intrinsic pathway factors or presence of an inhibitor of coagulation
Activated partial thromboplastin time (aPTT)	Intrinsic pathway activated by an 'activator' (e.g. kaolin); platelet phospholipid is substituted for by a 'partial thromboplastin' (e.g. cephalin)	Deficiency of intrinsic or common pathway factors (XII, XI, prekallikrein, HMWK,[*] IX, VIII, X, V, II) or presence of an inhibitor of coagulation
Prothrombin time (PT)	Extrinsic pathway activated by a 'complete thromboplastin' (usually extract of brain of rabbit, ox or human) which replaces tissue factor	Deficiency of extrinsic or common pathway factors (VII, X, V, II, severe deficiency of I) or presence of an inhibitor of coagulation
Thrombin time (or calcium-thrombin time)	Fibrinogen is converted to fibrin by added thrombin	Deficiency or defect of fibrinogen; presence of inhibitor of thrombin (e.g. heparin, FDPs)
Reptilase time	Fibrinogen is converted to fibrin by venom from a snake of the genus *Bothrops*	Deficiency or defect of fibrinogen or high level of FDPs
Russell's viper venom (Stypven) time	Factor X is activated by venom from Russell's viper	Deficiency of factor X, V or II or severe deficiency of I
Fibrinogen/fibrin degradation products (FDPs)	Immunological detection of fibrinogen/fibrin breakdown products in serum	*In vivo* fibrinolysis or fibrinogenolysis (including streptokinase/urokinase therapy)
Fibrinogen assay	Biochemical assay or heat-precipitation or immune-precipitation or timing of clot formation after the addition of thrombin to dilute plasma	Fibrinogen deficiency
Solubility of clot in 5 molar urea	Non-cross-linked fibrin clots are soluble in 5 molar urea	Factor XIII deficiency
Bleeding time	Duration of bleeding from skin punctures is timed	Defect of platelet numbers or function or severe deficiency of some coagulation factors

[*] High molecular weight kininogen.

Table 9.3 Inherited defects of coagulation factors

Deficient coagulation factor	Inheritance	Laboratory defect	Clinical manifestations
Factor XII (Hageman factor)	Autosomal recessive	Very prolonged activated partial thromboplastin time (aPTT); bleeding time long, whole blood clotting time (WBCT) prolonged	Nil
Factor XI	Autosomal recessive (incompletely recessive)	Prolonged aPTT; prolonged WBCT	Mild or no bleeding disorder
Prekallikrein (Fletcher factor)	Autosomal recessive	Prolonged aPTT but shortens on prolonged incubation; aPTT normal if ellagic acid used as activator; WBCT prolonged	Usually nil
High molecular weight kininogen* (Fitzgerald factor)	Autosomal recessive	Prolonged aPTT; WBCT prolonged	Nil
Factor IX (Christmas factor)	Sex-linked recessive	Prolonged aPTT; in some patients prolonged Thrombotest†	Severe bleeding disorder
Factor VIII (anti-haemophiliac globulin)			
Haemophilia	Sex-linked recessive	Prolonged aPTT	Severe bleeding disorder
Von Willebrand's disease	Autosomal dominant or recessive	Prolonged aPTT; prolonged bleeding time	Mild to severe bleeding disorder
Factor X	Autosomal recessive (incompletely recessive)	Prolonged prothrombin time (PT); coagulation time with Russell's viper venom normal (factor X Friuli) or abnormal (Stuart and Prower kindreds); aPTT somewhat prolonged	Moderate to severe bleeding disorder
Factor VII	Autosomal recessive (incompletely recessive)	Normal aPTT; prolonged PT; prolonged Thrombotest† except in the case of factor VII Padua; normal Russell's viper venom time	Mild to severe bleeding tendency
Factor V	Autosomal recessive	PT and aPTT prolonged; bleeding time often prolonged[18]	Moderate to severe bleeding tendency
Factor II	Autosomal recessive	PT and aPTT slightly prolonged	Moderate bleeding tendency
Afibrinogenaemia	Autosomal recessive	Bleeding time prolonged in about half of patients; fibrinogen concentration similarly reduced in immunological, biochemical and functional assays	Moderate bleeding tendency
Dysfibrinogenaemia	Autosomal recessive	PT usually prolonged; aPTT less often prolonged; WBCT normal or prolonged; prolonged thrombin time (rarely shortened thrombin time); prolonged reptilase time; fibrinogen concentration may appear normal in biochemical or immunological assays but reduced in functional (clotting) assays	Haemorrhagic disorder (about half) ± defective wound healing or clinically normal or thrombotic tendency (minority)
Factor XIII	Autosomal recessive	PT, aPTT and thrombin time all normal; increased clot solubility in 5 molar urea	Mild bleeding tendency; poor wound healing; spontaneous abortions

*The Reid trait is similar to Fitzgerald factor deficiency; in Flaujeac trait and Williams trait all species of kininogens are missing.[17]

†Thrombotest uses ox brain as a complete thromboplastin and tests for deficiency of factors VII, X and II (factor V and fibrinogen are included in the reagent).

± With or without.

of factor XII, XI, II, VII, IX or X). Specific factor assays can be performed which are based on the ability of the patient's plasma to correct the defect in a plasma known to be lacking only in the single factor which is being assayed. Certain factors, which when activated are proteases, can be estimated by an assay based on their ability to release a dye from a synthetic peptide substrate, designated a chromogenic substrate.

INHERITED DEFECTS OF COAGULATION

Inherited defects of coagulation usually affect a single coagulation factor. The coagulation factor may be totally absent, reduced in amount but apparently normal both structurally and functionally, or present as a defective molecule with reduced function. The inheritance, laboratory features, and clinical features of inherited defects of coagulation factors are shown in Table 9.3. Rarely an inherited coagulation disorder may result from excessive activation of fibrinolysis (plasminogen-activator excess)[19] or defective inhibition of fibrinolysis (α_2-antiplasmin deficiency).[20]

HAEMOPHILIA (HAEMOPHILIA A)

Definition

Haemophilia is a congenital haemorrhagic disorder with sex-linked inheritance occurring almost exclusively in males and characterized by a reduction or absence of factor VIII clotting activity (factor VIII:C). 20–30% of patients have no family history of the disorder and in them the disorder may result from a recent mutation or from passage through many generations of female carriers.

Incidence

Haemophilia is the commonest inherited coagulation factor deficiency with a prevalence of the order of 1 per 10 000 males.

Pathophysiology

Factor VIII:C is absent or reduced; factor VIII:CAg may be proportional to VIII:C, or may be present at a higher level indicating a structurally abnormal molecule with defective function. Factor VIIIR:Ag and von Willebrand factor activities (including factor VIII:RiCoF) are present in normal amounts. As a consequence of the deficiency of factor VIII, the intrinsic pathway of coagulation is defective. Following replacement therapy, between 5 and 10% of haemophiliacs develop inhibitors of factor VIII. The severity of the disease is not aggravated thereby, but therapy becomes relatively ineffective.

Clinical features

Excessive bleeding may follow circumcision in infancy but otherwise pathological bleeding is not usually noted in the first six months of life. Bleeding is noted when crawling starts and subsequently with teething. The most characteristic haemorrhages in the child are haemarthroses and soft tissue haematomas occurring spontaneously or after minor trauma. Haematuria and bleeding into internal organs, and gastrointestinal bleeding are somewhat less common. Intracranial bleeding is not common but is a major cause of death.[21] Excessive bleeding may occur following trauma or surgery and in milder haemophiliacs may be the only manifestation of the disease; bleeding may be immediate or delayed.

Laboratory features

The aPTT is prolonged whereas the PT is normal. In severe cases only, the whole-blood clotting time is prolonged. Factor VIII:C and factor VIII:CAg are reduced, the former sometimes more than the latter. Factor VIIIR:Ag is normal. The bleeding time is often somewhat increased.[22]

Therapy

Haemophilia is treated by replacement therapy at the time of bleeding, prophylactic therapy generally not being feasible because of the short in vivo half life of factor VIII. Replacement therapy is with a cryoprecipitate (containing fibrinogen and fibronectin in addition to factor VIII) prepared from fresh plasma, or with more purified factor VIII concentrates. Patients with mild haemophilia may also be treated in some circumstances with 1-desamino-8-D-arginine vasopressin (DDAVP), a vasopressin analogue which causes release of factor VIII from endothelial cells. With the replacement therapy which is now available, the life expectancy of patients with haemophilia is little different from that of other people.[21]

Pathology

The pathological lesions of haemophilia include: (1) acute haemorrhagic manifestations; (2) chronic tissue damage from previous or recurrent haemorrhage; and (3) lesions consequent on therapy. With increasingly effective therapy the mean age of death has increased and the proportion of haemophiliacs dying of unrelated disease has increased.[23] Nevertheless, haemorrhage remains the major cause of death, with intracranial haemorrhage becoming relatively more important as intra-abdominal and gastrointestinal haemorrhage has been more readily controlled.[24, 25]. Haemorrhage following trauma remains a significant cause of death. Death from respiratory obstruction secondary to haemorrhage is rare. A minority of haemophiliacs die of renal failure, or of therapy-related liver disease (see below).

Intracranial and intraspinal haemorrhage

Intracranial haemorrhage may be apparently spontaneous or may follow head injury, often of a minor nature. There may be a symptom-free interval of several days after the injury. Haemorrhage may be intracerebral, subarachnoid or subdural.[26] Intraspinal haemorrhage may also occur[27, 28] and may cause paraplegia. Mortality of intracranial haemorrhage is of the order of 30%. Those who survive commonly have moderately severe sequelae.

Joints and bones[29]

Haemarthrosis occurs most often in knees (Fig. 9.3), ankles and elbows. Bleeding occurs into the

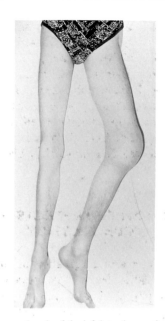

Fig. 9.3 Haemarthrosis of the left knee in a patient with haemophila A. The knee is flexed as a consequence of the haemarthrosis. The muscles of the left calf are wasted following immobilization consequent on previous haemarthroses. The right leg also shows muscle atrophy.

joint space and periarticular tissues. Blood is an extreme irritant to the synovium. Within a few hours of a haemarthrosis neutrophils accumulate in the synovium and there is hyperplasia of synovial cells; within the next few days, lymphocytes, plasma cells and histiocytes appear and haemosiderin is deposited. Severe intra-articular haemorrhages may be followed by organization of blood clot and intra-articular adhesions.

Recurrent bleeding leads to persistent chronic inflammation of the synovium which becomes thickened, increasingly villous with nodular projections, vascular, and increasingly prone to bleeding. Extreme vascular hyperplasia may give an angiomatoid appearance. The synovium and joint fluid of damaged joints have an increased content of hydrolytic enzymes. There is proliferation of subsynovial fibrous tissue with heavy haemosiderin deposition in periarticular tissues; haemosiderin deposits may cause the synovium to be opaque on X-ray. Multinucleate giant cells appear in the synovium. Chronic joint effusion often follows recurrent haemarthrosis.

Recurrent haemorrhage also leads to destruction of cartilage. Cartilage may be partially cov-

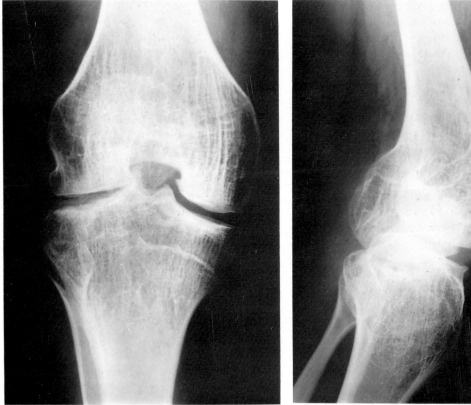

(a)   (b)

Fig. 9.4 Radiographs of the left knee in a patient with chronic haemophilic arthropathy. Features demonstrated are bone resorption, subchondral cyst formation, widening of the intercondylar notch, irregular joint surfaces, loss of joint space and osteophyte formation. The widening of the intercondylar notch is a result of chronic synovitis, while the other changes reflect osteoporosis and osteoarthritis.

ered by fibrous tissue containing haemosiderin and chronic inflammatory cells. Destruction of cartilage may leave pigmented eburnated bone ends exposed. The subchondral bone plate may suffer vascular invasion leading to mechanical weakness and bone collapse. Intraosseous haemorrhage causes bone necrosis and cyst formation. Bone cysts are usually lined by a single layer of synovial cells, and communicate with the joint cavity. Disuse of joints consequent on frequent acute haemarthrosis leads to osteoporosis, more marked in the epiphysis than the diaphysis. Preferential absorption of fine trabeculae gives an open lattice-work pattern on radiographs (Fig. 9.4). Transverse lines due to an arrest of bone growth may also be observed. Recurrent haemarthrosis in children and adolescents may lead to accelerated maturation with overgrowth

of epiphyses and premature ossification; these changes are probably mediated by the hyperaemia of chronic inflammation.[30]

The epiphyses may also fragment as in osteochondritis; X-rays of the hip may resemble those of Perthes' disease and similar changes may be seen in the head of the radius.[30]

In the long term, joints damaged by recurrent haemarthrosis develop osteoarthritic changes, visible radiologically as loss of joint space, irregular joint surfaces, cysts, sclerosis and osteophyte formation (Fig. 9.4). In the knee, posterior subluxation, lateral shift of the tibia, and valgus deformity are characteristic, the latter being consequent on hyperactivity of the tensor fascia lata when the quadriceps is severely wasted. Osteoarthritic changes may be accompanied by atrophy and contracture of muscles and oesteoporosis.

Uncommonly, fibrous and bony ankylosis may follow. Fractures may occur in osteoporotic bones.

Bleeding into muscles

Intramuscular bleeding is most commonly into flexor muscles. The blood spreads diffusely between the muscle fibres. Histologically, anuclear muscle fibres are seen embedded in blood clot. Neutrophil infiltration occurs within hours and is followed by the appearance of histiocytes and fibroblasts. Healing occurs by formation of granulation tissue and fibrosis; degenerating muscle fibres with central migration of sarcolemmal nuclei may be seen within the fibrous tissue.[29] Uncommonly, large intramuscular haemorrhages may leave residual cysts containing inspissated blood clot. Major intramuscular haemorrhages may be followed by ischaemic contractures, particularly when bleeding is into the calf or the forearm. Myositis ossificans can occur.

Peripheral nerve lesions

Peripheral nerve lesions are usually consequent on compression secondary to haemorrhage into surrounding tissue. However, lesions of the sciatic nerve may be due to bleeding from the vasa nervorum. About a quarter of haemorrhages into muscles are accompanied by peripheral nerve lesions; there is a particularly high incidence of femoral nerve lesions in association with iliacus haemorrhage. Other relatively common nerve lesions are those of the sciatic, common peroneal, median and ulnar nerves. Recovery may be slow, particularly from femoral nerve lesions.

Haemophiliac cysts and pseudotumours

Haemorrhage into confined spaces (either in bone or muscle) may be followed by the formation of simple intraosseous or intramuscular cysts or alternatively by the formation of pseudotumours originating either in bone (intraosseous or subperiosteal haemorrhage) or in muscle (haemorrhage into a muscle with wide periosteal attachments). In adults, pseudotumours are most often intrapelvic or in the upper thigh involving bulky muscles. They expand progressively, eroding bone and soft tissue and sometimes ulcerating through the skin. The radiological appearance may simulate a malignant tumour of bone with bone destruction, periosteal elevation, and new bone formation; there is a characteristic cyst-like trabeculated space with a 'soap-bubble' margin. Haemorrhages into small joints, e.g. metacarpophalangeal or tarsometatarsal, if inadequately treated may lead to complete destruction of the bone with rupture of soft tissue and skin. Successful conservative management of haemophiliac pseudotumors by factor VIII replacement is sometimes possible and is followed by bone remodelling.

Histological examination[29] shows blood clot, fibrous tissue with inflammatory cells, including haemosiderin-laden macrophages, and bone resorption and formation of new bone.

Other soft tissue haemorrhage

Haemorrhage may occur into any soft tissue. Haemorrhage into the intestinal wall may cause intestinal obstruction or intussusception. Intramesenteric haemorrhage also occurs. Pulmonary, pleural and mediastinal bleeding is uncommon. Rarely, sublingual and peritonsillar haemorrhage causes respiratory obstruction and death.

The kidneys and the urinary tract

The renal lesions of haemophilia are mainly a consequence of haemorrhage and obstruction. Microscopic haematuria is common and macrocopic haematuria not uncommon. Intrarenal haematomas occur. Rarely haemorrhage into the kidney may be followed by pseudotumour formation.[31] Passage of clots may cause clot colic. Bilateral or unilateral ureteric obstruction may be due to a clot in the ureter or renal pelvis (commonly but not exclusively in those given inhibitors of fibrinolysis) or due to retroperitoneal haemorrhage and fibrosis. Bilateral obstruction by clots causes acute oliguric renal failure. Recurrent obstruction may lead to hydronephrosis and chronic renal failure. Intravenous pyelography has shown, in addition to hydronephrosis, intracalyceal accumulation of contrast medium, a finding which is suggestive of papillary necrosis.[26]

Some renal lesions in haemophiliacs are not clearly related to haemorrhage. Diffuse renal enlargement has been observed, the pathological basis being glomerular hypertrophy with endothelial cell proliferation.[32] A potential cause of renal damage is deposition of immune complexes consequent on either hepatitis B infection or the development of antibodies to infused foreign proteins. Circulating immune complexes are often detectable. Four cases of renal amyloidosis have been reported in haemophilia or Christmas disease,[33, 34] an immunological basis being suspected. Renal calculi may be increased in incidence since two were observed among 35 patients.[34] Overall, abnormalities of renal function or structure are common, being found in 27 of the same series of 35 patients:[34] four had proteinuria, four had an elevated blood urea and nine had diminished creatinine clearance. Renal failure is responsible for approximately 1% of deaths in haemophiliac patients.[25] In some studies, the prevalence of hypertension has been found to be increased. In two series of relatively young haemophiliacs, hypertension was found in 8%[23] and 14%[33] of cases respectively. In the latter series its occurrence did not correlate with a history of haematuria, but obstructive uropathy was the commonest underlying lesion. However, in another study of 57 haemophiliacs in Britain, hypertension was no commoner than in a control population.[31] The occurrence of hypertension may be of grave import since intracranial haemorrhage may occur.

Liver

Haemophiliacs may suffer acute hepatitis consequent on the transmission of hepatitis B or non-A non-B hepatitis by blood products. More than one episode of non-A non-B hepatitis may occur,[35] suggesting that more than one agent may be responsible for this condition. Haemophiliacs who have not had an episode of clinical hepatitis may be found to have antibodies to hepatitis B virus, indicating previous exposure. A chronic carrier state for hepatitis B may occur, often without preceding clinical hepatitis. Chronic liver disease may follow hepatitis B and, probably, non-A non-B hepatitis. Abnormal liver function tests are common. The most frequent abnormalities are elevated transaminase levels and increased bromsulphthalein retention and less frequent abnormalities include elevated bilirubin, alkaline phosphatase and γ globulin levels, and reduced albumin levels.[36] Liver biopsy in patients with abnormal biochemical tests has shown chronic persistent hepatitis, granulomas, chronic active hepatitis, portal fibrosis, and cirrhosis (which is accompanied by ascites and oesophageal varices).[37] Such histological abnormality strongly correlates with the presence of the hepatitis B virus or antibody against the hepatitis B surface antigen (anti-HB_SAg). Indirect immunofluorescence studies have shown HB_SAg and hepatitis B core antigen (HB_CAg) in the livers of patients with anti-HB_SAg, an unexpected finding.[38] Biopsies from intensively treated patients who were not selected for liver complications has also shown a high incidence of subsiding hepatitis and chronic persistent and active hepatitis. The death of one haemophiliac has been reported as due to hepatocellular carcinoma superimposed on cirrhosis due to hepatitis B.[39] Superinfection with the defective RNA virus, the delta virus, has been reported in haemophiliacs who were carriers of hepatitis B; the incidence of chronic liver disease is higher in HB_SAg carriers who also have anti-delta virus antibodies. Although liver disease is mainly related to hepatitis viruses it is theoretically possible that infusion of foreign proteins could contribute.

Splenomegaly

Occasional patients with haemophilia have developed splenomegaly as a result of haemolysis caused by the presence of anti-A or anti-B isoagglutinins in therapeutic materials (see below). Splenomegaly may also be consequent on chronic liver disease in association with hepatitis B infection; splenectomy may be required to relieve hypersplenism.[40] A fluctuating splenomegaly not apparently related to either of these factors was noted in as many as 26% of a group of North American patients with haemophilia but was not noted in a group of somewhat less intensively treated British patients.[41] The cause of the splenomegaly was not readily apparent. Its occurrence could not be related to titres of antibodies to cytomegalovirus nor to abnormalities of liver function tests. There was some correlation with intensity of therapy and it may be hypothesized that splenomegaly was consequent on reticuloendothelial hyperplasia following repeated antigenic stimulation. Few histological observations are available, but reticuloendothelial hyperplasia was observed in one patient.[42] Splenomegaly and lymphadenopathy may sometimes be related to the acquired immunodeficiency syndrome (see below).

Other adverse effects of factor VIII infusions

Factor VIII infusions may cause febrile, allergic or anaphylactoid reactions. Acute pulmonary oedema has followed infusion of fresh-frozen plasma and was attributable to antibodies in the donor against white cells or plasma proteins. The presence of anti-A and anti-B isoagglutinins in factor VIII concentrates may cause overt haemolytic anaemia when large doses of concentrate are infused. Subjects on prophylactic therapy with moderate doses of high-purity concentrate have been observed to have low levels of haptoglobin; since patients with factor VIII inhibitors who were not receiving any therapy had normal levels[43] it is likely that chronic low-grade haemolysis was responsible for the reduced haptoglobin levels. This view was supported by the occurrence of a slow rise of haptoglobins when concentrate with a low titre of isoagglutinins was substituted.

Amyloidosis

It is possible that amyloidosis is a complication of therapy, relating to the frequent infusion of foreign proteins. Four patients suffering from either haemophilia or Christmas disease who developed amyloidosis have been reported.[33] The two patients reported in detail had both suffered frequent and severe reactions to plasma or blood transfusions. Both died of progressive renal failure, one patient also having had the nephrotic

syndrome.[42, 44] Both patients had amyloid in the liver, kidneys and adrenals, one had amyloid in the pituitary gland, and one had amyloid in blood vessels of the thyroid. Within the liver, the amyloid was present between the sinusoidal lining cells and the parenchymal cells;[42] within the adrenal glands, it was present mainly in the zona glomerulosa.[42] In the kidneys, amyloid was found in the glomeruli, tubules, blood vessels and interstitial tissues.

Acquired immunodeficiency syndrome

The acquired immunodeficiency syndrome (AIDS), now well-recognized in homosexual men and drug addicts, has also been observed in haemophiliacs. Of the first 2157 cases reported in the USA, 0.8% were in haemophiliacs.[45] Subsequently, further cases among haemophiliacs have been reported from the UK and other European countries. In haemophiliacs, AIDS appears to be related particularly to intensive treatment with lyophilized factor VIII concentrates rather than to treatment with cryoprecipitate. Immunological abnormalities have been noted in haemophiliacs with AIDS, and also in apparently healthy patients who had been intensively treated with lyophilized concentrates.[46–49] In the latter group, total T-cells and cells with the suppressor/cytotoxic phenotype (OKT8 positive) were increased, while cells with the helper phenotype (OKT4 positive) were normal. In addition to a decreased helper/suppressor ratio there were reduced responses to mitogens, reduced natural killer activity[46] and increased levels of immunoglobulin G.[47] One immunologically abnormal patient had marked generalized lymphadenopathy and splenomegaly and another had generalized lymphadenopathy. It is now known that the acquired immunodeficiency syndrome in haemophiliacs is due to transmission in blood products of the human T-cell lymphotropic virus, HTLV III. This virus may also cause splenomegaly and lymphadenopathy.

Idiopathic thrombocytopenia purpura

Idiopathic thrombocytopenic purpura appears to be associated with haemophilia under treatment with factor VIII concentrates more frequently than would be expected by chance.[50] As some of these patients have a reduced ratio of OKT4/OKT8 lymphocytes[50] and as homosexuals appear to have an increased incidence of idiopathic thrombocytopenic purpura, it may be speculated that there is some relationship between AIDS and ITP.

Thrombosis

Even severe haemophiliacs do not escape thrombosis and death may be due to the thrombotic consequences of severe atherosclerosis. Cerebral venous thrombosis has also been reported and may be related to hyperfibrinogenaemia following therapy with cryoprecipitate or low antithrombin III levels due to liver disease.

VON WILLEBRAND'S DISEASE

Definition and pathophysiology

Von Willebrand's disease (VWD) is an autosomally transmitted, congenital haemorrhagic disorder in which there is prolongation of the bleeding time in addition to reduction of factor VIII coagulation activity and factor VIII:VWF-related activities (Table 9.4). The underlying abnormality is an absence or reduction of the very high molecular weight multimeric forms of the factor VIII/VWF complex, which are necessary for platelet adhesion to subendothelium, for maintenance of a normal bleeding time, and for ristocetin-induced platelet aggregation in vitro. Small multimers of factor VIII/VWF are also reduced in the classical (type I) form of the disease, whereas in type II von Willebrand's disease there is selective reduction of large multimers (Table 9.4).[51, 52, 53] Factor VIII:C is usually also reduced but it can be synthesized if material containing factor VIIIR:Ag is infused. The abnormalities of platelet function are correctable in vivo and in vitro by infusion or addition of fresh plasma containing factor VIII/VWF. In pseudo-von Willebrand's disease (platelet-type von Willebrand's disease)[54, 55, 56] a lack of large multimers of VIII/VWF in plasma appears to be consequent on increased uptake by platelets.

Inheritance

Various patterns of inheritance occur. In the most severe cases of the classic (type I) form of the disease in which all factor VIII-related activities are reduced below 2–3%, inheritance is autosomal recessive. In the much commoner mild form of the disease, both type I and type II, inheritance is usually autosomal dominant but with the exception of type IIC in which it is autosomal recessive. Pseudo-VWD (platelet-type VWD) also has an autosomal dominant inheritance.

Incidence

Severe homozygous VWD is rare. The prevalence of the less severe heterozygous form is difficult to determine since mild cases may be unrecognized but it is probably similar to the prevalence of haemophilia. In Sweden, the prevalence of VWD is 1 in 20 000, with 1 severe case in 250 000.[57]

Laboratory tests

In mild VWD the results of relevant tests are variable over time, and not all of them are always abnormal. In a moderately severe or severe case there is prolongation of the bleeding time, reduction of factor VIII:C, factor VIII:CAg, factor VIIIR:Ag and factor VIII:RiCoF. Ristocetin-induced platelet aggregation is absent or reduced (see Fig. 7.6 on p. 284), except in type IIB and pseudo-VWD (see Table 9.4). In severe type I VWD (in contradistinction to haemophilia A) there is a similar degree of reduction of factor VIII:C and factor VIIIR:Ag. In type II and pseudo-VWD the selective reduction of large multimers and the more rapid migration of small multimers leads to an abnormality on crossed immunoelectrophoresis of factor VIIIR:Ag. More rapid migration of small multimers also leads to higher assayed values for VIIIR:Ag with the Laurell rocket technique (quantitative electroim-

Table 9.4 Laboratory findings in subtypes of von Willebrand's disease

	Essential features			Ristocetin-induced aggregation of platelets	Other laboratory features
Type I	Factor VIII/VWF is reduced in quantity but qualitatively normal (small, intermediate and large multimers proportionately reduced)*			Reduced	CIEP normal
Type II	Qualitative abnormality of factor VIII/VWF characterized by a selective lack of large multimers	II A	Reduced ability to synthesize large and intermediate multimers, which are lacking both in plasma and in platelets	Reduced	CIEP abnormal
		II B	Increased rate of removal of large multimers from plasma but normal levels of all multimers in platelets	Increased at low ristocetin concentrations; patient's platelets show normal (rather than enhanced) ability to absorb normal factor VIII/VWF	CIEP abnormal
		II C	Reduced ability to synthesize large multimers, which are lacking both in plasma and platelets; aberrant structure of smaller multimers	Reduced	CIEP abnormal
Pseudo-von Willebrand's disease (platelet type VWD)	Qualitative abnormality of factor VIII/VWF characterized by reduction of levels of multimers in plasma but with normal levels in platelets; differs from II B in that normal plasma causes aggregation of patient's platelets. May be essentially a platelet defect			Increased at low ristocetin concentration; patient's platelets show enhanced ability to absorb normal factor VIII/VWF	CIEP abnormal

* In severe homozygous VWD, VIIIR:Ag is absent in platelets and endothelial cells as well as in plasma; in classical autosomal dominant VWD, VIIIR:Ag appears normal in platelets and is present in endothelial cells.[51]

CIEP = crossed immunoelectrophoresis of factor VIIIR:Ag

munoassay) than with immunoradiometric assay (IRMA) in type II VWD, and the dose response curve on IRMA is non-parallel with normal samples.[53] Thrombocytopenia is sometimes observed in type IIB VWD and in pseudo-VWD.[53, 56]

Clinical features

VWD shows features consequent on the secondary defect in platelet function, in addition to features due to reduction of factor VIII:C. Thus, in addition to the type of bleeding which occurs in haemophilia with a comparable reduction of factor VIII:C, there is also cutaneous bleeding and mucosal bleeding, such as epistaxis, gastro-intestinal bleeding, gingival bleeding, menorrhagia (which has been fatal), and sometimes postpartum haemorrhage. The rise of factor VIII level which occurs during pregnancy gives some protection against bleeding. As the severe, homozygous disease is rare, VWD is generally milder than haemophilia.

Therapy

VWD may be treated by infusion of fresh-frozen plasma, cryoprecipitate, or factor VIII concentrates. Fresh-frozen plasma and cryoprecipitate give a better correction of the secondary defect of platelet function than the more purified concentrates. The correction of the prolonged bleeding time is more transient than the correction of factor VIII:C levels and a secondary rise of the latter, attributable to synthesis, usually occurs in the next 24 hours. The vasopressin analogue, desmopressin (DDAVP), is also of use in increasing factor VIII levels; it is contraindicated in type IIB disease where it may cause platelet aggregation[53] and thrombocytopenia.

Pathology

The pathological lesions of VWD are similar to those of haemophilia with a comparable level of factor VIII:C and, therefore, are generally less severe. Pathological lesions secondary to the infusion of therapeutic products are also less common. In severely affected patients, arthropathy similar to that of haemophilia occurs.[57]

Two apparently unrelated lesions appear to have an increased incidence in VWD. Angiodysplastic lesions resembling hereditary haemorrhagic telangiectasia have been reported;[58, 59, 60] in some of these cases VWD may have been acquired.[61, 62] The incidence of mitral valve prolapse may also be increased.[63]

In pigs, VWD offers protection against atherosclerosis but this does not appear to be so in man.[64] It might be postulated that only the rare severe disease would offer protection in man.

CHRISTMAS DISEASE (HAEMOPHILIA B)

Definition

Christmas disease is a congenital, sex-linked haemorrhagic disorder due to the absence, reduction, or functional abnormality of factor IX.

Incidence

The prevalence of Christmas disease is approximately 1 per 50 000 males.

Pathophysiology

Factor IX coagulation activity is absent or reduced; immunological studies show that in the majority of patients a defective molecule is present which is non-functional or dysfunctional. As a consequence of factor IX deficiency, the intrinsic pathway of blood coagulation is abnormal. 1–3% of patients with Christmas disease develop an inhibitor of factor IX.

Laboratory features

The aPTT is prolonged and the PT is normal. In some patients the Thrombotest gives an abnormal result (see Table 9.3).

Clinical features

The clinical features do not differ from those of classical haemophilia (see Fig. 9.5 and p. 324).

Therapy

Optimal therapy is with factor IX concentrate, which also contains factors X and II and sometimes factor VII. In the absence of factor IX concentrates, fresh-frozen plasma may be efficaceous. Some factor IX concentrates have been responsible for thrombotic lesions, particularly in patients whose Christmas disease has been complicated by liver disease.[25]

Pathological features

The pathological features are similar to those of classical haemophilia (see p. 324). The acquired immunodeficiency syndrome which may occur in haemophilia A appears to be much less common in Christmas disease and patients with Christmas disease have not generally shown the imbalance of T-cell subsets which has been found in haemophilia.[65]

FACTOR XII 'DEFICIENCY'

Factor XII 'deficiency' is an *in vitro* abnormality of coagulation with no clinical manifestations de-

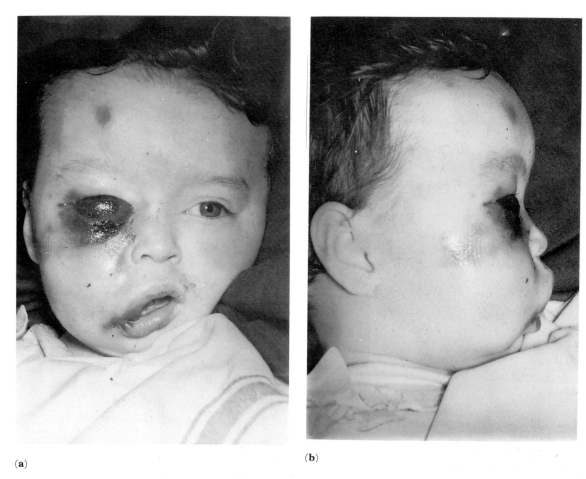

(a)

(b)

Fig. 9.5 Extensive soft tissue haemorrhage following a dog-bite in a child with Christmas disease.

spite homozygotes having less than 1 per cent of factor XII. The condition provides no protection against venous or arterial thrombosis.

FACTOR XI DEFICIENCY

Factor XI deficiency is a congenital haemorrhagic disorder with incompletely recessive, autosomal inheritance; it is rare except in Ashkenasic Jewish populations. Homozygotes may have up to 10–20% factor XI activity and the bleeding disorder is mild, or in some cases absent. There is a poor correlation between factor XI levels and the haemorrhagic tendency; some individuals with less than 10% factor XI do not bleed following surgery or trauma.

OTHER CONTACT FACTOR DEFICIENCIES

The essential features of these deficiencies are summarized in Table 9.3.

FACTOR X DEFICIENCY

Factor X deficiency is a rare, congenital haemorrhagic disorder of autosomal recessive inheritance; the term deficiency is applied when there is deficient factor X clotting activity due either to a true deficiency of factor X or the presence of a dysfunctional factor X molecule. Bleeding may be manifest from birth. Subcutaneous haemorrhages may occur as may bleeding from mucosal surfaces. Severe menorrhagia is seen in some factor-X-deficient women (Table 9.3).

FACTOR VII DEFICIENCY

Factor VII deficiency is a rare, congenital haemorrhagic disorder, of autosomal recessive inheritance, resulting from lack or dysfunction of factor VII. Bleeding characteristically affects the skin and mucous membranes but haemarthroses may also occur. The severity of bleeding does not appear to be closely related to the measured level of factor VII. Perinatal intracranial haemorrhage appears to be particularly common in factor VII deficiency[66] (see also Table 9.3).

FACTOR V DEFICIENCY

Factor V deficiency is a rare, congenital haemorrhagic disorder of autosomal recessive inheritance, consequent on lack or dysfunction of factor V. Bleeding may commence at birth with haemorrhage from the umbilical cord and thereafter is often from mucous membranes.

FACTOR II DEFICIENCY

Factor II deficiency is a very rare, autosomal recessive, congenital haemorrhagic disorder consequent on a lack (hypoprothrombinaemia) or dysfunction (dysprothrombinaemia) of factor II (prothrombin). Bleeding may start at birth with umbilical cord haemorrhage and subsequently there is subcutaneous and mucous membrane bleeding, together with haemarthroses.

ABNORMALITIES OF FIBRINOGEN

Afibrinogenaemia is a rare, congenital haemorrhagic disorder with an autosomal recessive mode of inheritance. Bleeding is of moderate severity. Haemarthroses are less common than in haemophilia and mucosal bleeding is more common. Umbilical cord haemorrhage has occurred in

about half of the reported cases. The results of laboratory tests are shown in Table 9.3. The lack of fibrinogen causes an erythrocyte sedimentation rate of virtually zero. Hypofibrinogenaemia may represent the heterozygous state for this disorder.

Dysfibrinogenaemia is the occurrence of a structurally and functionally abnormal fibrinogen as an inherited (codominant) characteristic. About half the reported cases have had an associated haemorrhagic disorder. A minority show thromboembolic phenomena and the remainder are clinically normal. Wound healing may be poor with a risk of wound dehiscence. The incidence of spontaneous abortions may be increased. Functional abnormalities reported include abnormal release of fibrinopeptide A or B, delayed or disordered polymerisation of fibrin monomer, defective cross-linking, abnormal resistance or sensitivity to degradation by plasmin and shortened half-life. It is likely that abnormal fibrinogens result from substitution of a single amino acid; some have abnormal mobility on immunoelectrophoresis.

The results of laboratory tests are shown in Table 9.3. The addition of calcium may shorten the thrombin time to a greater extent in plasma from patients than in that from controls. The plasma of patients with dysfibrinogenaemia may interfere with coagulation tests when mixed with normal plasma.

FACTOR XIII DEFICIENCY

Factor XIII deficiency is a rare, congenital haemorrhagic disorder, the inheritance of which is probably autosomal recessive. The bleeding tendency is usually apparent from birth (cord haemorrhage); intracranial haemorrhage is relatively common but otherwise the disorder is usually mild. Bleeding may be delayed and may be followed by the formation of pseudotumours (see p. 327). Wound healing is defective and delayed and women show a high incidence of spontaneous abortion unless replacement therapy is given during pregnancy. A concentration of a few per cent of factor XIII is adequate for normal haemostasis. The results of laboratory tests in factor XIII deficiency are shown in Table 9.3.

ACQUIRED DEFECTS OF COAGULATION

Acquired defects of coagulation may be due to: (1) failure to produce normal coagulation factors, e.g. in acute and chronic liver disease, in vitamin K deficiency and following administration of oral anticoagulants; (2) abnormal consumption of coagulation factors, e.g. in disseminated intravascular coagulation or following some snake bites; (3) absorption of clotting factors from the circulating blood, e.g. in amyloidosis; (4) loss of clotting factors from the body, e.g. in the nephrotic syndrome; (5) production of an inhibitor of coagulation; (6) heparin administration; (7) massive blood transfusion with failure to replace labile factors; and (8) a defect of platelet function or number (see Chapter 7).

Acquired defects of coagulation most often affect multiple coagulation factors. The factors affected and the usual abnormalities found in coagulation tests are shown in Table 9.5. Some abnormalities are dealt with in more detail below.

Liver disease

Coagulation abnormalities are due to: (1) failure of synthesis of all clotting factors except factor VIII, which is usually elevated; (2) synthesis of a defective fibrinogen molecule which has increased sialic acid and which polymerizes poorly (acquired dysfibrinogenaemia); (3) low-grade disseminated intravascular coagulation, fibrinogen survival being improved with low doses of heparin;[68] (4) failure of γ-carboxylation of factors II, VII, IX or X in liver disease *per se*, but to a greater extent if there is intra- or extrahepatic biliary obstruction; (5) defective synthesis of antithrombin III (ATIII) so that a thrombotic tendency may coexist with a bleeding tendency; and (6) thrombocytopenia due to hypersplenism accompanying portal hypertension. Factor V falls early in liver disease, in advance of the vitamin-K-dependent factors, whereas a fall of factor XIII occurs later and is a bad prognostic sign. Dysfibrinogenaemia is characteristic of hepatoma and of parenchymal liver disease, but not of obstructive jaundice or secondary carcinoma.[69]

Disseminated intravascular coagulation (DIC)

DIC is the conversion of fibrinogen to fibrin within the circulation, with consumption of coagulation factors. DIC results from the release of thromboplastins resembling tissue factor into the circulation, damage to endothelial cells causing contact activation, and activation of platelets. Thromboplastic substances may be released by tumour cells (e.g. carcinoma cells or the promyelocytes of hypergranular promyelocytic leukaemia) or from burnt or traumatized tissues, or may be generated by the interaction of bacterial endotoxin with monocytes. Amniotic fluid and ascitic fluid contain thromboplastins so that amniotic fluid embolism and the insertion of a Le Veen shunt to return ascitic fluid to the blood stream are potent causes of DIC. Ascitic fluid and amniotic fluid may also contain particulate material capable of causing activation of contact factors. The entry of activated coagulation factors into the blood stream is the likely mechanism of DIC associated with antepartum haemorrhage. In trauma, burns, shock, and sepsis, damage to endothelial cells is likely to contribute to activation of coagulation.

DIC may be acute (e.g. in obstetric complications, trauma and shock) or chronic (e.g. when a dead fetus is retained or when there is disseminated malignancy). The laboratory manifestations are determined by: (1) the rate of intravascular coagulation; (2) the rate of production of coagulation factors; and (3) the degree of activation of fibrinolysis. Activation of coagulation is invariably accompanied by some degree of activation of fibrinolysis (see Fig. 9.2) but the balance between the rates of deposition and of lysis of fibrin varies. If fibrinolysis is very active, fibrin/fibrinogen degradation products (FDPs) are high and at autopsy there may be little evidence of thrombosis. A lesser degree of activation of fibrinolysis is associated with: (1) a lesser elevation of FDPs; (2) microangiopathic haemolytic anaemia due to damage to red cells by contact with intravascular fibrin (see p. 150); (3) organ damage due to microvascular obstruction, and (4) more frequent thrombi at autopsy. The major clinical feature of DIC is a generalized bleeding

Table 9.5 Acquired abnormalities of coagulation

Primary disorder	Abnormality	Laboratory tests
Vitamin K deficiency or antagonism Dietary lack or malabsorption of vitamin K (coeliac disease, biliary obstruction); haemorrhagic disease of the newborn; coumarin or indanedione therapy	Failure of γ-carboxylation of factors II, VII, IX, X	Long PT; lesser prolongation of aPTT
Liver disease	Failure of synthesis of factors II, V, VII, X, IX, XI, I, XIII and antithrombin III and plasminogen	Long PT and thrombin time; lesser prolongation of aPTT. FDPs slightly increased
Disseminated intravascular coagulation (DIC)	Consumption and consequently low levels of any or all clotting factors plus ATIII, complement, plasminogen and α_2 antiplasmin	Long PT, aPTT, thrombin time; low fibrinogen; increased FDPs; thrombocytopenia. Occasionally a short aPTT may be seen because of the presence of activated coagulation factors
Amyloidosis	Binding of factor X by amyloid tissue[67]	Prolonged PT and aPTT
Nephrotic syndrome	Renal loss of factors IX, II, X, XII and sometimes loss of plasminogen and ATIII	Prolonged PT and aPTT; sometimes prolonged TT
Heparin administration	Inhibition of factors	Prolongation of aPTT and thrombin time; lesser prolongation of PT
Massive transfusion	Failure to replace platelets, and factors V and VIII, which are unstable in bank blood	Thrombocytopenia; long PT and aPTT

aPTT = activated partial thromboplastin time   PT = prothrombin time

ATIII = antithrombin III   TT = thrombin time

FDP = fibrin/fibrinogen degradation products

tendency. In very severe cases, when virtually complete defibrination occurs, the shed blood does not clot. The laboratory features of DIC are shown in Table 9.5.

Pathological features of DIC are haemorrhage and the presence of microthrombi in capillaries, arterioles and venules. Less often arterial or venous thrombi may be found. In patients with active fibrinolysis, thrombi may be difficult to find: special methods for demonstrating fibrinogen (e.g. immunohistochemistry or electron microscopy) may be necessary to demonstrate intravascular coagulation. The thrombi contain both fibrin and platelets. They are found in the lungs, kidneys, liver, adrenals, spleen, heart and brain. Thrombi may be mainly in the liver when the course is acute; when the course is longer, thrombi are usually mainly in the kidneys and may be organized.[70] In fulminant cases, haemorrhage into the adrenal glands may occur. A petechial rash, ecchymoses and dermal necrosis may occur. In chronic DIC, particularly that associated with malignant disease, non-bacterial thrombotic endocarditis may be present, mainly affecting the mitral and aortic valves; this lesion may give rise to arterial emboli.[71]

Nephrotic syndrome[72]

Clotting factors of low molecular weight are lost in the urine in cases of the nephrotic syndrome. Plasminogen and antithrombin III may also be lost and this may contribute to the thrombotic tendency which has been observed. Factor VII deficiency has been observed but an elevation is more common. Factor VIII, fibrinogen and α_2 macroglobulin (which has antithrombin activity) are usually increased. A long thrombin time is sometimes observed, suggesting that a dysfibrinogenaemia may occur.

Inhibitors of coagulation factors (Table 9.6)

Inhibitors of coagulation may develop spontaneously in otherwise healthy people, and may also develop in patients with various diseases, or with congenital coagulation factor deficiencies. Coagulation factor inhibitors are generally antibodies. The antibodies are usually polyclonal in origin but of restricted heterogeneity; they may be monoclonal when occurring in association with lymphoproliferative disorders. Inhibitors may act against single coagulation factors, in which case laboratory findings are similar to those seen in congenital deficiency of the same factors and a haemorrhagic disorder usually occurs. Factor VIII inhibitors are the commonest of this group. The inhibitor is detected by failure of the prolonged clotting test to be corrected by admixture with normal plasma, and by the ability of the test plasma to cause inactivation of the specific factor. Diseases which have been associated with coagulation factor inhibitors are shown in Table 9.6; the commonest concomitants are congenital factor deficiencies, pregnancy and the puerperium, systemic lupus erythematosus (SLE) and therapy with certain drugs. Inhibitors may disappear spontaneously or with immunosuppressive therapy.

Patients with SLE may also develop an inhibitor which prolongs the aPTT and the PT and which is not directed against a particular coagulation factor. This type of inhibitor does not inactivate coagulation factors and may be directed against phospholipid. Although the 'lupus anticoagulant' produces abnormal coagulation tests it is rarely associated with a haemorrhagic tendency. There is a paradoxical association with thrombosis, which is predominantly venous in type. An association with recurrent abortion, fetal growth retardation and fetal death has also been recognized.[73] The lupus-type inhibitor is not restricted to SLE (see Table 9.6); it may disappear spontaneously or following therapy of SLE or withdrawal of a causative drug.

Table 9.6 Inhibitors of coagulation

Factor inhibited	Clinical associations
Factor XII	SLE, procainamide-induced lupus
Factor XI	Factor XI deficiency, SLE,* procainamide-induced lupus, WM, following upper respiratory tract infection, carcinoma, previously healthy people
Factor IX	Christmas disease (1–3% incidence of inhibitor), SLE*, postpartum, AIHA plus thrombocytopenia, following hepatitis
Factor VIIIC	Haemophilia (5–10% incidence of inhibitor), pregnancy and postpartum,* drug reactions (penicillin,* sulphonamides, arsenicals, phenylbutazone, nitrofurazone), reaction to horse serum, multiple myeloma, WM, SLE, rheumatoid arthritis, Crohn's disease, ulcerative colitis, dermatitis herpetiformis, carcinoma, previously healthy people
Factor VIII/VWF	VWD (rare), paraproteinaemias, lymphoma, ? SLE
Factor VII	SLE
Factor V	Factor V deficiency, streptomycin* and other aminoglycosides, penicillin,* bullous pemphigoid, tuberculosis, carcinoma, cirrhosis, previously healthy people
Factor II	Procainamide-induced lupus
Fibrinogen	Afibrinogenaemia, previously healthy people, Down's syndrome
Factor XIII	Factor XIII deficiency, isoniazid,* drug-induced lupus, practolol

* Common association
AIHA = autoimmune haemolytic anaemia
SLE = systemic lupus erythematosus
VWD = von Willebrand's disease
WM = Waldenström's macroglobulinaemia

ORAL ANTICOAGULANTS AND THEIR PATHOLOGICAL EFFECTS

Oral anticoagulants (coumarins and indanediones) are vitamin K antagonists and prevent a post-translational vitamin-K-dependent γ-carboxylation of glutamic acid residues of the precursors of factors II, VII, IX and X (see p. 319).

Haemorrhagic effects of oral anticoagulants

The haemorrhagic effects of coumarins and indanediones are similar. Bleeding is related largely to excessive dosage or coexisting lesions (e.g. peptic ulcer). Bruising and gastrointestinal haemorrhage are relatively common. Bleeding may also occur at unusual sites (e.g. corpus luteum, adrenal glands).

Spontaneous splenic rupture occurs and is largely related to an excessive degree of anticoagulation. Spontaneous renal rupture has also been reported. Recurrent haemarthrosis, as observed in congenital haemorrhagic disorders, uncommonly occurs and may lead to destructive arthropathy.[74]

Non-haemorrhagic pathological effects of coumarins

All non-haemorrhagic effects of coumarins are rare.

Skin necrosis is a rare complication which is seen particularly in obese women and occurs early in treatment. The breasts, abdomen, buttocks, legs and genitalia are preferentially affected. Discrete erythematous and oedematous patches appear, become blue-black and then frankly necrotic. Necrosis involves all layers of the skin and may extend into the subcutaneous fat. Breast lesions may be severe enough to require mastectomy.[75] Microscopically there is vasculitis with thrombosis, particularly in capillaries, and also in veins.

Alopecia may occur.

The purple toe syndrome[76] is a rare complication of warfarin therapy. The toes are painful and discoloured with normal capillary blood flow. The condition is reversible with little or no permanent tissue damage.

Warfarin embryopathy and other effects on the fetus

Administration of warfarin (a coumarin) in the first trimester of pregnancy may cause a very characteristic fetal syndrome.[77] As the syndrome has also been described following phenindione, it is possible that it may result from any vitamin K antagonist. The syndrome is a phenocopy of an inherited condition, chondrodysplasia punctata. The characteristic skeletal abnormalities particularly affect the vertebrae and sacrum, but may also affect the femora, patellae, calcanei, carpal bones, phalanges and ribs. Radiology shows multifocal punctate calcification of epiphyseal cartilages. Histological studies of the epiphyses show acellular myxomatous material, chondrocyte proliferation and thin-walled vascular channels. With growth, the stippled areas become reabsorbed or incorporated into normally developing bone; some stippled areas ossify later. Other features of the syndrome which have been observed following the administration of vitamin K antagonists are nasal hypoplasia, short limbs or fingers, congenital dislocation of the hips, cataracts, optic atrophy, mental retardation, deafness, high-arched palate, agenesis of the corpus callosum, midline cerebellar atrophy, congenital heart disease, asplenia, and malrotation of abdominal viscera. Vitamin K antagonists given in the second and third trimesters of pregnancy may be associated with microcephaly and mental retardation; when given in the week before delivery they may cause neonatal haemorrhage.

Non-haemorrhagic pathological effects of indanediones

Indanediones may also rarely cause skin necrosis. Hypersensitivity reactions occur in 1–3% of patients and may include fever, a rash, eosinophilia, granulocytopenia, thrombocytopenia, hepatitis and nephritis. The affected liver shows both hepatocellular and cholestatic lesions.

REFERENCES

1. Aronson DL, Mustafa AJ. Thromb Haemost 1976; 36: 104.
2. Østerud B, Rapaport SI. Proc Natl Acad Sci 1977; 74: 5260.
3. van den Besselaar AHMP, Ram IE, Alderkamp GHJ, Bertina RM. Thromb Haemost 1982; 48: 54.
4. Østerud B, Laake K, Prydz H. Thromb Diath Haemorrh 1975; 33: 553.
5. Mertens K, Bertina RM. Thromb Haemost 1982; 47: 96.
6. Gallop PM, Lian JB, Hauschka PV. N Engl J Med 1980; 302: 1460.
7. Muller HP, van Tilburg NH, Bertina RM, Veltkamp JJ. Thromb Res 1980; 20: 85.
8. Nachman RL, Jaffe EA. Thromb Haemost 1976; 35: 120.
9. Stead NW, McKee PA. Blood 1979; 54: 560.
10. Wall RT, Counts RB, Harker LA, Striker GE. Br J Haematol 1980; 46: 287.
11. Jaffe EA. N Engl J Med 1977; 296: 377.
12. Nemerson Y. Thromb Haemost 1976; 35: 96.
13. Ratnoff OD. Blood 1980; 57: 55.
14. Estelles A, Aznar J, España F. Thromb Haemost 1983; 49: 66.
15. Schapira M, Silver LD, Scott CF, et al. N Engl J Med 1983; 308: 1050.
16. Kaplan JE, Snedeker PW, Baum SH, Moon DG, Minnear FL. Thromb Haemost 1983; 49: 217.
17. Donaldson VH, Kleniewski J, Saito H, Sayed JK. J Clin Invest 1977; 60: 571.
18. Sixma JJ. Thromb Haemost 1978; 40: 163.
19. Booth NA, Bennett B, Wijngaards G, Grieve JHK. Blood 1983; 61: 267.
20. Yoshioka A, Kamitsuji H, Takase T, et al. Haemostasis 1982; 11: 176.
21. Rizza CR, Spooner RJD. Br Med J 1983; 286: 929.
22. Eyster ME, Gordon RA, Ballard JA. Blood 1981; 58: 719.
23. Lewis JH, Maxwell NG, Brandon JM. Transfusion 1974; 14: 203.
24. Forbes CD, Prentice CRM. In: Frantanoni JC, Aronson DL, eds. Unsolved therapeutic problems in hemophilia. US Department of Health, Education and Welfare, 1977: 15.
25. Aledort LM. In: Frantanoni JC, Aronson DL, eds. Unsolved therapeutic problems in hemophilia. US Department of Health, Education and Welfare, 1977: 9.
26. Kerr CB. J Neurol Neurosurg Psychiatry 1964; 27: 166.
27. Beck P, Evans KT. Clin Radiol 1972; 23: 349.
28. Eyster ME, Gill FB, Blatt PM, et al. Blood 1978; 51: 1179.
29. Duthie RB, Matthews JM, Rizza CR, Steel WM, Woods CG. The management of musculoskeletal problems in the haemophilias. Oxford: Blackwell Scientific Publications, 1972.
30. Caffey J, Schlesinger ER. J Pediatr 1940; 16: 549.
31. Small M, Rose PE, McMillan N, et al. Br Med J 1982; 285: 1609.
32. Dalinka MK, Lally JF, Rancier LF, Mata J. Radiology 1975; 115: 337.
33. Gralnick HR, Coller BS, Shulman NR, Andersen JC, Hilgartner M. Ann Intern Med 1977; 86: 598.
34. Prentice CRM, Lindsay RM, Barr RD, et al. Q J Med 1971; 40: 47.
35. Craske J, Spooner RJD, Vandervelde EM. Lancet 1978; ii: 1051.
36. Mannucci PM, Capitanio A, del Ninno E, Colombo M, Pareti F, Ruggeri ZM. J Clin Pathol 1975; 28: 620.
37. Lesesne HR, Morgan JE, Blatt PM, Webster WP, Roberts HR. Ann Intern Med 1977; 86: 703.
38. Spero JA, Lewis JH, van Thiel DH, Hasiba U, Rabin BS. N Engl J Med 1978; 298: 1373.
39. Dalldorf FG, Taylor RE, Blatt PM. Arch Pathol Lab Med 1981; 105: 652.
40. Hilgartner MW, Giardina P. Transfusion 1977; 17: 495.
41. Levine PH, McVerry A, Segelman AE, Cranford CM, Zimbler S. Arch Intern Med 1976; 136: 792.
42. Sharma HM, Geer JG. Arch Pathol 1970; 89: 473.
43. Egberg N, Blombäck M. Thromb Haemost 1981; 46: 554.
44. Prentice CRM, Izatt MM, Adams JF, McNicol GP, Douglas AS. Br J Haematol 1971; 21: 305.
45. Curran JW, Lawrence DN, Jaffe H, et al. N Engl J Med 1984; 310: 69.
46. Lederman MM, Ratnoff OD, Scillian JJ, Jones PK, Schacter B. N Engl J Med 1983; 308: 79.
47. Menitove JE, Aster RH, Casper JT, et al. N Engl J Med 1983; 308: 83.
48. Luban NLC, Kelleher JH, Reaman GH. Lancet 1983; i: 503.
49. Lee CA, Janossy G, Ashley J, Kernoff PBA. Lancet 1983; ii: 158.
50. Ratnoff OD, Menitove JE, Aster RH, Lederman MM. N Engl J Med 1983; 308: 439.
51. Mannucci PM. Eur J Clin Invest 1978; 8: 201.
52. Ruggeri ZM, Pareti FI, Mannucci PM, Ciavarella N, Zimmerman TS. N Engl J Med 1980; 302: 1047.
53. Holmberg L, Nilsson IM, Borge L, Gunnarsson M, Sjörin E. N Engl J Med 1983; 309: 816.
54. Takahashi H. Thromb Res 1980; 19: 857.
55. Miller JL, Castella A. Blood 1982; 60: 790.
56. Weiss HJ, Meyer D, Rabinowitz R, et al. N Engl J Med 1982; 306: 326.
57. Ahlberg A, Silwer J. Acta Orthop Scand 1970; 41: 539.
58. Ramsay DM, Macleod DAD, Buist TAS, Heading RC. Lancet 1976; ii: 275.
59. Ahr DJ, Rickles FR, Hoyer LW, O'Leary DS, Conrad ME. Am J Med 1977; 62: 452.
60. Conlon CL, Weinger RS, Cimo PL, Moake JL, Olson JD. Ann Intern Med 1978; 89: 921.
61. Wautier J-L, Caen JP, Rymer R. Lancet 1976; ii: 973.
62. Rosborough TK, Swain WR. Am J Med 1978; 65: 96.
63. Pickering NJ, Brody JI, Barrett MJ. N Engl J Med 1981; 305: 131.
64. Silwer J, Cronberg S, Nilsson IM. Acta Med Scand 1966; 180: 475.
65. Luban NLC, Kelleher JH, Reaman GH. Lancet 1983; i: 503.
66. Matthay KK, Koerper MA, Ablin AR. J Pediatr 1979; 94: 413.
67. Greipp PR, Kyle RA, Bowie EJW. N Engl J Med 1979; 301: 1050.
68. Coleman M, Finlayson N, Bettigole RE, Sadula D, Cohn M, Pasmantier M. Ann Intern Med 1975; 83: 79.
69. Francis JL, Armstrong DJ. J Clin Pathol 1982; 35: 667.
70. Shimamura K, Oka K, Nakazawa M, Kojima M. Arch Pathol Lab Med 1983; 107: 543.

71. Sack GH, Levin J, Bell WR. Medicine 1977; 56: 1.
72. Thompson AR. Thromb Haemost 1982; 48: 27.
73. Lubbe WF, Butler WS, Palmer SJ, Liggins GC. Lancet 1983; i: 1361.
74. Andes WA, Edmunds JO. Thromb Haemost 1983; 49: 187.
75. Davis CE, Wiley WB, Faulconer RJ. Ann Surg 1972; 175: 647.
76. Akle CA, Joiner CL. J R Soc Med 1981; 74: 219.
77. Hall JR, Pauli RM, Wilson KM. Am J Med 1980; 68: 122.

Index